An Introduction to

HEALTH
SERVICES
RESEARCH

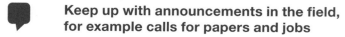
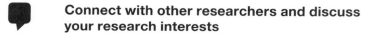
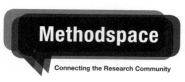
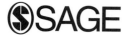

An Introduction to

HEALTH SERVICES RESEARCH

edited by
Dawn-Marie Walker

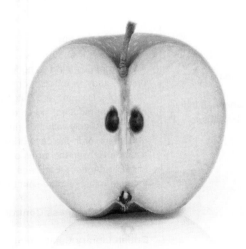

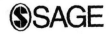

Los Angeles | London | New Delhi
Singapore | Washington DC

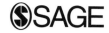

Los Angeles | London | New Delhi
Singapore | Washington DC

SAGE Publications Ltd
1 Oliver's Yard
55 City Road
London EC1Y 1SP

SAGE Publications Inc.
2455 Teller Road
Thousand Oaks, California 91320

SAGE Publications India Pvt Ltd
B 1/I 1 Mohan Cooperative Industrial Area
Mathura Road
New Delhi 110 044

SAGE Publications Asia-Pacific Pte Ltd
3 Church Street
#10-04 Samsung Hub
Singapore 049483

Editor: Jai Seaman
Production editor: Ian Antcliff
Copyeditor: Jane Robson
Proofreader: Clare Weaver
Marketing manager: Tamara Navaratnam
Cover design: Francis Kenney
Typeset by: C&M Digitals (P) Ltd, Chennai, India
Printed and bound in Great Britain by Ashford
Colour Press Ltd

First published 2014

Library of Congress Control Number: 2013937333

British Library Cataloguing in Publication data

A catalogue record for this book is available from the British Library

ISBN 978-1-4462-4739-6
ISBN 978-1-4462-4738-9 (pbk)

CONTENTS

NOTES ON CONTRIBUTORS

Andrew Barton has an academic background in psychology but has been working as a generalist in health services research for thirty-five years. He has worked as a lecturer and senior lecturer at the medical schools in Newcastle and Cardiff and is currently Associate Professor in Health Services Research at Plymouth University Peninsula Schools of Medicine and Dentistry.

Dr Leonardi-Bee completed an MSc and PhD in medical statistics, and is an Associate Professor in medical statistics. Her areas of expertise focus on systematic review and meta-analysis of epidemiological studies and randomised controlled trials, and analysing large databases. She is the Statistical Editor of the Cochrane Collaboration Skin group, and has published widely in the areas of tobacco control, dermatology, and respiratory medicine.

After eleven years as a speech and language therapist within the NHS, Dr Benford was awarded a PhD in 2008 for her investigation of the use of the internet as a communication medium by people with Asperger syndrome. Since its completion, she has been working as a researcher within the School of Community Health Sciences at the University of Nottingham.

Dr Peter Blair has a background in medical statistics and a particular interest in infant and childhood epidemiology and is now a Senior Research Fellow at the University of Bristol. From his work on several major observational studies he is a recognised expert in Sudden Infant Death Syndrome and was made an honorary fellow and advisor to UNICEF, is the vice chair of the International Society for the Study and Prevention of Perinatal and Infant Death (ISPID) and chair of the epidemiological working group.

Dr Helen Close is a health research methodologist with the Research Design Service (North East) and an academic trialist in Durham Clinical Trials Unit at Durham University. Helen has a clinical background in community and palliative care, and her research interests focus on end-of-life care. Her current research focuses on mixed-methods approaches to cardiovascular disease and gastrointestinal disorders.

Dr Sarah Damery is a research fellow in clinical epidemiology at the Department of Primary Care Clinical Sciences, University of Birmingham. She has expertise in the use of both qualitative and quantitative methodologies, and her research interests focus on the prevention and early diagnosis of cancer, and interventions to improve the uptake of cancer screening. She is a senior adviser for the West Midlands Research Design Service.

Abdel Douiri is an applied mathematician by background, MSc in 1998 and PhD in 2002. He is currently a Lecturer in Medical Statistics at King's College London. His research interests focus mainly on statistical and mathematical models and methods applied to medical research, with a current application in stroke and cognitive impairment.

Jane Dyas is a Senior Research Fellow with the NIHR Research Design Service for the East Midlands based at the University of Nottingham. In this capacity she has developed experience of, and insight into, the process of applying for funding. Her methodological experience is qualitative and her current research activity includes research on insomnia and health care in care homes.

Mary Edmunds Otter has been a librarian and information specialist in pharmaceutical and health fields since the 1980s. She currently works for the NIHR Research Design Service East Midlands. She gives advice on the design and methodology of systematic reviews, developing search strategies and critical appraisal, and conducts literature searches.

Adrian Gheorghe, MSc, trained as a health economist and has since been working in clinical trials. He has expertise in clinical trials methodology, evidence synthesis, decision modelling and economic evaluation, and has been involved in trial methodology research on topics such as the generalisability of trial results and clinician recruitment.

Laura J. Gray is a medical statistician currently working as a Lecturer at the University of Leicester. The main focus of her research is in the area of type 2 diabetes, focusing on early detection and prevention, including developing and validating clinical risk scores, meta-analyses, and clinical trials (in particular ordinal outcomes, complex interventions and cluster randomised trials).

Gill Green is the Regional Director of the Research Design Service East of England. She is a Professor of Medical Sociology at the University of Essex, and has been researching aspects of chronic illness since the early 1990s with a particular interest in the experience of long-term illness and the impact it has on self-identity. She has also conducted research related to socially excluded groups such as offenders with mental health problems and people living in poor-quality housing.

Helen Hancock is a methodologist in the Research Design Service (North East) and an academic trialist in Durham Clinical Trials Unit at Durham University. Her main area of interest is cardiovascular disease, with a current research focus in the diagnosis and management of heart failure.

Jonathan Ives is a Senior Lecturer in Bioethics in the University of Birmingham. He has expertise in applied ethics (bioethics) and the use and application of qualitative research methods. His primary research interests lie in the methodological integration of ethical and empirical research methods. He currently co-chairs the Wellcome Trust Interdisciplinary and Empirical Ethics Network (IEEN), and sits on the Royal College of General Practitioners Ethics Committee.

Matthew Jones is a PhD student in the Division of Primary Care at the University of Nottingham, with his thesis investigating the cost-effectiveness of smoking cessation during pregnancy. He studied economics before undertaking an MSc in health economics, both at the University of York. On completion of his masters, he worked at the East Midlands Research Design Service, giving advice on health economics and designing economic evaluations.

Christine Keen is an information officer for East Midlands Research Design Service, where her main role is searching for literature on health and health-related databases. She provides guidance and advice in the use of electronic databases and undertaking systematic reviews. A former public librarian Christine began working in health information after gaining an MSc in health information management.

Paul Leighton is a Senior Research Fellow in the NIHR Research Design Service for the East Midlands based at the University of Nottingham. Through his role at the RDS he has worked with researchers from a range of settings in designing studies and seeking funding. He maintains research activity in a number of clinical areas, contributing to funded studies in audiology, rheumatology, pain management and orthopedic surgery.

Louise Marsland is based in the School of Health and Human Sciences at the University of Essex. She has an eclectic mix of research interests including complementary therapies, cancer care, brain injury, women's health and vulnerable young people. Methodologically, she specialises in qualitative methods but also has expertise in longitudinal survey research.

Victoria Hall Moran is a Reader in Maternal and Child Nutrition at the University of Central Lancashire. Her research has focused on the nutritional intake of women during pregnancy and lactation. Her methodological expertise is in quantitative research design and systematic review. She is Senior Editor of *Maternal and Child Nutrition* (Wiley-Blackwell).

Puja Myles is a public health specialist and epidemiologist. She is an Associate Professor at the University of Nottingham. Her main area of interest is infectious disease, with a current research focus in influenza and other respiratory diseases.

Caitlin Notley is a Senior Research Fellow in the Norwich Medical School at the University of East Anglia. She has expertise in qualitative research methodologies applied across health and social sciences and extensive experience in running qualitative studies alongside clinical trials. She has been researching in the field of addiction and substance misuse for over ten years. Her research has focused particularly on opiate addiction, exploring populations in and out of treatment. Her current research on smoking relapse prevention targets at-risk groups.

Raksha Pandya-Wood works for the Research Design Service East Midlands as the Regional Lead for Patient and Public Involvement in Research. Raksha is a Senior Research Fellow who is based at De Montfort University. Raksha is currently in the middle of her PhD looking into the impact of patient and public involvement in cancer research. Raksha's previous teaching and research projects have been on women and children living with HIV, substance misuse in minority populations and promoting independence for young people living with disabilities.

Katherine Payne is Professor of Health Economics in the University of Manchester. She has eighteen years' experience working as an academic health economist with a main research interest focusing on the economic evaluation and valuation of healthcare technologies and services. She is a senior methodologist for the North West Research Design Service.

Roy Powell has worked in health services research for the past twenty years, based at the Royal Devon and Exeter Foundation NHS Trust and the University of Exeter Medical School. He has a zoology and biostatistics background, with further training in medical statistics and epidemiology, and has co-authored over seventy peer-reviewed publications. He currently works in the NIHR Research Design Service – South West and has served on ethics committees for over ten years. His current research interest is in the prevention of skin lacerations in people with fragile skin and the elderly, using novel protective leg and arm hosiery.

Casey Quinn is a health economist and econometrician with experience in health economic analysis, economic evaluation and decision analysis, and expertise in econometrics and modelling methodologies. Casey is an associate at the University of Nottingham, where he was a lecturer for three years. There, he worked on economic evaluation alongside clinical trials and complex interventions, as well as being part of the NICE Technology Appraisal Committee. He has a PhD from the University of York.

Carol Rivas is the NIHR Research Design Service Regional (London) Lead for Qualitative Research Methods. She is also trained in cognitive neuropsychology and her research interests are ethnicity, communication and cognition, gender and identity, mental health and behaviour change. She currently runs an NIHR programme grant on smoking cessation. Carol also teaches qualitative research methods and lectures in medical sociology at Barts and the London School of Medicine and Dentistry. In the past she has worked as a medical journalist and as a writer for a medical communications agency.

Andrew Robinson is Patient and Public Involvement Lead for Research Design Service North East. His experience of patient and public involvement spans many years, in contexts including NHS primary and secondary care, the voluntary sector and, more recently, health and social care research. Andrew has developed a particular interest and specialism in the development of community-based models of involvement, including involvement of disadvantaged and marginalised groups and communities.

After graduating in medicine, Paul Silcocks trained originally as a pathologist, later developing an interest in epidemiology. Previously he was a Clinical Senior Lecturer at the University of Nottingham, working for the NIHR Research Design Service East Midlands and helped to set up the Clinical Trials Unit at the University. Since retirement he works at the Cancer Research UK Liverpool Cancer Trials Unit as a senior statistician, and is currently working on trials in pancreatic cancer, melanoma, head and neck cancer and chronic lymphatic leukaemia.

Roz Sorrie has worked in the NHS for over 22 years in the fields of clinical audit and effectiveness, clinical governance and research. She joined Leicestershire, Northamptonshire and Rutland Comprehensive Local Research Network (LNR CLRN) in 2008 as Lead Research Management and Governance Manager. Her role involves overseeing the research governance reviews of National Institute for Health Research Portfolio studies and ensuring that studies are resourced appropriately before they start. She also works closely with local LNR investigators and CLRN colleagues to ensure that studies can be delivered within a timely way in the NHS.

Nick Taub is a medical statistician with the NIHR Research Design Service for the East Midlands and a Research Fellow at the University of Leicester. He has collaborated on studies in a wide range of areas of medicine, currently concentrating on musculoskeletal and public health research.

Gordon Taylor is a Reader in Medical Statistics at the University of Bath, and spends part of his time working for the NIHR Research Design Service South West. He has experience of being a member of grant funding panels, as well as ethics committees. His research interests are in the health and well-being of the NHS workforce, older adults and those with high cardiovascular risk.

Doreen Tembo is a Senior Research Officer working with the NIHR Research Design Service for the East of England and the University of Essex. Dr Tembo specialised in global health policy and policy making in the field of HIV/AIDS with a focus on resource poor countries for both her MSc and Doctorate at the University of Oxford. She is a mixed-methods specialist whose research experience lie in health policy, health promotion, patient and community experiences of health and health care.

Mary Tully is Reader in Pharmacy Practice in the University of Manchester. She also works one clinical day per week. She has served on and chaired research ethics committees for the past thirteen years. Her main research interests are about prescribing, especially hospital and non-medical prescribing, including patient safety and the measurement of the outcomes.

Dawn-Marie Walker currently works at the NIHR Research Design Service for the East Midlands. After an undergraduate degree in psychology and an MSc in research methods and statistics in psychology, Dr. Walker went on to complete a PhD looking at the cognitive function in early-onset psychosis. She is a mixed-methods researcher, with vast experience of conducting research concerning mental health, complementary medicine and studying complex interventions. She is also very interested in emergent online research technologies and public, patient involvement.

Olwyn M. R. Westwood is Professor of Medical Education and the Associate Dean (Education Quality) at Barts and The London School of Medicine and Dentistry and has worked for around twenty years in medical and health care education. She is recognised for her work in integrated medical curricular design, and her expertise has led to her being called upon as an adviser in Europe, China, Brunei and Australia. She has a keen interest in making biomedical sciences education accessible and relevant in medicine.

Diane Whitham is Deputy Director of the Nottingham Clinical Trials Unit based at University of Nottingham. She has over twenty years of commercial and academic clinical trials management experience. Her trial methodology research interest is site identification and selection.

To all of those people throughout my life who believed in me when sometimes I didn't believe in myself. I am forever grateful for your support and kindness. Thank you x

PREFACE

The teacher who is indeed wise does not bid you to enter the house of his wisdom but rather leads you to the threshold of your mind. (Khalil Gibran)

I wish this book had been around when I was first starting out in research. I am not a born nerd (although I guess I would be described as one now), and did not find research easy initially. I remember after a further statistics masters class I would go home and pull out three or four textbooks and have to read the section regarding that analysis in them all. Bits would make sense in one, other bits in another, and so on ... together giving me an overall understanding. I think that this lack of innate ability to understand research methods and analysis has enabled me to be able to communicate the complex process of research in a manner which my former self would have understood and appreciated, and I hope you do too.

I strongly believe that the best way to learn about research is to actually do it (hence the quote above)! However, from my experience as an academic working within health services research, I noticed that there were no easy-to-engage-with textbooks to take students and health service professionals through their projects from start to finish. I designed this book to be a 'guide' through the process, which mirrors the steps that one takes in a project, from 'Asking the Right Question' right through to 'Dissemination' with lots of examples and case studies, so that the topic comes alive and is more tangible. The book is not written in a theoretical, academic or intimidating way. My experience has taught me that often people do not want to know the theory behind the methodology, just how to do it! If you do wish to explore any area further, we have incorporated a further reading section in each chapter. My aim is to get you thinking broadly about all of the issues that need to be considered when embarking on a project, and then prompting you to access further resources and support to enable you to produce a good study.

This book will be useful for any student project, whether undergraduate or postgraduate, and any health service professionals who would like to conduct a study who are new, or fairly new, to research, and who have little knowledge of how to conduct health services research. Maybe this book will support you in your first ever journey into a piece of health services research, and you will go onto become an eminent professor! Some of you might try and decide it is not for you:

research definitely has the 'marmite factor'; people either love it, or hate it. However regardless of whether you enjoy the experience or not, at some stage you may need a research portfolio for career progression, or you may have a good idea to improve patient care that you need 'evidence' for in order to be able to implement it. This book will provide enough information for you to make an informed decision whether you would like to take your idea forward, and whether it is possible to do so.

Part I

GETTING STARTED

1

ASKING THE RIGHT QUESTION

Peter S. Blair and Andy Barton

- Appreciate the importance of a clear and focused research question
- To be able to use criteria such as PICO (Population, Intervention, Comparison, Outcome) to frame an answerable question
- Understand the need for primary and secondary questions and the process of refinement
- To understand what a hypothesis is and how it differs from the aims and objectives of a study
- Be aware of over-interpreting the findings, post-hoc assumptions and spurious associations
- Understand the answer and appreciate negative results

Introduction

In health services research, asking the right question is important because everything else hinges upon it, such as your choice of study design, the interpretation of your results and their impact on clinical practice. Often when a researcher is having difficulty with designing the research, it is either because the methodology is inappropriate for answering the question, or the question itself is inappropriate. The focus and nature of these questions vary according to the perspective of the individual asking them. Patients and carers focus on issues often of immediate personal relevance such as the relief of symptoms or where to get treatment; clinicians bear in mind the broader issues, taking into account, for instance, the range of interventions available and the wider implications of choosing different treatments; whilst funders and researchers seek justification for an intervention and whether clinical care can be improved and/or money saved with it. For example, if a child had a sore throat, their question may be: 'When will I feel better so that I can play out?' The parent may ask: 'Should I take him to the doctor?' The doctor may ask: 'Is it a bacterial or viral infection? Are antibiotics needed?' The funder of the health care may ask: 'Can we afford to routinely analyse throat swabs?' The researcher may then ask: 'Can we formulate an algorithm from signs and symptoms of illness to predict hospitalisation from bacterial infection?' Given the different perspectives, all of these questions are equally valid.

Questions do not just vary depending on the perspective from which they are being asked; they can often be multi-layered and interdependent. Breaking the overarching question down into what is known and unknown will help, but this is partly reliant on one's own current knowledge and the lengths one is prepared to go to read and critically appraise the peer-reviewed published literature on that topic (please see Chapter 3: 'Critical Appraisal'). With the exponential growth in the number of medical journals in recent years (Smith, 2006), online literature searching is now an important element of the clinician's and researcher's armoury and it has become relatively easy to find out if a particular question has already been asked in full, or in part, and whether the methodology was robust enough to inform clinical practice (please see Chapter 2: 'Finding the Evidence to Support your Research Question'). Although this step seems initially a lot of effort, several purposes are served by it; it increases your knowledge of the field in general, starts to delineate the frontiers of what is known and not known at the present time and thus helps develop or refine your research question. Your literature search will also provide references for when you start to write up your protocol, grant or ethics applications, or findings, and can provide you with templates of good-quality research design. It is important to distinguish between when there is no evidence because a study has posed the question and come up with a negative result and no evidence because no study has actually asked the question yet. However not every question requires evidence. There has never been a single randomised controlled trial proving that parachutes are a safe intervention when you jump out of a plane at a great height (Smith and Pell, 2003) for example, but that does not mean we should not use them!

The culture of enquiry and collecting evidence in clinical practice has moved through a series of stages from early descriptive pioneering work on individual patients, such as the work of Edward Jenner who tested the smallpox vaccine initially on one person in 1796, through to more population-based evaluative studies in recent times (please see Chapter 10: 'Epidemiology'). The importance of evidence-based medicine has slowly gained momentum, challenging the idea that health care professionals, by the simple virtue of reading medical texts and their own anecdotal experience, have some sort of unique insight or unquestionable 'clinical judgement' into the social causes of disease (*The Lancet*, 1995). In 1747, the Scottish physician James Lind conducted the first clinical experiment, in which he researched treatments for scurvy. The results clearly showed that including citrus fruits in the diet produced the best recovery, but the medical establishment and Lind himself was wedded to the idea that scurvy was a disease of putrefaction, curable by the administration of elixir of vitriol (sulphuric acid) and other remedies designed to 'ginger up' the system such as mustard, or horseradish. It was another 50 years before the British Admiralty accepted the evidence of the first trial and recommended that lemon juice should be issued routinely to the whole fleet (Vale, 2008).

With the emerging disciplines of statistical techniques in the early part of the 20th century and computing technology in the latter, evidence-based medicine has thrived and become more sophisticated in terms of research designs and methodologies, together with an increased understanding of the complexity of the different issues involved in the research process, for example, sources of potential bias, missing values, etc. However in essence, evidence-based medicine is founded on a simple bottom–up approach that integrates the best external evidence with individual clinical expertise and patient choice (Sackett et al., 1996), and which begins with a clinical question. It might be a new treatment that needs testing, a particular problem that needs solving or a more general desire to improve the patient's well-being.

What is a good question?

A good question in health services research is one that is important and which will give a meaningful answer. For example, there would be no importance in researching a superseded medication or technique, or researching something when the definitive answer for it already exists from previous research. For people new to research, many of their initial questions are aimed at solving the problems of the world, which by their very nature are largely unanswerable. Although this enthusiasm is commendable, there needs to be a degree of 'funnelling' whereby a large topic is broken down into smaller more manageable ones, to generate an answerable clinical research question. By breaking the topic down to answer individual key questions elegantly and robustly, your results will remove the uncertainty about those parts, and so the knowledge about the larger topic slowly moves forward. An answerable question in research terms is one which seeks specific knowledge, is framed to facilitate literature searching and therefore follows a semi-standard structure (Bragge, 2010). This process is critical because if a methodological approach is used to address a question that is too broad, lacks rigour, would be difficult to rerun or refine, and would create inefficiencies once the research process is under way, it would fail to answer the research question. Conversely a question that is too narrow may generate more questions than answers, findings would be less generalisable and therefore not worth the time of the researchers or the money of the funders.

It seldom happens that a researcher gets the question right first time. Indeed, most research questions undergo a series of iterations before the team are certain that the question they have framed is appropriate and timely. After reviewing the literature or discussions with colleagues and patients, aspects of your research question may change, such as the population, intervention or comparison. This sort of refinement and transformation of the question is common but does not happen quickly. Discussions are often frequent and lengthy before the whole team is agreed that they have an important and answerable question. Do not underestimate the importance of involvement of patients and public in this step, as your research needs to be meaningful and acceptable to those whom it will affect (please see the case study and Chapter 16: 'Patient and Public Involvement in your Research').

Case study

A study is being conducted regarding the effectiveness of steroids in children with asthma. The research team identified 'coughing at night' and 'days lost at school' as important outcomes to be measured. However, after discussing the study with parents of these children at the planning stage, it was revealed the most serious concern of the parents was the effects of long-term steroid use. Thus, research about the effectiveness of steroids would be redundant as, regardless of their efficacy, the intervention would not be acceptable to the parents of the children. The research team therefore refocused their question, to ascertain the minimum dose regimen of steroids and its relationship to efficacy. Due to their involvement strategy, they know that this information would be welcomed by the patients and their parents, and therefore more likely to influence clinical practice.

Research question criteria

There have been several criteria formulated to ease the process of drafting a good research question, such as the FINER criteria (Hulley et al., 2007):

Feasible	Adequate number of participants available and adequate skill mix in the research team. Also is the project manageable within the specified time frame, and budget?
Interesting	The answer will be interesting to other researchers in the field, health professionals and patients.

Novel   Confirms, refutes or extends previous findings (whether yours or published).

Ethical   No reason why ethical approval could not be obtained.

Relevant   To current scientific knowledge, policy, future research and patients.

Whereas the FINER criteria outlines the important aspects to consider in general, the PICO criteria; Population, Intervention or Indicator, Comparison (if relevant) and Outcome (Richardson et al., 1995) is useful for the development of a specific research question. A clear, answerable research question has three or four of these PICO components. The general format of a PICO question is: 'In [Population], what is the effect of [Intervention] on [Outcome], compared with [Comparison]?'

P: Population/Patient/Problem

I: Intervention or indicator

C: Comparison/control (if relevant)

O: Outcome of interest

Your population is who your research will affect. Be precise, because if you put your sample as 'asthmatics', for example, this is a huge and variable population. However you may particularly be interested in asthmatics who smoke. This therefore is your population. The intervention is whatever treatment it is you will be studying, whereas an indicator is whatever risk factor you are interested in, such as smoking as the indicator in your study of asthma (for more discussion on risk factors please see Chapter 10: 'Epidemiology'). A comparator or control depends upon what type of study you are conducting. Is there an alternative to your intervention/indicator? For example, you could compare asthmatics who smoke with those who do not, or from the previous example, you could compare outcomes from different steroid regimens. The outcome is what you hope to accomplish with this research, such as asthma control. In general, the more precise you are in defining the components, the more focused the study.

Case study

A cardiologist proposes the initial simple question: whether placing antibiotic sponges into the chest cavity at the end of heart surgery will prevent infections?

After discussion with various groups, amendments to the question are made:

- 'heart surgery' is too broad and it might be sensible to pick a specific procedure;
- different types of sponges are on the market so it is decided to stick to one type;

(Continued)

(Continued)

- the sponges are not free, so cost and cost-effectiveness need to be considered;
- getting out of hospital and home as soon as possible is seen as a priority by patients.

Thus the question became: in patients undergoing coronary artery bypass grafting, what is the effectiveness and cost-effectiveness of inserting a gentamicin-impregnated collagen sponge into the chest cavity at closure on wound infection rates and length of stay?

Thus the PICO format for this question would be:

P: Patients who are undergoing coronary artery bypass grafting

I: Gentamicin-impregnated collagen sponge

C: No gentamicin-impregnated collagen sponge

O: Wound infection rates and length of stay

Clarity in articulating the question not only helps you in designing the research, but helps the reader to understand what the research is about and what to expect upon further reading about the project. Different question types can follow similar formats, but the key principle in this 'criteria' approach is that important components of the question are identified and defined (please see Chapter 2: 'Finding the Evidence', for examples of criteria for other research designs). Using a strategy such as this to break down the question determines the question type and thus determines the most appropriate study design to answer it.

Mnemonics like PICO are used in an evidence-based literature search, and in the conduct of a systematic review (please see Chapter 14: 'Systematic Reviews'), where the components of the systematic review question will set the criteria for selecting studies to appraise. The PICO components of the question may directly translate into medical subject headings or key words guiding the literature searches. Thus, well-formulated questions are directly linked to the data collection process which will not only help you design your literature search strategy, but also improve the citation rate associated with any ensuing publications stemming from your research.

There is also a wider element to 'framing' a question that goes beyond the particular format used. Often in health services research there is a flux of particular issues that need to be addressed which are sometimes highlighted in the media or manifest themselves in theme-specific calls from funding bodies. The general area of a themed call, for example, obesity, smoking, etc., may be clear to a funder, but by using a framework such as PICO, it allows you to crystallise what you are actually looking at, and how your question relates to those issues/themes and, if appropriate, is framed in order to meet the needs of resolving them.

Primary and secondary questions

The primary question serves as the main focus of a particular study, although it is rarely that only one question is being answered. So, although there are often several questions driving an investigation, there is a need, especially with intervention trials, for one primary question to be resolved. This achieves the required focus in order to design an investigation that will provide a definitive answer for at least one particular question. It also means the primary question can be used to calculate the number of people we might require in some study designs. For instance, a sample size calculation is required in a randomised controlled trial (RCT) in order to obtain sufficient power to test the intervention without oversampling patients and wasting resources and the patient's time (see Chapter 17: 'Sampling'). This calculation is conducted by using an estimate obtained from previously published results which have used the same/similar outcome measure as the one you propose using in your primary question, Alternatively you may have previously gathered the data to inform your sample size calculation from a pilot study, i.e. a small-scale preliminary study to test if the chosen design works. Having several questions, all requiring sample size calculations and then choosing the largest sample calculated to cover all the questions can often be an inefficient approach to use.

In studies, not only is a primary question answered, but often ancillary data are collected and studied to answer secondary questions. The study design is centred on the primary question, and any causal claims of the study are specifically in regards to this primary question, as the main outcome measure will be chosen in order to answer this primary question, and the sample size will be based on this also. Therefore the power of the study is to detect a change in that one main outcome. Secondary questions are generally instrumental in defining future research projects, as they may be based on underpowered samples, due to the fact that the sample size calculation was conducted on another measure. There is an argument, however, that in some intervention studies, especially the more complex ones, the role of secondary questions should be more prominent, especially if the study is powered to adequately test these questions. In observational studies such as case-control or cohort studies (please see Chapter 6: 'Quantitative Data Collection') these rules can be slightly more relaxed and the intention is often to test a set of primary and secondary hypotheses.

Number of questions

A common error is overloading a study with too many questions and too much data collection. Life is a fairly complex thing and trying to replicate the many variants by collecting lots of data to answer a battery of questions often leads to simplistic assumptions and an over-reliance on modelling techniques that are not sensitive enough for the task. Given a certain number of observations in a data set, there is an upper limit to the complexity of the model that can be derived with any acceptable degree of uncertainty (Babyak, 2004). Therefore the more questions you are answering, the more there is likely to be the introduction of error. You also need to be sensitive to the work load of your participants, which in turn can have an effect on your recruitment and retention. For example, if your research involved post-operative care, not many patients recovering from an operation would like to complete a huge stack of questionnaires for the purpose of your project. In instances like these, obtaining as much data as you can from notes or staff would be preferable to burdening the patient.

Using the study design to simplify comparisons by choosing a particular group of patients or matching on certain factors should reduce the many potential variants, and therefore remove the need to ask questions about that variant, for example, for a case control study investigating cot death you may restrict the age limit from birth to 12 months, as few cot deaths occur after this age, and also age-match the controls so that questions on infant care practices such as breastfeeding take into account the age-related variability of the practice you wish to measure. Modelling the remaining variants will bring further clarity but only up to a point. Sometimes a programme of work is needed which may require more than one study, often building on what is learnt, to provide a more definitive answer. Therefore, if it becomes apparent that you have many research questions, it would be wiser to dissect the work into separate work packages or projects. As a rule of thumb, especially in RCTs, you may have one primary, but no more than seven secondary questions (Cresswell, 2009).

Hypothesis, aims and objectives

Qualitative research is often regarded as hypothesis generating, whilst quantitative is regarded as hypothesis answering. Therefore in qualitative work research questions (rather than hypothesis) are posed. However in reality the contrast is not as stark as this. Quantitative studies can often generate many hypotheses whilst qualitative studies can often provide complex answers to questions that are difficult to measure.

Whereas a research question is just that: 'What', 'Why', 'When', 'How', 'Where' and 'Who', a hypothesis is a statement of prediction of what you believe will happen in your study. A simple hypothesis contains one predictor and one outcome, for example, 'patients with Crohn's disease who take the new medication X, will have less abdominal pain than those on usual care'. You could design a complex hypothesis with more than one predictor or outcome variable, for example, 'patients with Crohn's disease who take the new medication X, *and do not have a stressful life,* will have less abdominal pain than those on usual care'. Here there are two predictors, i.e. medication and stress, with one outcome, less abdominal pain. However, complex hypotheses cannot be easily tested, so ideally you would split these hypotheses into two: (i) Those who take the new medication X will have less abdominal pain than those on usual care; and (ii) Those who do not have a stressful life will have less abdominal pain.

As you can see, hypotheses can describe the direction of the difference, for example, you are not only expecting there to be a difference in abdominal pain between those who are on the new medication X when compared to those on usual care, but you are predicting a direction, that those on the new medication X will have *less* abdominal pain. This therefore is a one-tailed hypothesis (as you are specifying the direction of the association). If your research question was however, 'Those who take the new medication X, will have a *different* level of abdominal pain compared to those on usual care', this is a two-tailed hypothesis, as you are not predicting the direction of the association, just that there will be one, either negative or positive. A null hypothesis is the statement that there will be no association between the intervention and the outcome, for example, 'Those who take the new medication X will not have a different level of abdominal pain compared to those on usual care.' The null hypothesis is usually the default position when analysing quantitative data, i.e. you set out to disprove the null hypothesis (thereby proving an association).

Your hypotheses should always be drafted prior to the research commencing as this will help prevent too much *post-hoc* (from the Latin 'after this') analysis being conducted, which is the investigation of data after the collection has concluded for patterns that were not specified *a priori* (from the Latin 'what comes before'). Sometimes described as data dredging, in that the more one looks, the more likely something will be found, i.e. the more comparisons are made, the more likely you will get a type I error, which is the incorrect rejection of a true null hypothesis and instead reporting a false positive finding. For example, if there was a 5% chance of incorrectly rejecting a true null hypothesis per test, if you did 100 tests where the null hypothesis is true for them all, the expected number of incorrect rejections would be 5, with a probability of 99.4% for at least one incorrect rejection! Post-hoc analyses should always be explicitly labelled in any publication or report, the idea being to strike a balance between limiting the chance of obtaining false positives and the use of post-hoc analyses to inform and generate hypotheses that may be worth investigating in the future.

Your research objectives and aims should be linked to your hypothesis or research question. Aims are broad statements about what you hope your research will achieve, for example, to evaluate the efficacy of the new medication X in patients with Crohn's disease. Objectives on the other hand are the steps you need to take in order to meet your aims and so are usually more specific and are usually numbered in sequence, for example, your first objective may be to assess effectiveness of new medication X in lowering abdominal pain in patients with Crohn's disease, as measured with the McGill Pain scale (Melzack, 1975). Objectives should be 'SMART':

Specific	clear about what will be achieved
Measurable	you have a measure of when objectives have been achieved
Achievable	are the objectives feasible?
Realistic	they can be achieved using the resources available
Timed	they can be achieved within the timescales specified.

Obtaining a good answer

When you are determining the most appropriate research question/s for your project, you must bear in mind what the answer may be, as this will ensure that you understand what it means to evidence-based medicine, and also help you in the formulation of your hypothesis if you are conducting quantitative work. Moreover, if you anticipate presenting your work at a peer-reviewed conference or publishing in a scientific journal, you may have to defend your work, therefore you do not merely have to know what the answer is, you have to *understand* it and be confident that your project was conducted as robustly as possible.

When writing up the findings of an investigation after a sustained period of often laborious work, there can always be a temptation to overinterpret what has been found. This can be driven by a need to justify the effort, to increase the chances of publication, to argue a particular point for which you are a keen proponent, or simply just from enthusiasm. It should be remembered that publications are peer-reviewed and, if published, the findings will be further scrutinised by a discerning audience. It is far better to interpret your findings with a critical eye and ask 'why might my findings be wrong?' and proactively seek alternative interpretations and limiting factors to your findings. In qualitative studies, any derived themes should be substantiated with quotes which will enable your reader to ascertain whether your conclusion is warranted or whether there could be an alternative explanation. In quantitative studies, we rely on statistical inference to determine whether an association or an effect is really 'true', i.e. that our observed association or effect is not due to chance (please see Chapter 19: 'Quantitative Analysis'). If we can say chance is very unlikely, our results are positive, if chance is a distinct possibility, then we report a negative result, like the case study shows.

Case study

Faced with an association between dental flossing and obesity (lack of daily flossing is associated with being morbidly obese), the authors of a cross-sectional survey in the US (Hujoel et al., 2006) adjusted for potential confounding variables (other factors that may be responsible for the association) as they thought the association was spurious. However, even after adjustment for socio-demographic variables, age, sex, smoking status, and diabetes, they still found a dose-dependent relationship between dental flossing and obesity. They explained this as good oral health being an indicator of general health awareness, which is why the participants who floss more are also more likely to have a normal weight.

It is therefore important to not just report the associations or themes found, but also report any suspected error by investigating how robust your results are in terms of the strength of the association, and the consistency with other findings in the literature. A good answer is not necessarily a positive answer, as long as the study is robust and valid. There are many instances when a failure to demonstrate that a new treatment works can be a benefit to both patients and health care providers. In the case of a new and more expensive treatment, there is a temptation to assume it must be better for the patient. However, if rigorous research demonstrates that the new treatment is no better than the presently used, cheaper one, this will save the health care provider money that can be diverted to more useful treatments. There are numerous examples of interventions that have been routinely performed in clinical practice until rigorous research evidence has demonstrated that they are entirely useless or even harmful. For example, for many years women in labour who were about to deliver would routinely have their pubic hair shaved off in the belief that this would lessen the chances of infection, in particular if there was any tearing during delivery. It was only the negative results from well-designed trials that provided evidence that the practice was completely unnecessary. Even when there was perineal damage, the practice appeared to increase the rate of infection rather than prevent it (Basevi and Lavender, 2001)!

Summary

- The bedrock of good research is in asking the right questions and then designing a study that will provide meaningful answers to these questions.
- The larger and often unanswerable questions can often be broken down into smaller ones and should go through a refinement process involving the different perspectives of a multi-disciplined team including patients.
- The question should be structured using criteria such as PICO which breaks down an individual question into components which may directly translate into keywords that inform the design and literature search of any study. Using a criterion also ensures that any publications resulting from your project will be found during a literature search on the same subject.
- The primary question serves as the main focus of a particular study. Secondary questions can be used to define future studies or can be answered in the current study (if quantitative these need to be suitably powered).
- In general, a qualitative project will have a research question and is hypothesis generating. A quantitative project will have a hypothesis, including the expected direction of the association. Projects should detail the aims and objectives of the research.
- Any answers to a question should be interpreted with a critical eye; associations, whether part of the analytical plan or spurious, should be robustly tested and viewed in a wider context, and in qualitative work, themes should be assessed for alternative explanations.
- Negative findings are usually just as useful as positive ones and can be of equal benefit to the patients and health care providers.

Questions for Discussion

1. A themed call has come out to address the growing pandemic of obesity in children. Researchers have found a strong association between obesity in children and lack of sleep.

   i. How could the primary question be framed to provide a meaningful answer?

   ii. Would you need any secondary questions?

2. What are the differences between 'research question', 'hypotheses', 'aims' and 'objectives'?

Further Reading

Bragge, P. (2010) 'Asking good clinical research questions and choosing the right study design', *Injury, International Journal of Care of the Injured*, S3–S6.

Cross, N.B., Craig, J.C. and Webster, A.C. (2010) 'Asking the right question and finding the right answers', *Nephrology*, 15: 8–11.

Lees, J., Manning, N. and Rawlings, B. (2004) 'A culture of enquiry: research evidence and the therapeutic community', *Psychology Quarterly*, 75 (3): 279–93.

References

Babyak, M.A. (2004) 'What you see may not be what you get: a brief, nontechnical introduction to over-fitting in regression-type models', *Psychosom Med*, 66 (3):411–21.

Basevi ,V. and Lavender, T. (2001) 'Routine perineal shaving on admission in labour', Cochrane Database Syst Rev. 2001;(1):CD001236. Review.

Bragge, P. (2010) 'Asking good clinical research questions and choosing the right study design', *Injury, International Journal of Care of the Injured*, S3–S6.

Cresswell, J. (2009) *Research Design: Qualitative, Quantitative and Mixed Methods Approaches*. London: SAGE.

Hujoel, P.P., Cunha-Cruz, J. and Kressin, N.R. (2006) 'Spurious associations in oral epidemiological research: the case of dental flossing and obesity', *Journal of Clinical Periodontology*, 33 (8): 520–3.

Hulley, S.B., Cummings, S.R., Browner, W.S., Grady, D.G. and Newman, T.B. (2007) *Designing Clinical Research* (3rd edn). Philadelphia, PA: Lippincott, Williams & Wilkins.

Melzack, R. (1975) 'The McGill Pain Questionnaire: major properties and scoring methods', *Pain*, 1: 277–99.

Richardson, W.S, Wilson, M.C, Nishikawa, J. and Hayward, R.S. (1995) 'The well-built clinical question: a key to evidence-based decisions', *ACP Journal Club*, 123 (3) A12–13.

Sackett, D.L., Rosenberg, W.M.C., Gray, J.A.M. et al. (1996) 'Evidence based medicine: what it is and what it isn't', *British Medical Journal*, 312: 71.

Smith, G.C. and Pell, J.P. (2003) 'Parachute use to prevent death and major trauma related to gravitational challenge: systematic review of randomised controlled trials', *British Medical Journal*, 20: 327 (7429): 1459–61.

Smith, R. (2006) 'The trouble with medical journals', *Journal of the Royal Society of Medicine,* 99: 115–19.

The Lancet (1995) Editorial: 'Evidence-based medicine, in its place', 346: 785.

Vale, B. (2008) 'The conquest of scurvy in the Royal Navy 1793–1800: a challenge to current orthodoxy', *The Mariners' Mirror*, 94 (2): 160–75.

2

FINDING THE EVIDENCE TO SUPPORT YOUR RESEARCH QUESTION

Mary Edmunds Otter and Christine Keen

Learning Objectives

- How to use evidence throughout the research process, from formulating your research question to dissemination
- How to develop a search strategy and conduct your searches
- Where you can find the literature with an introduction to health databases
- How to manage your references

Introduction

Following on from the previous chapter which looked at asking the right question, this chapter will discuss finding the evidence to support that question. Finding relevant information is an important part of the research planning process as it

- Provides a background and context to your research proposal.
- Illustrates why the planned research is important.
- Ensures that no one else has done, or is currently working on, the same project.
- Helps define your research question by identifying gaps or inconsistencies within the existing research literature.
- Gives you an idea of how much research has already been published on the proposed topic.
- Helps you develop an appropriate methodology, including choosing outcome measures.
- Identifies experts in the field who might be recruited as consultants, collaborators or reviewers.

Evidence and information is required throughout the research process and as the body of research literature grows, it is important for researchers to gain and maintain the skills to search for it effectively. This includes searching the literature for good-quality health care information, and accessing some of the newer electronic information resources increasingly being used by the health and social care research community. Literature can be found in a number of places, such as in journal articles and books. Although books do not contain the most up-to-date material (owing to the length of time it takes to write and publish them), information found in books can provide useful background material to a research topic, including ascertaining the historical development of a field. Traditionally available in print, they are now increasingly available online as electronic books (e-books) which can be accessed through an institution's library with a password, or purchased for download from an internet bookstore. Peer-reviewed journals, on the other hand, provide access to the latest published research and give more in-depth and up-to-date information than books. There is, however, an ever increasing number of journal titles and articles, which means that searching for the evidence requires a systematic and thorough approach. Although journals are published in print, many are also available via the internet using a personal subscription or through your institution's library.

Literature can also be found in less obvious places, such as conference proceedings, dissertations or government reports, i.e. grey literature. As well as these traditional forms of grey literature, other media available on the internet may be included within the term such as podcasts, videos, blogs or open access repositories (also known as digital repositories). Podcasts (audio or video files which can be downloaded) are an emerging information resource (Peoples and Tilley, 2011) as they can include output from scholarly journals and research organisations, such as the *New England Journal of Medicine* or British Medical Journal Publishing Group. An open access repository is a concept which has developed in recent years and is '...one whose mission is to provide reliable, long-term access to managed digital resources to its designated community, now and in the future' (RLG/OCLC, 2002: 5). They contain research works, often from an academic institution, including student dissertations, research articles and reports. Many funding bodies, for example, Research Councils UK, now have a policy that supports open and unrestricted access to published research, and 'are encouraging researchers to place their papers in digital repositories' (JISC, 2005: 2).

Finding the evidence to support your research

A good starting point is getting to know your local health librarians which many institutions such as universities and hospitals will employ. They have knowledge regarding which resources to search and the best way to search them. They will also be able to help you obtain materials not held in the library, and may run training sessions to improve the skills needed to conduct literature searches and critically appraise the retrieved information (please see Chapter 3: 'Critical Appraisal'). If your research includes a systematic review (please see Chapter 14: 'Systematic Reviews'), having an information specialist or health librarian named on the research proposal, although not necessarily as a co-applicant, will add weight to your application.

Using the most effective techniques for searching for information is important for several reasons:

1. A haphazard approach may mean that the searches done are not thorough and so important literature is omitted.
2. Time can be wasted by forgetting which resources have previously been searched, which keywords have been used, or by getting distracted by irrelevant items of interest.
3. You may need to describe your methods to others, or in a protocol, publication or report.

Preliminary searches (sometimes known as scoping searches) should identify some key papers which can be incorporated into the background and methodology sections of your research proposal, and form a basis for further literature searches as your protocol develops. Searching is an iterative process and additional keywords might be needed once some initial searching has been done.

Developing a search strategy

The first step in developing your search strategy is to write down your research question in full, from which the key concepts of the search can be identified. To do this it may help to think about how your research question could be explained to someone else in a precise and specific way. The second step is to break down your question into its key elements or concepts. A number of mnemonics can help us to do this. For example, you might choose the PICO framework (Richardson et al., 1995) when thinking about a quantitative research question (please see Chapter 1: 'Asking the Right Question' or the next case study). If your research is using qualitative methodology or is considering a health management or social care topic, it may be more appropriate to use either the SPICE (Booth, 2004) or the ECLIPSE (Wildridge and Bell, 2002) framework. For example, if you were exploring the question, 'How effective are nurse-led antenatal breastfeeding education programmes for first-time mothers, in increasing breastfeeding rates?'

Table 2.1 uses the ECLIPSE framework.

TABLE 2.1   ECLIPSE framework

E	Expectation (what is the information for?)	To improve access to antenatal breastfeeding programmes
C	Client Group	First-time mothers
L	Location	Antenatal classes
I	Impact (what is the impact of the change in service?)	Breastfeeding rates
P	Profession	Nurses
SE	SErvice	Breastfeeding education

Table 2.2 presents the same example using the SPICE framework.

TABLE 2.2   SPICE Framework

S	Setting	Antenatal classes
P	Perspective / Population	First-time mothers
I	Intervention/ Interest	Breastfeeding education
C	Comparison	No breastfeeding education
E	Evaluation	Breastfeeding rates

When developing a search strategy, two elements of a framework are needed but not necessarily more as there will not always be a comparison with the intervention.

Once the key concepts of your research question and their associated keywords, such as 'breastfeeding' from this example, have been chosen, adding synonyms, i.e. alternative phrases, terms or spellings which describe the same concept, will improve your search. Sometimes this is due to concepts having different names or spellings according to country, for example, American/English. These keywords and synonyms will then be used as your search terms. Your search terms will then be combined together to form your search strategy, by the use of AND/OR/NOT (known as Boolean operators) to group the terms so that the search will find the most relevant results for you. Boolean logic is a way of performing a database search that combines keywords and synonyms to either narrow or widen a search. Major health databases use this way of constructing a search which is unlike using a generic internet search engine, in which you type some terms of interest in the search box without connecting them. 'OR' is used when combining synonyms together, for example, stroke OR cerebrovascular accident (here either, or both, words will be present in the list of results retrieved); 'AND' combines two concepts, for example, animals AND asthma (both concepts will be present in the list of results retrieved); 'NOT' is used to exclude terms from a search, for example, depression NOT anxiety (the list of results would include articles about depression but exclude articles which mention anxiety). 'NOT' should be used with care however, as relevant results can be lost as there may be some useful articles about depression which also mention anxiety. Finally, you can add limits to make your search even more relevant. These can include participant age groups; year range of search; country of interest; type of publication; study design; or language of article. You can see how Boolean operators may work in a project in the next case study.

Case study

A physiotherapist working in a hospital rheumatology clinic has anecdotally noticed that patients with osteoarthritis who take some exercise, such as walking or swimming, have better mobility and less pain than those who do not. She would like to know whether patients with osteoarthritis would have an improvement in mobility, a reduction in pain, and/or an improvement in their quality of life, if they have some kind of prescribed exercise programme. The physiotherapist uses the PICO criteria to develop her search strategy which she extends with synonyms and Boolean operators as can be seen in Table 2.3.

TABLE 2.3 PICO example of a search strategy

PICO	Keywords	Boolean operator	Synonyms
P Patient/ Population	Osteoarthritis	OR	OA, degenerative arthritis
Boolean operator: 'AND'			
I Intervention	Exercise	OR	Exercise therapy, exercise programme/ program
Boolean operator: 'AND'			
C Comparison	Not applicable		
Boolean Operator: 'AND'			
O Outcome	Pain reduction, Improved mobility, Quality of life	OR	Pain, movement, QoL, wellbeing, well-being

Choosing resources to search

Which databases or resources you search will depend upon what information is needed. For example, when thinking of a new research project it is important to find out what current research is taking place to make sure that similar research is not in progress, or that existing research does not already answer the question. If there is a recent systematic review on the topic, this can suggest whether further research is needed or not. Primary research articles which report original findings may also help with writing the background to your proposal, or writing up the project once finished.

- Databases

Bibliographic databases index the content of articles published in academic journals, (such as reports of primary research) which can be searched to find articles on a given topic. Many of the medicine and health databases are found in the invisible, deep or hidden web, i.e. content on the web which is not accessible through general search engines and which requires passwords to access it. Primary research such as publications in peer-reviewed journals, are usually held online as electronic journals and can be accessed via their website or bibliographic databases both of which usually require a subscription. Many academic institutions and other organisations use an authentication system which uses password protection, for example, Athens, Shibboleth, etc. to control access to the range of databases and electronic information sources they subscribe to.

There are also databases of secondary research such as the Cochrane Database of Systematic Reviews. Secondary research is the synthesis of existing research into systematic reviews, health technology assessments, economic evaluations or guidelines. For details of this database, as well as other databases for secondary and primary research please see Table 2.4 in the further reading section at the end of this chapter. This comprehensive list also has suggestions for searching for ongoing research. Details for ongoing research are not usually part of the invisible web but rather are freely available on the internet. Not only do these resources help establish what research is currently being undertaken, but because they include who is funding the research can provide useful information about who is likely to fund your research if you find a similar trial to the one you propose. If a researcher is conducting a clinical trial, registering it is considered a 'scientific, ethical and moral responsibility' (World Health Organisation, 2013) and the Declaration of Helsinki (2008: para. 19) stated that 'Every clinical trial must be registered in a publicly accessible database before recruitment of the first subject'.

If you are conducting a systematic review where the intention is to review all literature on a topic (please see Chapter 14: 'Systematic Reviews'), you should also have a strategy to identify grey literature. A variety of databases and websites help you find grey literature such as Open Grey (formerly known as the System for Information on Grey Literature in Europe) or the Web of Science databases which include Conference Proceedings Citation Indexes for Science and Social Science and are a useful way of finding proceedings from conferences, symposia and seminars. You may also find grey literature by using a more generic search engine such as Google Scholar which will find scholarly literature including theses, books, pre-prints and technical reports, as well as research output in digital repositories. If you would like to search the open access digital repositories there are some specialist resources, for example, OAIster (OCLC – Digital Collection Services). Details of grey literature databases and open repositories are in Table 2.4 in the further reading section at the end of this chapter. When searching a particular topic area, it is also worth checking for reports from leading charities such as Cancer Research, as these charities may conduct their own research and publish their findings on their websites, rather than via the more usual ways of dissemination.

Case study

The physiotherapist needs to find information for the background to her research such as the size of the problem, and the cost of osteoarthritis to the health care provider. She also wants to make sure that no other researchers are working on the same hypothesis currently. She decides which would be the most appropriate databases to search to find information about exercise therapy for patients with osteoarthritis.

Databases of primary research:

Medline, the major database for health and biomedical information

CINAHL, good for information on allied health practices including physiotherapy

Databases of secondary research:

The Cochrane Library

PEDro, the physiotherapy evidence database

Database of ongoing research:

Current Controlled Trials

Grey Literature:

As she is not conducting a systematic review, she will not conduct a special search for grey literature.

Hand searching

Hand searching is a technique of looking through the indexes of relevant journals for further articles, letters or editorials which meet your search criteria, and can be particularly useful for finding conference proceedings or book chapters which are not always indexed in the databases or missed due to the publication not being represented by the databases you are searching. Additionally indexing, even in the major databases, is not always foolproof. You should develop a hand search strategy if a systematic review is being conducted (Hopewell et al., 2007), but is not usually necessary otherwise.

Conducting a literature search

There are several ways of searching a bibliographic database. The first is by using free text terms, which simply looks for the word or phrase in the abstract or title of the article. The difficulty with this method is in making sure that all of the different spellings and terms are covered. Many of the major health databases include an index of terms (in Medline this is called MeSH: Medical Subject Headings). Each article added to a database will have been indexed with its appropriate terms or medical subject headings. It is possible to search just using the medical subject headings within the database; however in most cases it is best to use a combination of both free text and medical subject headings to get the best results.

Once you have conducted a preliminary search, it can be useful to see how the relevant papers you find have been indexed, and include their keywords in your search, i.e. citation pearl searching. Additional articles can also be found by searching the reference lists of your key papers, known as snowball searching, or for papers written by authors who are known specialists in the field. The danger with these final two methods is that it can lead to a biased set of references as the articles cited in reference lists are likely to support the original argument, as are papers written by the same researcher.

You can also use methodological filters or 'hedges' (or in PubMed 'Clinical Queries'), which are lists of terms that can be added to a completed subject search. This will narrow down your results to retrieve only references which use a particular methodology, such as randomised controlled trials. These filters have been tested rigorously to ensure that they retrieve all of the papers that use that methodology (Glanville et al., 2008), therefore it is a reliable way of limiting the results. Additionally, there is often a facility to vary the sensitivity or specificity of the filter. The more sensitive the filter, the more results will be retrieved, but the number of irrelevant studies will increase also, whilst a highly specific filter will reduce the number of results found, and the ones that are found should be more relevant, though some papers on the topic may be missed. A group of information professionals (InterTASC Information Specialists' Sub-Group), who support health research for the National Institute for Health and Clinical Excellence in the UK, have compiled a search filter resource which provides access to search filters for many study designs useful for health services research, such as qualitative methodology, therapy and diagnostic studies: www.york.ac.uk/inst/crd/intertasc/index.htm (accessed Jan. 2013).

Documenting the search

Whilst performing your search of the databases it is useful to keep a record of the searches completed and how you conducted them. This documentation will make writing up your reports easier and will be useful if it is necessary to rerun the same search at a later date. When documenting your search, keep a record of the:

- title of the databases searched, e.g. Medline;
- date the search was done;
- the date range you searched;
- the number of references retrieved from each database;
- the search strategy used including keywords and subject headings.

Keeping this kind of record is particularly important if a systematic review forms part, or all of the research project, as it will be required when writing up the review.

Case study

The physiotherapist conducted her search via Ovid SP (authorised access platform for databases). She documented her search as follows:

Database	Date searched	Date Range	No. of Results	Notes
Medline	27/02/12	1996-date	57	Imported into reference software
CINAHL	27/02/12	1996-date		

Search strategy

Searches		Results	
1	exp osteoarthritis/	7740	Subject heading
2	osteoarthritis.tw.	7549	Free text term
3	OA.mp.	4083	Synonym
4	degenerative arthritis.tw.	99	Synonym
5	1 or 2 or 3 or 4	11207	Combining OA related headings, free text terms and synonyms
6	exp Exercise/ or exp Exercise Therapy/	28061	Subject headings
7	exercise program*.tw.	1507	Free text term
8	6 or 7	28371	Combining exercise subject headings and free text term
9	5 and 8	560	Combining the OA and exercise results

Note: Gives too many results about exercise causing OA therefore refine search to include exercise therapy

(Continued)

(Continued)

10	exercise therapy.mp. or exp Exercise Therapy/	6641	Keyword or subject heading
11	7 or 10	7369	Exercise program or exercise therapy
12	5 and 11	287	Combing OA related results with exercise program or therapy
13	quality of life.mp. or exp 'Quality of Life'/	44918	QoL free text or subject heading
14	QoL.tw	5126	Synonym
15	well being.tw.	8079	Well-being free text term
16	wellbeing.tw.	1430	Synonym
17	13 or 14 or 15 or 16	51844	Combining all quality of life terms
18	12 and 17	57	OA, exercise and QoL

Note: Fewer, more appropriate, results

Key:

exp   exploded subject heading, (you are searching the subject heading 'osteoarthritis' but also for any narrower and more precise terms)

tw   searching for a text word in the title or abstract

mp   searching for the term as a keyword in the title, abstract, subject heading and other fields

*   the word with any ending after the asterisk (truncation symbol)

Managing your references

Reference management is a term used to describe any systematic method of organising the references found while conducting literature searches. Careful and exhaustive referencing of the literature and citations in the research proposal, report or dissemination is important to avoid plagiarism, i.e. passing someone else's words or ideas off as your own by not crediting the original author/s (Council of Writing Program Administrators, 2003). Thorough referencing will also enable the reader to find the sources cited if required. A reference management system will help you to keep track of which studies have been found already, and whether they have been obtained either electronically or ordered via inter-library loan. The reference management system you use could be manual, though there are now many different types of bibliographic reference software, for example, Refworks, Endnote, Mendeley, which can be time-saving and efficient. References found while searching can then be imported into your own personal reference library, and the cite-while-you-write feature, which can be added to Microsoft Word, enables you to insert references from your library into your document at the click of a mouse. A bibliography can then be generated automatically at the end of your text which will save you a lot of time.

Managing references will take place at several points in the research process: first when the scoping searches have been conducted and key papers identified; again when the research project is under way and you conduct a systematic literature search that will find additional papers; finally, when the research is being written up and citations used and a bibliography drafted.

Summary

- Good evidence and information is required throughout the research process from developing the research idea, to writing the final report.
- There are many sources of information to consider when searching for good-quality information including books, journal articles, government reports, and conference proceedings.
- It is important to know the best resources to search, have a clear plan of keywords to use, and an appropriate method for combining them.
- Make notes about the databases searched and the keywords used at the time the searching is done, as this will save time when writing up the research, as will using some clear system to manage the references found.

Questions for Discussion

1. Why is it important to document your search?
2. Using a PICO grid, devise a search strategy for the following research question: Is using unfractionated heparin more effective than compression therapy for deep vein thrombosis (DVT) prophylaxis, in patients who have just undergone surgery?
3. Why is it important to look for any systematic reviews on your research topic?

Further Reading

Booth, A., Papaioannou, D. and Sutton A. (2012) *Systematic Approaches to a Successful Literature Review*. Los Angeles, CA, and London; SAGE.

Brunton, G., Stansfield, C. and Thomas, J. (2012) 'Finding relevant studies', in D. Gough, S. Oliver and J. Thomas (eds), *An Introduction to Systematic Reviews*. Los Angeles, CA,and London: SAGE.

Centre for Reviews and Dissemination (2009) *Systematic Reviews: CRD's Guidance for Undertaking Reviews in Health Care*. York: CRD, University of York.

Haynes, R.B. (2010) 'Acquiring the evidence: how to find current best evidence and have current best evidence find us', in S.E. Straus, W.S. Richardson, P. Glasziou and R.B. Haynes (eds), *Evidence-Based Medicine: How to Practice and Teach it*. Edinburgh: Churchill Livingstone, Elsevier.

Lefebvre, C., Manheimer, E. and Glanville, J. (2008) 'Searching for studies', in J.P.T. Higgins and S. Green (eds), *Cochrane Handbook for Systematic Reviews of Interventions*.

Version 5.1.0. Cochrane Collaboration, 2011: www.cochrane-handbook.org (accessed April 2012).

Ridley, D. (2012) *The Literature Review*. London: SAGE.

There are also some online tutorials for literature searching, about the methodology of constructing a literature search:

www.youtube.com/watch?v=QlgWG10RMgg (ScHARR Library, 2010) (accessed April 2012).

www.thecochranelibrary.com/view/0/HowtoUse.html (Cochrane Library, 2012) (accessed April 2012).

TABLE 2.4   Databases of Research

Resource	Website	Access
Clinical Trials.gov ClinicalTrials.gov is a registry of federally and privately supported clinical trials conducted in the United States and around the world	http://clinicaltrials.gov/	Free
Current Controlled Trials Current Controlled Trials allows users to search, register and share information about randomised controlled trials worldwide	http://www.controlled-trials.com/	Free
Europe PubMed Central Grant Lookup Tool Searches for grants information provided by UKPMC funders (these include NIHR and well known charities	http://europepmc.org/GrantLookup/	Free
UK Clinical Research Network Portfolio The portfolio is a database of high-quality clinical research studies that are eligible for support from the NIHR Clinical Research Network in England	http://public.ukcrn.org.uk/search/	Free
UK Clinical Trials Gateway The UK Clinical Trials Gateway provides information about clinical research trials running in the UK. Intended for public and clinicians	http://www.ukctg.nihr.ac.uk/default.aspx	Free
WHO International clinical trials registry platform Provides access to a central database containing the trial registration data sets provided by national registries. It also provides links to the full original records	http://apps.who.int/trialsearch/default.aspx	Free
MRC/Clinical Trials Unit Website provides information on ongoing trials and research areas	http://www.ctu.mrc.ac.uk/research_areas.aspx	Free

Databases of Published research

Database/Resource	Website	Access
AMED Coverage includes alternative and complementary therapies	http://www.evidence.nhs.uk	NHS Athens/ Institution
ASSIA (Applied Social Sciences Index & Abstracts) Coverage: health, social services, psychology, sociology, economics, politics, race relations and education	Check your institution's database subscriptions	Institution
British Nursing Index (BNI) Coverage: mainly nursing literature	http://www.evidence.nhs.uk	NHS Athens/ Institution
Campbell Library Systematic reviews in education, justice and social care	http://www.campbellcollaboration.org/library.php	Free
CINAHL (Cumulated Index of Allied Health Literature) Coverage: Nursing and Allied Health	http://www.evidence.nhs.uk	NHS Athens/ Institution
Cochrane Library Secondary research including systematic reviews, health technology assessments and economic evaluations, and a database of clinical trials	http://www.thecochranelibrary.com/view/0/index.html	Free in UK
DARE (Centre for Reviews and Dissemination) Systematic reviews that evaluate the effects of health care interventions, delivery and organisation of health services	http://www.crd.york.ac.uk/CRDWeb/HomePage.asp	Free
Embase Coverage: drugs and pharmacology, general health and medicine	http://www.evidence.nhs.uk	NHS Athens/ Institution
EPPI-Centre Databases A number of databases containing primary research studies and evidence reviews, many of which have been used in EPPI-Centre systematic reviews	http://eppi.ioe.ac.uk/cms/	Free
Google Scholar Searches the internet for theses, books, articles, abstracts, grey literature and online repositories	http://scholar.google.co.uk	Free

(Continued)

TABLE 2.4   (Continued)

Databases of Published research

Health Business Elite Coverage: Health management and administration, full text journal articles	http://www.evidence.nhs.uk	NHS Athens/Institution
Health Technology Assessments Completed and ongoing health technology assessments from around the world. Source for identifying grey literature – much of the information it contains is only available directly from individual funding agencies	http://www.crd.york.ac.uk/CRDWeb/HomePage.asp	Free
HMIC Health service management, social care services, NHS organisation grey literature	http://www.evidence.nhs.uk	NHS Athens/Institution
Medline via PubMed Premier source of biomedical literature, health and life sciences	http://www.evidence.nhs.uk http://www.pubmed.gov	NHS Athens/Institution
NHS EED (Centre for Reviews and Dissemination) Focuses primarily on the economic evaluation of health care interventions and aims to help decision makers interpret an increasingly complex and technical literature	http://www.crd.york.ac.uk/CRDWeb/HomePage.asp	Free
OT Seeker Contains abstracts of systematic reviews and randomised controlled trials relevant to occupational therapy	http://www.otseeker.com/	Free
PEDro Coverage: Physiotherapy, includes systematic reviews, RCTs and practice guidelines	http://www.pedro.org.au/	Free
PsycInfo Coverage: Psychology and mental health	http://www.evidence.nhs.uk	NHS Athens/Institution
ProQolid Patient reported outcomes and quality of life instruments	http://www.proqolid.org/	Free basic search
Scopus Coverage: Science, social science and medicine	Check your institution's database subscriptions	Institution
Social Care online Coverage: Social care	http://www.scie-socialcareonline.org.uk/	Free
Sociological Abstracts Coverage: Sociology, social and behavioural sciences	Check your institution's database subscriptions	Institution

Databases of Published research

Europe PubMed Central Coverage: Pubmed Central archive, European patents; NHS clinical guidelines and grant information	http://europepmc.ac.org	Free
Web of Science Coverage: Science, social science, medicine, conference proceedings and grey literature	Check your institution's database subscriptions	Institution

Grey Literature Resources	**Website**	**Access**
Conference Proceedings Citation Index (Science and Technology) Is an index to the published literature of the most significant conferences, symposia, seminars, colloquia, workshops, and conventions in a wide range of disciplines	Check your institution	Institutional
Dissertations and Theses (WorldCat) All dissertations, theses and published material based on theses catalogued by OCLC members	Check your institution	Institutional
Google Scolar Provides a search of scholarly literature across many disciplines and sources, including theses, books, abstracts and articles	http://scholar.google.co.uk/	Free
HMIC (Health Management Information Consortium) Coverage includes official publications, journal articles and grey literature on: health service policy, management and administration	http://www.evidence.nhs.uk/	NHS Institutional
OpenGrey (System for Information on Grey Literature in Europe) Provides open access to 700,000 bibliographical references of grey literature (paper) produced in Europe	http://www.opengrey.eu/	Free
Official-documents.gov.uk Official Documents is the official reference facility for Command and departmentally sponsored House of Commons Papers. All Command Papers and House of Commons Papers published from May 2005 onwards, as well as key Departmental papers, are available for free on the site in PDF format	http://www.official-documents.gov.uk/	Free

(Continued)

TABLE 2.4   (Continued)

Grey Literature Resources	Website	Access
PsycExtra A database of grey literature produced by the American Psychological Association (APA) in the field of psychology and behavioural science. Documents indexed in PsycEXTRA include newsletters, magazines, newspapers, technical and annual reports, government reports, consumer brochures, and more	check your institution	Institutional
Institutional Repositories		
DRIVER (Digital Repository Infrastructure Vision for European Research) Search portal provides access to over 295 digital repositories in Europe	http://www.driver-repository.eu	Free
Google Scholar Will find research output deposited in digital repositories	http://scholar.google.co.uk/	Free
OAIster OCLC Digital Collection Services Contains records of digital resources from open archive collections worldwide	http://www.oclc.org/oaister/	Free
OpenDOAR (Directory of Open Access Repositories) Provides a listing of open access repositories around the world	http://www.opendoar.org	Free

References

Booth, A. (2004) 'Formulating answerable questions', in A. Booth and A. Brice (eds), *Evidence-Based Practice for Information Professionals: A Handbook*. London: Facet Publishing, pp. 61–70.

Council of Writing Program Administrators (2003) *Defining and Avoiding Plagiarism: The WPA Statement on Best Practices*: www.wadsworth.com/english_d/special_features/plagiarism/WPAplagiarism.pdf (accessed April 2012).

Declaration of Helsinki (2008) 'WMA Declaration of Helsinki: ethical principles for medical research involving human subjects', 59th WMA General Assembly, Seoul, Oct.

Glanville, J., Bayliss, S., Booth, A., Dundar, Y., Fernandes, H., Fleeman, N.D., Foster, L., Fraser, C., Fry-Smith, A., Golder, S., Lefebvre, C., Miller, C., Paisley, S., Payne, L., Price, A. and Welch, K. (2008) 'So many filters, so little time: the development of a search filter appraisal checklist', *Journal of the Medical Library Association*, 96 (4): 356–61.

Hopewell, S., Clarke, M.J., Lefebvre, C. and Scherer, R.W. (2007) 'Handsearching versus electronic searching to identify reports of randomized trials', *Cochrane Database of Systematic Reviews*: http://onlinelibrary.wiley.com/doi/10.1002/14651858.MR000001. pub2/pdf/standard (accessed April 2012).

JISC (2005) 'Opening up access to research results: questions and answers': www.jisc.ac. uk/publications/generalpublications/2005/pub_qanda.aspx (accessed April 2012).

Peoples, B. and Tilley, C. (2011) 'Podcasts as an emerging information resource', *College and Undergraduate Libraries,* 18 (1): 44–57.

Research Libraries Group/OCLC (2002) 'Trusted digital repositories: attributes and responsibilities': www.oclc.org/research/activities/past/rlg/trustedrep/repositories.pdf (accessed April 2012).

Richardson, W.S, Wilson, M.C, Nishikawa, J. and Hayward, R.S. (1995) 'The well-built clinical question: a key to evidence-based decisions', *ACP Journal Club,* 123 (3) A12–13.

Wildridge, V. and Bell, L. (2002) 'How CLIP became ECLIPSE: a mnemonic to assist in searching for health policy/management information', *Health Information and Libraries Journal,* 19 (2): 113–15.

World Health Organisation (2013) *International Trials Registry Platform*: www.who.int/ictrp/ trial_reg/en/index.html (accessed Jan. 2013).

3

CRITICAL APPRAISAL

Christine Keen and Mary Edmunds Otter

Learning Objectives

- Understand what is meant by critical appraisal
- Why critical appraisal is crucial for research and clinical practice
- Understand the concepts of validity and reliability
- How to locate and use resources regarding critical appraisal including checklists
- Know what key questions should be asked of which methodology

Introduction

Critical appraisal is the structured process of examining a piece of research in order to determine its strengths and limitations. Put simply, critical appraisal focuses on whether we can 'believe' a study, i.e. whether it is sufficiently free of bias. This is also known as 'internal validity'. Bias technically means a systematic error, where a particular research finding deviates from a 'true' finding. The design of the research and how it has been carried out, i.e. the methodology, will also have a bearing on whether the results can be considered 'true' or valid, and therefore we need to look critically at the methodology for flaws that may invalidate the findings. Thus, critical appraisal weighs up the evidence critically in order to assess its validity (closeness to the truth) and its usefulness (clinical applicability) (Sackett and Haynes, 1995). Therefore the relevance, or weight, you give a piece of research, either as part of the evidence base for your own project, or to inform your clinical practice, will be the result of critical appraisal, and so being able to critically appraise literature is an important skill for researchers and clinicians to develop.

It is worth noting that no research is perfect but the process of critical appraisal should help you identify any bias so that a judgement of their effects on the outcomes can be made. Bias might come about through, for example, errors in the manner of collecting the data, or by how the participants are selected to take part in a study which results in a non-representative sample. In practice, good research aims to minimise bias, such as by blinding the researcher who is collecting the participant data to the participant's trial arm allocation (please see Chapter 11: 'Clinical Trials'). Other terms may also be used instead of critical appraisal, such as 'quality assessment', 'critical evaluation or reading', or 'critiquing'. All of these terms, however, are describing the same critical appraisal process.

Critical appraisal to inform clinical practice

Many of you will already be familiar with critical appraisal in relation to informing your clinical practice, as you may have been asked to critically appraise pieces of research as a student, or at work, and the importance of critical appraisal cannot be over-emphasised. The controversy surrounding the measles, mumps and rubella (MMR) combined vaccination illustrates this well (please see the case study).

Case study

In 1998 *The Lancet* published a paper by Wakefield and colleagues which caused much concern and controversy. In this paper, Wakefield et al. described how they investigated a series of 12 children who had been referred to their paediatric gastroenterology unit with a history of normal development followed by loss of acquired skills including language, as well as suffering from diarrhoea and abdominal pains. The parents reported that the onset of symptoms was associated with the administration of the MMR vaccination in 8 of the 12 children and with a measles infection in another child. Wakefield and colleagues concluded that the potential link between autism and bowel disease with the MMR vaccination should be investigated (Aveyard, 2010).

Any practitioner who read Wakefield et al.'s (1998) original article would see that the evidence it provided for the argument that the MMR vaccination causes autism/ bowel disease was not strong. Given the small number of child participants and the lack of a comparison group, the researcher's conclusions would rank in the 'evidence pyramid' (please see Figure 6.1, p. 85) as little more than expert opinion or anecdotal evidence. After critically appraising the paper, you would conclude therefore, that the findings should not be acted upon in clinical practice and that further empirical primary evidence is needed. Unfortunately this did not halt the media scare that ensued, which resulted in many parents not allowing their children to have the MMR, resulting in the vaccination uptake rate dropping. Single vaccines were available but not free in the UK, which deterred many parents from accessing an alternative. Before Wakefield et al.'s publication, uptake of MMR was 92% in the UK; afterwards it fell to 80% (Thomas, 2010), having a detrimental effect on the nation's health. In 1998 there were 56 cases of measles in the UK, by 2012 there were 2,016 cases (Health Protection Agency, 2013). Further studies have since been undertaken and, as yet, no evidence has been found to substantiate Wakefield's claims. Eventually all of the primary studies were incorporated into a Cochrane systematic review, which is the highest rank on the 'evidence pyramid' that again found no link between the MMR vaccination and bowel disease or autism (Demicheli et al., 2012). Wakefield was subsequently stripped of his medical licence for unethical behaviour.

The MMR controversy illustrates the importance of the critical appraisal of research to identify how strong and relevant the evidence is to a particular topic/ diagnosis. Novices may perceive that a paper which is published in a reputable journal should be above critique, yet this is clearly not the case as the MMR paper was published in *The Lancet*, currently ranked as second best out of 153 general medical journals (following the General Medical Investigation, where Wakefield and two other colleagues were found guilty of abuse and dishonesty, *The Lancet* immediately retracted this publication). Therefore in evidence-based medicine, the ability to critically appraise a paper is imperative.

Critical appraisal in research

Critical appraisal is not only imperative to inform clinical practice, it is also an important integrated part of all research projects. Learned techniques for appraisal will be used throughout your research.

Refining your research question

During the design and development of a research project you will be looking at existing literature to help you focus and shape your own research question (please see Chapter 2: 'Finding the Evidence to Support your Research Question'). During this process you will need to appraise the papers you find to identify where gaps or inconsistencies exist around your topic of interest. It may also be that you find a study that is very similar to the one you are proposing, and critical appraisal will tell you if it is worthwhile conducting a study with the same research question. If there are serious flaws with the published paper, it is ethical and worthwhile to conduct this study again.

Designing better research

One of the key elements of the critical appraisal of a research paper is judging whether the study design and methods used were appropriate to answer the research question posed. By critically appraising published research you will gain an awareness of the various designs and methods which can be used, and which methodology is best to answer which type of questions. You will also become knowledgeable about possible problems with the various research designs, topics or populations, which will help prevent them in your own project. Therefore critical appraisal will be invaluable in deciding which will be the best methods to use for your own project.

Evaluation of your own research proposal

Critical appraisal can also be an extremely useful skill in reviewing your own project proposal prior to applying for ethical approval or funding. When applying for ethical approval your application is reviewed by a panel (please see Chapter 15: 'Designing and Conducting an Ethical Research Study'), and if you are applying for funding your research protocol will be reviewed by experts on your topic, who will make recommendations to the funding panel (please see Chapter 5: 'Budget and Funding'). Reviewers will be concerned with the quality of your research proposal, and in the case of commissioned research, how adequately it addresses the research question presented in the commissioning brief. It can be quite difficult to be objective about our own projects though, as we get so passionate about them. If you have time, it helps to put your protocol to one side for a few days, and critically appraise it again with fresh eyes, or ask someone external to the research team to review it for you. This can help highlight issues that you had not noticed.

Critical appraisal during the research project

Every research protocol has a background/introduction section. This section is where the most relevant papers to your research question found during your literature search are discussed. This informs the reader why you are asking this particular research question as it highlights gaps in existing knowledge due to either a lack of research, or serious flaws in the published research which was highlighted through your critical appraisal. If your research is a systematic review, or contains a systematic review as part of it, critical appraisal will be an extremely important part of your project (please see Chapter 14: 'Systematic Reviews').

Reporting of research

Your ability to critically appraise a paper is influenced by the quality of the reported information, such as an explicit description of the methods and analyses used, both of which can be highly variable in quality. Often there is insufficient methodological detail to be able to judge particular aspects. Any omissions should be recorded during the appraisal process, or if you are conducting a systematic review, by contacting the author of the paper for clarification. To minimise the effect of poor-quality reporting, in recent years several standards have been published regarding the quality of research reporting for certain specific study designs. The Consolidated Standards of Reporting Trials team (2010) for example, produced the CONSORT statement which is an evidence-based, minimum set of recommendations for reporting randomised controlled trials (www.consort-statement.org (accessed Sept. 2012)). It gives a standard way of reporting trial findings which is complete and transparent, which in turn aids interpretation. The CONSORT statement includes a flow diagram of each stage of the trial, with participant numbers at each stage, beginning with the number assessed for eligibility, through to the final data collection including detail about attrition and the reasons for this. Researchers can use this diagram for reporting their own figures. Other reporting statements are the PRISMA, which is a 27-item checklist and example flow diagram for reporting systematic reviews (www.prisma-statement.org, accessed Jan. 2013; Moher et al., 2000), or the STARD which is for reporting diagnostic accuracy studies (www.stard-statement.org, accessed Jan. 2013; Bossuyt et al., 2003).

Validity and reliability

To be able to critically appraise a document, you must first understand the concepts of *validity* and *reliability* which are principles that underpin the process.

- Validity asks whether the results of the study are true, i.e. valid, and report what they say it does, i.e. does the study truly measure what it sets out to, or is the study impaired by confounding factors or variables. This is when you cannot be sure whether another variable or factor (other than the one being studied) has influenced the results. Sensitive researchers will often draw attention to any possible confounders in the discussion of their publication and this helps you in judging its overall quality. For example, if your project was looking at smoking, if the only measure was a subjective, self-report scale your validity may be subject to confounding variables such as prestige bias, where the participant answers what they feel would reflect positively on them, or gives an answer which they feel is more socially acceptable. Often a good piece of research will also include an objective measure which validates the subjective one. In this case it could be by observation or from taking a breath carbon monoxide reading.

- Reliability refers to whether the same results/conclusions would be found if the research was repeated. There is often variability in the results from different studies, even if they are measuring the same thing with similar tools, which can be due to bias. If one considers the Wakefield MMR publication (please see the case study in this chapter), no ensuing trials have ever replicated his findings; therefore his research has poor reliability.

To illustrate this look at Figure 3.1 below. The bull's eye of the target represents the true risk of a disease in a sample. The holes symbolise the multiple objective measures of the risk for that disease. In target 1, the reliability is good in that it measures nearly the same value each time, but it has poor validity as it does not represent the true risk, as it is nowhere near the target. This may occur if you had a non-representative sample, or you are actually measuring something other than what you wished, such as the effects from a confounding variable. In the second target, the validity is good, in that you are measuring something that is centred

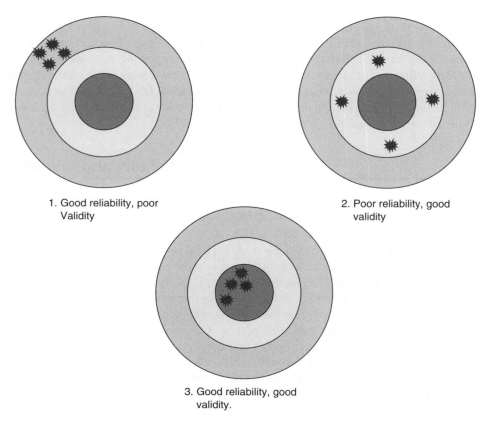

1. Good reliability, poor
   Validity

2. Poor reliability, good
   validity

3. Good reliability, good
   validity.

FIGURE 3.1   Validity and reliability

around the target. However, you have poor reliability, as there is a lot of variability in the scores as they are at a distance from each other. Target 3 is what you should be aiming for, where the results are reporting what the researcher thinks they are as the measures are in the target, therefore the validity is good, and so is the reliability as the measures report similar values each time.

The critical appraisal process

By this stage of the book, you may have refined your question after reading Chapter 1, and perhaps conducted a literature search to see if anyone else has answered your question, or to help develop your reasoning for wanting to conduct the research. Now you need to know whether the literature you retrieved is valid and reliable in order to support your argument. There are a series of points to consider when critically appraising an article.

Moving knowledge forward

Nowadays, with the huge volume of research being reported, seminal papers are scarce, although most research makes incremental steps forward, for example by researching a different regime for a medication already proven effective. Research can also validate results from prior studies by obtaining similar results.

Research question

First of all, is the topic discussed in the article relevant for your project? If not there is no point in appraising it as the information it contains will not be useful. If it is relevant, what is the research question it sets out to answer? Specifying this will help you determine whether the results are valid. A well-developed research question will have three parts: population or sample; parameter being studied, such as intervention; and the outcomes of interest (National Health and Medical Research Council, 2000) (please see Chapter 1: 'Asking the Right Question').

Study design

Identifying the specific research question will help you determine the optimal research design by which to answer it. Questions about effectiveness will usually use a quantitative method (please see Chapter 6: 'Quantitative Data Collection'), whilst research that 'explores' will usually be using a qualitative method (please see Chapter 7: 'Qualitative Data Collection'). Because you need to assess whether an appropriate study design was used, you need a general basic knowledge about different research methodologies to conduct an appraisal appropriately.

Acknowledgement of potential bias

Once you have determined the research design used, the best way to detect bias in a paper is to use an appropriate critical appraisal tool.

Critical appraisal tools

Critical appraisal tools are essentially checklists that help you ask appropriate questions of the evidence in order for you to determine how strong and relevant it is and help you maintain a consistent and systematic approach to the appraisal process. Using a critical appraisal tool helps prevent us from reviewing the paper with our own inherent bias through the use of the questions in the checklist to help us decide on the quality of each paper (rather than subjective opinion), and which prompts us to evaluate different aspects of the paper, that are considered in turn. You will then begin to determine the strengths, limitations and relevance of the information to your research question. Initially, a research paper you have found might appear to address your research question directly, but upon closer inspection the appraisal may reveal that the scope of the paper is very different, or that the methods used in the research have been poorly carried out.

There are many critical appraisal tools available, but it is best to stick to checklists that have been validated or are widely accepted in the health and social care field. If you are new to critical appraisal and looking for a generic checklist, Cottrell (2011) has developed one which you can use to evaluate any piece of academic writing. This is relatively straightforward and a good start. More specifically, many critical appraisal tools have been developed for reviewing different types of methodologies. The Critical Appraisal Skills Programme (CASP), originally developed by the University of Oxford Public Health Resources Unit, has developed tools for the most common types of studies, such as randomised controlled trials, systematic reviews, cohort and case control studies, and qualitative studies. With the qualitative appraisal tool the checklist is not designed to result in a numerical value which usually determines a cut-off point for inclusion (like on the quantitative appraisal tools), but rather it prompts you to consider different issues in the paper which can influence its validity and reliability. You may access these tools and information about CASP at: www.casp-uk.net (accessed Sept. 2012). Another website which is a good source of tools is Best Evidence Topics: www.bestbets.org (accessed Sept. 2012) which was developed by the Emergency Department of Manchester Royal Infirmary, UK. They hold tools for many research designs such as educational interventions, economic evaluations and surveys. There are details of other websites that host critical appraisal tools in the Resource Section of this chapter.

Case study

Following on from Chapter 2, the physiotherapist has been developing her research proposal around osteoarthritis and exercise. She has decided that one of the work packages in her research project will be a review of the literature about patients' attitudes towards exercise and any barriers to undertaking it. She will review qualitative literature on this topic and needs to decide which will be the most appropriate checklist to use to appraise the literature she finds. After a search, she chooses the CASP critical appraisal tool for qualitative research.

Key questions to ask when critically appraising research

Whether you are using a tool or developing your own, there are key questions that should be asked of all research papers regardless of research design:

Q.   What journal is the publication in?

You should be aware of the quality of the journal in which the research is published. Usually a journal is considered to be of good quality if it is peer reviewed, i.e. each paper is appraised by at least one recognised expert in the subject area, prior to acceptance for publication. It should be noted, however, that the peer-review process is not perfect. It is not always possible for the reviewer to know every aspect about any particular topic. It is also not uncommon for corrections or amendments to a paper to appear in later issues of the journal. In reality, the peer-review process takes place when the research paper is published (especially now that rapid responses can be made via the internet)! Individual journals have different levels of relative importance within their field. This is calculated by the frequency with which the average article has been cited (the journal's impact factor). The impact factor is basically the average number of citations in a year for articles published in the previous two years. Citable articles are somewhat loosely defined. In general, they include original research articles and review articles, however they may also include editorials, if the editorial contains a lengthy reference list. Impact factors are reported in individual journals. It might be assumed that the higher the importance of a journal (or its impact) the higher the standard of study. However, as can be seen in the Wakefield MMR example in the case study, this is not always the case as *The Lancet* is regarded as having an extremely high impact factor!
It must also be remembered that a journal will have a viewpoint in certain theoretical debates; therefore its reportage can be biased (i.e. publication bias).

Q.   Who are the authors of the paper?

Do the researchers have the necessary experience to undertake the research or the authority to write the article? It is argued that this is particularly important in qualitative research as the quality of the data collected is dependent upon the skills of the researcher. This can be assessed by reviewing the author's qualifications, which are usually listed after their names, together with their affiliations.

Q.   What is the purpose of the paper?

In a publication, the research question should be clearly stated and founded on argument and rationale, using information and evidence provided in the introduction to support the question. The paper's purpose needs to be established so that you can determine how to evaluate the paper.

Q. Is the sample representative of the population?

Have a look at the participant demographics; does the sample seem representative of the group of people it is meant to? For example, with Wakefield and the MMR study, one of the criticisms was that it was a very small sample of 12 children who had been pre-selected through MMR campaign groups. The children were also aged between 2.5 and 9.5 years (autism can usually be reliably diagnosed by age of 3 with symptoms appearing at 2). Moreover two were brothers, two others attended the same doctor's office, none of the 12 lived in London where the study was being carried out, and one of the children had to be flown in from the USA (not to mention that three of the participants did not even have clinically diagnosable autism)!

Q. Were ethical considerations observed?

Does the paper say that the researchers obtained ethical approval to conduct the study from an appropriate board? How did the researcher approach the patients and obtain their consent and was this ethical? Please see Chapter 15: 'Designing and Conducting an Ethical Research Study'.

Key questions to ask of quantitative studies (see Chapter 6)

Generally these studies use experimental methods or methods that involve the use of numbers in the collection of data. Quantitative studies include observational studies such as cohort studies, or case-controlled studies, whilst the randomised controlled trial (RCT) is considered the gold standard design for comparing treatments (or active treatment against usual care) (please see Chapter 11: 'Clinical Trials').

Q. If randomisation is a key feature of a trial, is the randomisation process used as free from bias as possible?

Is it possible to blind, i.e. hide, the participants, researchers or both, to which arm of a trial the person is in? If it is, did they do this? Is the randomisation procedure appropriate, such as using a method for allocating the randomisation sequence which is external to the research team, e.g. via a clinical trials unit, etc., which ensures concealment of allocation sequence?

Q. How were the study participants treated in the study and the follow-up?

In an RCT you would not expect there to be quantifiable differences in the characteristics of participants between the arms of the trial, or differences in their involvement in the study, such as different timings of data collection. If there is, it indicates systematic bias which can skew the data.

Q. What were the results and how have they been reported?

Since the CONSORT statement was published in 2001 by Moher et al., reporting of clinical trials has improved dramatically and bias is far easier to detect. The RCT should also conduct an intention to treat analysis to ensure that attrition was not due to a systematic reason. For instance, if you were testing a medication, analysis just of the end data might show that the treatment is effective, but the intention to treat analysis might show that attrition was due to side effects of the medication, which could change clinical opinion about using the treatment.

Key questions to ask of qualitative research (see Chapter 7)

The interfaces between the researcher and participant and the researcher and the data can both introduce bias, such as by asking participants leading questions or interpreting the data in a certain way. Although subjectivity is unavoidable, reflecting upon, and detailing areas of possible bias allows the reader their own interpretation. This concept of reflexivity acknowledges that the researcher plays a shaping role and that detachment from the focus of the research is neither desirable nor possible. For this reason, there is considerable debate around critical appraisal of qualitative research, although it is generally accepted that it should be done. Lincoln and Guba (1985) argue that the terms *credibility, transferability, dependability* and *confirmability* are more appropriate for assessing the rigour of a qualitative study than the terms validity and reliability.

Credibility focuses on the degree to which the findings make sense. This can be established by giving participants their interview transcripts and research reports so that they can agree or disagree with the researcher's conclusions. Credibility is also established by prolonged engagement in the field with persistent observation, and the triangulation of data (please see Chapter 20: 'Qualitative Analysis'). Transferability replaces the concept of external validity and qualitative researchers are encouraged to provide a detailed portrait of the setting in which the research was conducted. The aim of this is to give readers enough information for them to judge the applicability of the findings to other settings. Dependability replaces the concept of reliability. It encourages researchers to supply an audit trail (documenting data and methodology) which can be laid open to external scrutiny. Confirmability also invokes auditing as a means to demonstrate quality. For example, the author can offer a self-critical, reflexive analysis of the methodology they used in the research. In addition, techniques such as triangulation can be useful tools of confirmability.

Q.   What was the relationship between the researcher and participants?

By identifying the relationship, you will be able to ascertain the dynamics of the relationship such as power (Meara and Schmidt, 1991). Arguably as the researcher is the one who is leading the data collection, i.e. asking the questions, taping and transcribing the dialogue, etc., they are, by default, more powerful. There are techniques that can help minimise this effect, such as meeting somewhere neutral, or perhaps involving patients in collecting the data (please see Chapter 16: 'Patient and Public Involvement'). As a bare minimum one would not expect the researcher to be collecting data from someone currently in their care as this could not only bias the data by inhibiting openness, but may also be detrimental to the therapeutic relationship and impair ethical responsibilities.

Q.   Is there overt interpretation of the data by the researcher?

Not only should the data be adequately analysed, they should be reflected upon to add meaning, and in turn, provide new knowledge regarding the phenomena of interest. Furthermore, these interpretations of the data should be embedded in the literature outlined in the introduction. To help reduce bias here, it is good practice to have other team members involved in the analysis to ensure that the meaning remains the same, regardless of who is analysing the data.

Key questions to ask of a systematic review (see Chapter 14)

As a clinician, you may use systematic reviews (which may include a meta-analysis) to inform your clinical practice, as they are more powerful than single RCTs and so can give you a real authority in whether an intervention is efficacious. However, as the vast majority of reviews are conducted retrospectively, a risk of bias may be inherent, due to factors such as publication bias, i.e. studies showing positive results are easier to publish than those with non-significant or negative results. Therefore reviews need to also be critically appraised. Like any other piece of research written for publication, a systematic review will have a detailed methodology section, documented in a way that can be reproduced, such as detailing the search strategy and how the articles were appraised and selected. The paper will also have a results section which will sometimes include a meta-analysis, although more often than not just a description of the included studies. To ease the process of critically appraising a review, the QUORUM (Quality of Reporting of Meta-Analysis) statement provides a comprehensive framework for reporting reviews of RCTs and meta-analysis (Moher et al., 2000), whilst the MOOSE (Meta-analysis of Observational Studies in Epidemiology) may be used for reviews and meta-analysis of non-RCT studies (Stroup et al., 2000). If a review is described as a *Cochrane Review* you can be confident that it has been undertaken systematically, as the Cochrane Collaboration have their own internal review and support groups for any reviews it adopts. In general, questions you should ask of a review are as follows.

Q.   Have all of the relevant studies been included in the review?

Was the search in-depth, using an appropriate and exhaustive list of keywords, and a variety of databases? Due to publication bias, it is also important that ongoing and unpublished studies (grey literature) are identified as far as is possible. Without trying to identify grey literature, the systematic review may include an over-representation of positive studies, ultimately leading to a conclusion which is biased.

Q.   Were appropriate methods to prevent bias incorporated?

Not only would this include a grey literature search, but did the researchers use appropriate critical appraisal tools for the inclusion or exclusion of any identified papers? Critical appraisal tools for quantitative methodology allow for a score to be calculated. Therefore studies should be excluded that have a quality score below a predetermined threshold. This ensures that papers are included or excluded based solely on merit. Also, was a sample of the papers critically appraised by another member of the research team for quality assurance?

Q. If there is a meta-analysis, is it appropriate?

The results of a meta-analysis are only as robust as the data being entered into it. Poor-quality data in a meta-analysis will only lead to poor results. It is therefore important that the researchers have ensured the quality of the studies being input. There are two approaches for determining study quality for a meta-analysis. The first approach is to restrict the meta-analysis to include only high-level research data, for example the decision to only include RCTs, with weaker evidence trial designs such as case control (which are more prone to bias) being excluded. The second approach would be to include the quality score from the critical appraisal tool in the analysis, and check if there is an association between their quality and their effect size. Another question to ask is whether it was a reasonable decision to combine the results? The meta-analysis will be calculated using a summary measure that is common across papers. In the paper they may have assessed homogeneity, i.e. the similarities between the studies inputted, prior to the meta-analysis. The researchers may have also excluded papers with the extreme effect sizes (either high or low) until homogeneity was reached, therefore ensuring that the studies were not too heterogeneous, i.e. different.

Key questions to ask when appraising information on a website

Although this chapter mainly focuses on critical appraisal of research papers, the increase in the volume of information now available on the internet means that it is also important to consider the quality of websites. Anyone can publish on the web and there are few methods to control the validity or quality of the information found there. It is also easy to assume that websites are kept up to date, but this is not necessarily true. To make this process easier, there are some quality checklists with which to appraise websites such as Health on the Net (HON). HON was founded to encourage dissemination of quality health information via the web. Their website has information for website publishers, patients and health care professionals (www.hon.ch, accessed Sept. 2012). A good critical appraisal tool for consumers is the DISCERN Instrument: www.discern.org.uk, accessed Sept. 2012). This tool might also be useful for getting feedback from patients and the public regarding your research webpage. In general when you are appraising a web page, you should ask:

Q. Who is the author of the website or who owns the site? Can you find anything about their credibility?

Some websites have more authority to discuss certain topics than others, such as Mind for mental health issues, or Macmillan for cancer issues. Recognised charities such as these often have their own research grant schemes and so amass a body of data which they publish on their website. If the host is not a recognised charity, is it possible to ascertain who the author is and what is their affiliation? Perhaps there are links from the webpage to authoritative bodies such as other known charities or royal colleges, which confers credibility.

Q. Is the information provided accurate?

Does the webpage include references so that you can check the original source of the information or is it just personal opinion? Perhaps if it is data you are reviewing, there may be links to a scientific publication, or the webpage may give an author's email address for correspondence. If this information is missing be wary, as often seemingly informative websites can be biased, for example being owned by a company trying to sell a product.

Q. How up-to-date is the material?

On websites there is usually an indication of how current the website is, such as the last blog on the site, or a reference on the page to a dated article. If it is old, the theory around that topic may have moved on.

Practice makes perfect

Critical appraisal is an activity which needs to be practised on a regular basis. You should be using appraisal techniques every time you read some scientific information, which at first may seem an arduous process. However, if you think about the numerous times you read scientific information, these skills soon become 'second nature'. If you feel you need to further develop this skill there are various resources to help:

- Health libraries often have courses/workshops and may produce printed and online tutorials.
- Journal clubs are a great way of learning critical appraisal skills and can be found in health and university libraries and workplaces such as hospitals where they encourage the application of research in clinical practice. Essentially these comprise groups of individuals who get together to discuss and appraise papers in their particular field.

Summary

- Once mastered, critical appraisal skills can be applied not only in your research but also to evidence-based practice.
- Critical appraisal assesses the validity and reliability, and the level of bias in a study.
- Appraised studies are only as good as their reporting. The wider adoption of standards for reporting may help with the process of critical appraisal.

- There are many different tools and resources available to aid with critical appraisal to ensure that the process is systematic.

- Appraising different study designs will require different questions to be asked of it. There are different tools for different methods so it is important to understand which is the best tool to use.

Questions for Discussion

1. Why is it important to use critical appraisal skills in your research?

2. Which two concepts underpin the process of critical appraisal, and what might you look at in the paper to assess these?

Further Reading

Health Knowledge online tutorial including guided appraisals of an RCT and a systematic review:
http://www.healthknowledge.org.uk/interactive-learning/finding-and-appraising-the-evidence (accessed Aug. 2012).
A succinct guide to critical appraisal: http://www.whatisseries.co.uk/whatis.
Booth, A., Papaioannou, D. and Sutton, A. (2012) *Systematic Approaches to a Successful Literature Review*. Los Angeles, CA, and London: SAGE.
Harden, A. and Gough, D. (2012) 'Quality and relevance appraisal', in D. Gough, S. Oliver and J. Thomas (eds), *An Introduction to Systematic Reviews*. Los Angeles, CA, and London: SAGE.
Sutton, A.J., Abrams, K., Jones, D.R., Sheldon, T.A. and Song, F. (2000) *Methods for Meta-Analysis in Medical Research*. Chichester: Wiley.

References

Ajetunmobi, O. (2002) *Making Sense of Critical Appraisal*. London: Arnold.
Aveyard, H. (2010) *Doing a Literature Review in Health and Social Care* (2nd edn). New York and Maidenhead: McGraw-Hill.
Bossuyt, P.M., Reitsma J.B., Bruns, D.E., Gatsonis, C.A., Glasziou, P.P., Irwig, L.M., Moher, D., Rennie, D., de Vet, H.C., Lijmer, J.G. (2003) 'Standards for Reporting of Diagnostic Accuracy. The STARD statement for reporting studies of diagnostic accuracy: explanation and elaboration,' *Clinical Chemistry Jan*: 49(1):7 –18.
Cottrell, S. (2011) *Critical Thinking Skills* (2nd edn). Basingstoke: Palgrave Macmillan.
Demicheli, V., Rivetti, A., Debalini, M.G. and Di Pietrantonj, C. (2012) 'Vaccines for measles, mumps and rubella in children', *Cochrane Database of Systematic Reviews*, 2.
Health Protection Agency (2013) Public Health England press release: 'National MMR vaccination catch-up programme announced in response to increase in measles cases', 24 April 2013.
Lincoln, Y.S. and Guba, E.G. (1985) *Naturalistic Inquiry*. Beverly Hills, CA, and London: SAGE.
Meara, N.M. and Schmidt, L.D. (1991) 'The ethics of researching counselling/therapy processes', in C.E. Watkins, Jr. and L.J. Schneider (eds), *Research in Counselling*. Hillsdale, NJ: Lawrence Erlbaum Associates.

Moher, D., Cook, D.J., Eastwood, S., Olkin, I., Rennie, D., and Stroup, D.F. (2000) 'Improving the quality of reports of meta-analyses of randomised controlled trials: the QUOROM statement', *Onkologie,* 23 (6): 597–602.

Moher, D., Schulz, K.F. and Altman, D.G. (2001) 'The CONSORT statement: revised recommendations for improving the quality of reports of parallel group randomized trials', *BMC Medical Research Methodology,* 1: 2.

National Health and Medical Research Council (2000) *How to Review the Evidence: Systematic Identification and Review of the Scientific Literature.* Canberra: NHMRC.

Sackett, D.L., Haynes, R.B., Guyatt, G.H. and Tugwell, P. (1991) *Clinical Epidemiology: A Basic Science for Clinical Medicine.* London: Little, Brown & Co.

Sackett, D.L. and Haynes, R.B. (1995) 'On the need for evidence-based medicine', *Evidence-Based Medicine,* 1: 5–6.

Stroup, D.F., Berlin, J.A., Morton, S.C., Olkin, I., Williamson, G.D., Rennie, D., Moher, D., Becker, B.J., Sipe, T.A. and Thacker, S.B. (2000) 'Meta-analysis of observational studies in epidemiology: a proposal for reporting meta-analysis of observational studies in epidemiology (MOOSE) group. *JAMA,* 283 (15): 2008–12.

Thomas, J. (2010) 'Paranoia strikes deep: MMR vaccine and autism', *Psychiatric Times,* 27 (3): 1–6.

Wakefield, A.J., Murch, S.H., Anthony, A., Linnell, J., Casson, D.M., Malik, M., Berelowitz, M., Dhillon, A.P., Thomson, M.A., Harvey, P., Valentine, A., Davies, S.E. and Walker-Smith, J.A. (1998) 'Ileal-lymphoid nodular hyperplasia, non-specific colitis and pervasive developmental disorder in children', *The Lancet,* 351: 637–41 (paper now withdrawn).

Wakefield et al. (1998) 'Ileal-lymphoid-nodular hyperplasia, non-specific colitis and pervasive developmental disorder in children', *The Lancet,* 351: 637–41 (paper now withdrawn).

4

DEVELOPING AN EFFECTIVE RESEARCH PROPOSAL

Jane Dyas and Paul Leighton

Learning Objectives

- Understand the need for matching the research you propose to the requirements of the funding organisation
- Appreciate the importance of clear communication and targeted writing in funding applications.
- Be aware of the timescale and tasks involved in writing a proposal
- Gain useful tips and hints on what makes a good application

Introduction

Previous chapters have demonstrated that successful research starts with a meaningful and well worked out question; future chapters will consider the importance of well-founded and appropriate research methods, and will provide insight into designing studies which are scientifically robust. Here we consider the medium through which these elements are to be communicated when seeking funding and how best to make your case for support, indicating that effective writing is as important as well worked out science:

> The art of 'grantsmanship' will not turn mediocre science into a fundable grant proposal. But poor 'grantsmanship' will, and often does, turn very good science into an unfundable grant proposal. Good writing will not save bad ideas, but bad writing can kill good ones. (Kraicer, 1997: 1)

Writing grant applications is part of every research career, and understanding and developing the skills of grant writing is perhaps an integral part of success therein (Koppelman and Holloway, 2011; Goodman, 2011; Kraicer, 1997; Chung and Shauver, 2008; Aldridge and Derrington, 2012).

Funder remit

A critical part of your grant application is making sure that your research falls within the remit of the funding stream that you are applying to. It can be helpful to view your application from the perspective of the funding organisation; they want to 'buy' research with their funds, but also want to spend it wisely and get value for money. Above all, they have a clear picture of what they want to procure in terms of scope and quality, and the timescales within which the results will be worthwhile. It is highly unlikely that funding will be obtained if your study is not able to meet ALL of the requirements set out in the funding brief. The application is your opportunity to 'sell' them what they are looking for. It is perhaps productive to consider writing a grant application as a marketing exercise for your research ideas (Hickson, 2008).

Each funding stream will have a clearly set out funding brief which is usually located on their website. It is advisable that you search for a funding stream that is suitable for your project, rather than 'shoe horn' your project to fit a funding stream's remit. If you have any doubts whether your research matches their remit, it is wise to contact the programme administrators to ask them directly. Another useful activity which helps you assess whether you have applied to the right funding stream is to look at the details of previously funded projects, which will be hosted on their websites, to see if they are in a similar vein to yours.

In some cases, looking at the list of panel or board members of the programme you would like to apply to (once again on their website) can give you an indication of the expertise which will be judging your application. Some local panel members are willing to chat to applicants about their programme, though not at the project-specific level, which can provide insight regarding what is likely to be looked for in any particular application round. Investing time and effort in this step is a good idea because a great deal of time and goodwill within your team can be lost by putting an application to a funding programme which is out of scope and likely to be rejected early on.

Valuable and timely

Money for research is limited. In the case of health services research, where the sources of funding may often be from a charity or the health service provider, the funding bodies are answerable to the public who donate or contribute to the research budgets through paying taxes. So apart from being in scope, the knowledge, outcomes or findings must be important either because the research question needs answering now, or the answers will have a significant impact on health, health care or policy. If you can include these reasons in your application you are creating a strong case for why they need to fund your project. Although this does not necessarily mean that your study will get funded, by conveying the need and urgency it will indicate that your research is valuable to health care. In commissioned calls, the topic and/ or research question is identified by the funder, and applications are invited focusing on the given topic/question. Thus a strong case of *need* has already been established by the funder, which is the reason for the call being put out (please see the case study).

Case study

This case study is based on the National Institute for Health Research's (NIHR) commissioned call 12/133, September 2012, who wanted the research question answered: 'Which interventions maintain and/or increase physical activity in older people?' The need for this research can be analysed in terms of timing, policy driving and impact on both services and health.

Timing

Apart from the importance of exercise in preventing many chronic diseases, the overall number of older people in our society with health or care needs has risen and continues to rise.

Policy driving

This fact has led to older people being the biggest users of our health and care services, which means new responsibilities for health and social care providers to help older people stay healthy and active to maintain independence.

(Continued)

(Continued)

Impact on services

There are opportunities to reduce the financial burden on both the management and treatment of chronic diseases as a result of prevention, as well as preventing, or deferring, the ultimate costs of hospitalisation and residential care.

Impact on health

The benefits to the older people are better quality of life and well-being.

Quality

Once you have ascertained the need and urgency for your research you need to think about the research design in order to establish how best to generate the answers/findings/outcomes required to fulfil your research. This means funders must be able to see a clear link between the methods you plan to use to produce the results (the products they want to buy) in order to answer the research questions you have asked. Additionally, they will want to buy the best results they can for their money so you must justify why you are going to use the methods you propose. This way the judging panels can compare your research with those of other applicants. In the case of commissioned calls, this is a direct comparison, but in the case of the researcher-led bids, i.e. where the research question and topic are chosen by the researcher, this is more subjective; the way you design your research is an opportunity to show the quality of what you are 'selling'.

The structure of an effective proposal

The structure of your application will vary according to the funding stream you apply to; the headings used and the number of words or characters allowed may very well differ significantly between funders according to their priorities and the information that they deem necessary to judge your request for funding. Nowadays most funders use electronic application forms.

Complete the application form in full and do not leave sections blank. If it is not appropriate to complete a section indicate why this is so. Do not be tempted to stretch word/page limits by writing in a smaller font than requested or by submitting unsolicited appendices – a small font will only aggravate reviewers, and in many cases, administrators will not circulate additional materials. Most programmes give detailed guidance on how to complete the form and it is advisable to read this before you start to populate the document. Regardless of the form used, or the funder applied to, all good applications will contain similar core elements.

A concise, explanatory title

This is usually the first thing that reviewers read; it influences their understanding of the rest of the application form. Our advice would be to include a reference to the research design/methods that are being used as well as an indication of who the participants might be and the benefit that the research might lead to, or you may choose one of the question criterion such as PICO to help you determine your question (please see Chapter 1: 'Asking the Right Question'). A good acronym is a bonus! For examples of good research titles, below are some titles of projects funded by the NIHR Health Technology Assessment Programme (HTA) (project numbers are in brackets and full details are available from www.hta.ac.uk/research/index.shtml, accessed Jan. 2013):

- Managing Injuries of the Neck Trial (MINT): a randomised controlled trial of treatments for whiplash injuries (02/35/02)
- Systematic review and economic modelling of the relative clinical benefit and cost-effectiveness of laparoscopic surgery and robotic surgery for removal of the prostate in men with localised prostate cancer (09/14/02)
- The use of Melatonin in children with Neurodevelopmental Disorders and impaired Sleep: a randomised, double-blind, placebo-controlled, parallel study (MENDS) (05/14/02)

A statement of why the research matters

You might express this in terms of need – as discussed above – or it might be that you have to argue a case for your research. For example, your research may matter because although the problem affects only a small number of people, as might be the case with a new treatment for a very rare disease, the benefit to those individuals would be phenomenal, such as postponing death by several years. Whatever case you make, use the evidence from the most up-to-date literature that you can (please see Chapter 2: 'Finding the Evidence to Support your Research Question').

A statement of why your team should be chosen to do the research

In the application you are completing you may find a section dedicated to the role of each applicant in the team. In others you will need to make sure this information shines out in any section that you can. Quite often at the beginning of the application you will be asked for details of the co-applicants. One subsection is usually titled 'Role in Project'. It is rarely appropriate to just write 'lead' or 'statistician', instead consider something along the lines of 'She has worked with Professor Brains on previous studies using cluster randomised trials. She will be responsible for data quality and the quantitative analyses and the reporting of this in publications.' Sometimes there is a section that allows you to elaborate further, for example when they ask you for details regarding 'relevant expertise and experience'. Also do not forget opportunities such as citing applicant's work in the 'background' section either. Quite often co-applicants will have to state the percentage of their time that will be dedicated to the project; be honest, the panels can detect if the lead applicant is over-committing themselves. Remember they are trying to judge whether this study will be delivered on time and run according to plan – the amount of time the experts dedicate to this is an indicator of success.

Funders scrutinise the quality of the research team as closely as they do the research question and the science because this is the only way that they can assess the likelihood that they will get the research delivered to the standards that they want, in the time they expect it. It is therefore vital that you take time to build a team that will reassure the funding body. The team should include people with the expertise and experience in the methodologies that you are using, for example, statisticians or qualitative methodologists, as well as experts in the health field – both academics and clinicians. If your study involves a clinical trial, then a clinical triallist, or a clinical trial unit is also a must (please see Chapter 11: 'Clinical Trials').

The construction of the team should also reflect an ability to work with the necessary health or social care organisations to ensure smooth running of the study and for the implementation of outcomes if appropriate. The reality of these expectations is that most successful teams are led by, or have within them, people who have held research grants previously and published widely. Frequently, such people are academics; however clinicians or managers who are well placed to understand the needs of the research from a clinical or organisational perspective can, with the right partnerships within the team, lead and gain funding for research.

Clearly focused research aims, and questions or hypotheses

Although it seems fundamental, the methods you choose should answer the questions or hypotheses you pose and achieve your aims. There should be no aim given without appropriate methods, time and expertise factored in to accomplish it. The rationale for these should stem from your cited literature in the 'background' section.

A well thought out and justified research design

Tell the reviewers what you are going to do to deliver the outcomes that the funders are 'buying' and why the design you propose is the best way of doing it (in preference to any other). It is your chance to demonstrate that the research will be systematic and structured. Whether the design is fixed such as an experimental design, or flexible as in a qualitative design, show that you have considered what data are relevant and should be collected, and how best to analyse them. Keep designs elegant and simple. The more complicated your study the more the chance that a reviewer will spot flaws in it!

A detailed description of the methods

Many researchers find this a challenging section of the application form. The word count is rarely sufficient to allow a free description and justification of your choice of methods, thus your writing must be succinct without losing detail. Answer clearly and concisely and try to avoid too much repetition, although some is unavoidable. Whilst repeating key points can be important, be careful not to waste limited space by saying the same things time and again. Before writing, establish the key points that you want to make and work out where best (and where you have space) in the form to place them. Try to make a distinct point in each section of the form even if it seems to be asking for the same thing in other sections. However, do not fall into the trap of padding out sections so that you reach a word count, reviewers will not thank you for saying something in 500 words which could be said in 250. White space on the page can make an application seem less dense and easier to engage with.

Structuring your text using descriptive subheadings such as standard research protocol headings and bullet points can also help make a bid more understandable, and can make your application easier to navigate. It is important to remember that an application may be read by a reviewer in chunks, so writing in a way which accommodates this will help to promote a positive response (please see the case study for illustration).

Case study

In response to an NIHR commissioned call 12/133 (as in the previous case study); a sports therapist intends to submit a proposal investigating the value of yoga in a retired population. In drafting his 'plan of investigation', he intends to use the following headings:

Design: What type of study he will conduct, e.g. a trial, cohort, etc.

Participants: Description of the type of person he will recruit. He will also detail inclusion and exclusion criteria, such as including those who can communicate in English, and excluding those with certain co-morbidities such as inner ear problems which can affect balance.

Intervention: Here he will describe in full the yoga intervention and what the participants will be doing, who will be delivering the intervention, and the timings, i.e. length of session, frequency of sessions and the length of the course of yoga.

Outcomes: He will detail what measures will be used and when. He will also draw a flow chart with the participant's pathway through the study to help clarification.

Take little for granted, and presume that you need to explain and justify all elements of your research. Whether you are using quantitative or qualitative methods or a combination of both, your research plan should be described in detail and justified with regard to the generation of the type of data that you require to answer the question that you are posing. If you are using more than one method, give them equal status and balance. For example, in a mixed-methods study a researcher familiar with quantitative methods may give good, justified detail, regarding sample size, recruitment, randomisation, data collection, data management and data analysis. However when writing the paragraph outlining the qualitative methods, the information may be scant, just referring to the fact that the patients will be interviewed and the transcripts thematically analysed. This may indicate to the reviewer that not enough qualitative expertise is included in the team, or that the co-applicant, who is an expert in that methodology, has not been involved in the preparation of the application. Both would cause alarm to the panel regarding whether the team could deliver the promised outcomes. Another aspect where getting the balance in detail right lies between the descriptions of the methods and the analysis. Quite often researchers pay more attention to the data collection methods rather than what will be done once the data has been obtained. Therefore ensure that you have appropriate specialists to help write the analysis plan.

A demonstration that ethical issues have been considered

Many applications ask if ethical approval will be required, and if there are any ethical considerations. If it does not, you should mention this. This question is to ascertain whether your research is 'high-risk' or not. There is no point in a panel considering funding your research, if it is unlikely to take place due to an inability to obtain the required ethical approval (please see Chapter 15: 'Designing and Conducting an Ethical Research Study').

Address any anticipated difficulties

All studies have strengths and weaknesses. Researchers tend to 'sell' the strengths well. However, reviewers need to know that you are aware of areas where there may be difficulties. For example, if you are recruiting participants from an unusual setting and there are no previous studies that you can draw on to give confidence that you will be able to meet your recruitment targets, state this, and suggest a second recruitment strategy that can be used if the first is not successful.

An up-to-date bibliography

Chapter 2 explains how to make sure your bibliography is up to date and in-depth. In an application you may be limited in the extent to which you can use these references. Good advice is to make sure you have included all appropriate, critically appraised research whether it is published or ongoing in your subject, not just the important papers by the field leaders. Also, see if any panel members judging your research have relevant knowledge and make sure you include material that they will be bound to identify if it is omitted – you may even be able to cite their work!

Detail of your public involvement

Chapter 16 gives advice on developing an appropriate involvement strategy for your research. When including this in your application, it is advisable to integrate what you have done, and what you will do, throughout the proposal rather than only to refer to it in the section headed 'Public Involvement'. It is becoming increasingly important to outline how stakeholders have been involved in the development of the research as well as the contribution they will make during the study, if funded. Referring to named individuals is also a strengthening feature, such as a patient representative as a co-applicant.

A clear dissemination strategy

It is not the responsibility of the funding body to decide how the research findings will reach those making decisions about changes to clinical practice. This is another aspect of the research process that they are 'buying' from the researcher. When thought of in this way, it becomes easier to ensure that you provide the reviewers with sufficient detail for them to see that you have truly thought about who needs to get your findings and how they will get them. It is important to publish in peer-reviewed journals, but dissemination includes more, and depending on the nature of your research, you might consider how you will reach policy-makers, commissioners, practitioners, patients and other stakeholders (please see Chapter 21: 'Dissemination').

An outline of the project management and timescales

This section comes near the end of most application forms. Leave enough time to get this completed thoroughly. Understandably, researchers are not usually as passionate about management as they are their research interests, however funding programme managers are! Always include a Gantt chart, i.e. a type of bar chart that details the project schedule, such as Table 4.1 which is an example of a systematic review project which is being conducted over 18 months.

A statement of the anticipated impact of the research

It can be hard to describe and outline the impacts that the funder is going to have most interest in. Try using a research impact framework to ensure that you

TABLE 4.1   Example of a Gannt chart for a systematic review

Tasks	Feb-Apr 0–3	May-Jul 4–6	Aug-Oct 7–9	Nov-Jan 10–12	Feb-Apr 13–15	May-Jul 16–18
Advertise and hire staff	▓					
Determine data collecting tools, and write protocol	▓					
Searches		▓	▓	▓	▓	
Data extraction and critical appraisal			▓	▓	▓	▓
Meta-analysis				▓	▓	▓
Writing up, e.g. final report, publications, summary for policy-makers, etc.					▓	▓
Dissemination						▓

consider fully all of the relevant issues (Kuruvilla et al., 2006). For example, clinicians usually have a clear concept of how their research findings will have an impact on their clinical practice but may overlook the impact that the research may have on policy.

Supporting documentation

This has to be submitted in accordance with the programme's policies. It might include flow charts, pictures and letters of support. The latter can be of particular help in making the case that you are supported by key players in the health or social care organisation – a letter from a ward manager who has agreed to allow you to recruit participants on their ward for example. Do be selective in what you send; no reviewer wants to be swamped with unnecessary documentation.

Financial sections

These sections should be completed with the assistance of an appropriate finance officer; all universities and large health care organisations will have staff responsible for this (Chapter 5: 'Budget and Funding' adds more detail). Finances can be complex and it is advisable to start this process early.

Effective communication

Funding applications are invariably read quickly, reviewed by panel members reading multiple applications or by fitting a review into an already full diary. They are read by clinical experts, academic researchers, specialist methodologists and by members of the public. They are sometimes read alongside other bids addressing the same question, at other times they are compared with proposals derived from different clinical fields or academic traditions. Consequently, effective communication is critical and an application which is easy to read, and understood quickly by a wide readership, has succeeded in addressing a significant barrier to its potential success.

Avoid specialist, technical, clinical language, jargon and acronyms which may not be familiar to all readers. Instead, use short catchy phrases as labels for complex theoretical, clinical or economic phenomena. For example, the ultimate aim of the sports therapist in the case study is to produce an educational tool which will enable people to practise the yoga intervention at home. He labels this an 'interactive video', i.e. an electronic patient resource (consisting of information and exercises). Interactive video is straight-forward and understandable to most readers, and summarises, in an accessible fashion, a resource which is designed to be delivered via multiple formats (DVD, CD-ROM or webpage) with some degree of interactivity. The repetition of these labels can help to emphasise what is being proposed, and can help to generate a sense of coherence and consistency in the application. Using one simple phrase throughout reduces the potential for the reader to be confused by multiple variations on a theme, for example, interactive DVD, web tutorial, video pamphlet or short instructional film.

Long paragraphs and long, complex sentences may have the effect of hiding important information, and they can make an application harder to follow and interpret. Write in a fashion that is amenable to all and do not make the mistake of demonstrating your brilliance by writing an application which can only be understood by a small number of experts from your own clinical or academic field. In every application you are asked to describe your research for a lay reader or provide a plain English summary. Ask other people to read your proposal to make sure it is understandable to a wide audience.

Use a bold style of writing. Normal academic writing with a balanced argument and multiple perspectives can lack the punch to make an impact on a reviewer. Asserting that 'Many General Practitioners are uncomfortable managing prescriptions for strong opioid medications' is more likely to grab a reviewer's attention than comprehensively giving a range of arguments about the challenges of prescribing opiates. Make your point and then defend it, and do not lose focus in too much extraneous detail or debate. Present evidence and hard facts wherever possible, for example, 'Eighty thousand hearing aids each year are consigned to patients' bedside drawers, costing the NHS £25M per annum', makes a compelling case to justify research in this field. Connect what you propose to do with future benefits to health or health service delivery; understanding why hearing aids are abandoned will inform future audiology provision and contribute to better patient support, with the net result of improved patient outcomes and a more efficient use of NHS resources.

You can also help with the flow of your proposal by using sign-posting and summarising, such as 'here we ...', 'in the following section we ...', 'to conclude ...', etc., which can be used to emphasise the key elements of your study and can help a reviewer maintain a clear sense of the narrative that is being presented to them.

What the panel are looking for

Although you have the superimposed structure of the application form, you need to bear in mind what information the reviewer or panel member will be looking for so that you can ensure that you describe all of the information they require. To assist with this process it can be helpful to look on the website of the funding organisation to see if they provide any documentation they require their reviewers to complete when assessing an application. Below is an example of what the reviewer is asked to complete with regards to the research design in a proposed application for an NIHR Research for Patient Benefit grant (the full form can be found on their website: www.ccf.nihr.ac.uk/RfPB/Documents/Peer%20Review%20 Form_RfPB%20Sample.pdf, accessed Dec. 2012). You can see immediately that you are advantaged if you make it easy for the reviewer to find what they need; even though there is no section on the application form that asks you to provide this information directly.

1. *QUALITY of the proposed work*
    i. *Research design*
        a. *Is the proposed research of high quality and does it address the stated objectives?*
        b. *How convincing and coherent is the proposed rationale and approach?*
        c. *Is the proposed design and methodology for all elements of the research well defined, appropriate, valid, robust and feasible within the timeframe and resources requested?*
        d. *What are the strengths and weaknesses of the research design as proposed?*

Process of proposal construction

The tradition of bid writing alone late at night with a deadline pressing may not be totally extinct but effective grant writing is increasingly conceived of as a collaborative venture which requires a great deal of time, commitment and planning. The completed proposal is the endpoint of a process which may require consultation with the public, the generation of pilot data, negotiation with institutions (academic and clinical), drafting the budget, as well as the design of a study and the plan of its dissemination and implementation. The act of filling in the form and finalising the study design may well take place in the weeks leading up to a competition deadline, but the preparation and groundwork is likely to have taken place for many months preceding this. If you are new to research, or exploring a new clinical or academic field, then expecting to spend up to 12 months developing a major research funding application may not be unrealistic. Funding applications may involve several stages (outline to full) or a single full application. The following timeline offers some indication of the key tasks that you need to consider when starting from scratch.

Up to 12 months ahead of submission

Before you commit to develop a major funding application it is sensible to discuss your idea with some of your clinical and/or academic colleagues. Establishing through these discussions that what you are considering is both interesting and worthwhile will ensure that you do not waste time preparing a study that only you are interested in, and which consequently is unlikely to be supported by a funding body. To substantiate this, you should also conduct a brief literature review to ensure that the research you are thinking about has not already been done, or is being done currently, and in order to consider the sort of research that has previously been undertaken. This type of reflection will start the process of refining your broad research idea into a more clearly focused project through identifying where the gaps in the current knowledge are, and will also help you identify the most appropriate methods for answering your question.

You also need time for a realistic assessment of whether what you propose is feasible, and whether there is sufficient foundation on which to build a plausible and convincing proposal for research funding. This may mean collecting some pilot or audit data prior to applying. A research idea regarding a diagnostic procedure, for example, may require a comprehensive local audit of diagnostic accuracy before a full study of clinical efficacy and cost effectiveness can be proposed. Or you may need to conduct a feasibility study to establish that the research question and proposed study design is acceptable. For example, a precursor to a clinical trial of glaucoma surgery may be a focus group with the patients of a glaucoma clinic to ensure that the surgical study would be acceptable to them, and that they would be likely to consent to participate in it. Completing, reporting and even publishing the outcomes of any pilot or feasibility research should be finalised before moving on as these can be cited in the main application, and thus can remove any uncertainties about a proposed study to the reviewers and can make it seem far less speculative.

Considering the range and scope of funding opportunities in your field at this early stage can also help to focus research ideas and establish what is possible for your chosen topic. For example, the British Heart Foundation offer project grants (up to £300,000), programme grants (to support multiple interconnected projects), clinical study awards (for clinical research) and new horizons grants (to encourage researchers new to cardiovascular research). An initial look at sources of funding at this stage can provide insight into 'hot topics' for which funders are explicitly seeking project proposals, or help to identify those broad areas which seem to have a greater chance of being funded. Again, this type of early preparation can help you to think about how best to frame and focus your research idea, and how best to sell it to those that have money to support research.

Up to 6 months ahead of submission

Presuming that the outcomes of the preliminary research are supportive, now is the time to pull together an initial outline for the research and to identify the core team that will assist you in putting the submission together. The core team should be made up of both clinical and academic colleagues who have an interest and track record in the field where you propose the research, or bring methodological expertise. The initial outline should include the key research question, aims and objectives and a broad summary of the research plan which will form the basis for the team to work on. Once revised and refined, the research outline can subsequently be used as a focus for consultation with other stakeholders, e.g. service commissioners, to ensure that any findings from your research will, in principle, inform clinical practice; or patient groups and/or other interested members of the public, so that all perspectives are incorporated into the development of your proposal. Starting at this early stage will enable patient and lay representatives to be fully engaged in the process of bid development, which will directly inform the nature and scope of the proposed study. By now you should have a clearer idea of the focus for your research and some notion of the scale (size, budget and time) of the study that you are proposing. Once you have established this, you can think in more detail about the application process for your chosen funder and can establish deadlines for various aspects of the bid development up to the point of submission.

Up to 3 months ahead of submission

Now you should become fully familiar with the funding competition. Download guidance notes and application forms and take time to consider them. Discuss any issues that you have with competition administrators and, if you can, identify colleagues who have previously been successful, or colleagues who sit on the funding panel, and talk to them about the funding competition and take advice on what they feel makes an attractive proposal.

Prior to completing the application form, a full and comprehensive literature review will be required. Responsibility for constructing a first draft of the form should be shared amongst the research team with the research lead acting as a central point to coordinate and combine the different sections as they are completed by the most appropriately qualified team member. Once a complete first draft has been achieved, this should be circulated amongst the research team for comment and reflection. At this stage it is perhaps important to finalise: (i) the research question, aims and objectives; (ii) the plan of investigation; and (iii) expected outcomes/dissemination.

With these sections close to completion, it is possible to consider a detailed research budget. This should not be left until the last minute, and establishing a dialogue with the relevant research and/or finance offices a month or more before the submission is advisable. It takes time to establish how much research will cost and sometimes more time still to allocate these costs to the appropriate research, support or treatment budgets (please see Chapter 5: 'Budget and Funding'). You also need to begin discussions with local service managers and directors as you will need their permission to undertake research within their settings.

The final month before submission

At this stage you are likely to be still finalising: (i) the budget; (ii) the justification for resources sought; and (iii) the timetable and Gantt chart. The abstract/summary should be the final section that you write once you are content that all revisions to the application have been made.

With the deadline getting closer it is important to have a fully worked up draft application which you can expose to informal peer review. Doing this several weeks before the submission deadline will allow your reviewers time to consider the application in full, and will allow you time to make amendments in a well-thought-out, rather than hurried, fashion. A final proofread by several members of the research team, will help ensure that all corrections have been made and that no typographical errors remain. Sloppy applications which are full of grammatical and typographical errors suggest a sloppy researcher, hardly an impression likely to gain a positive response. Draft and redraft your application until it is a polished piece of writing, read it several times to ensure that you are happy with the message it communicates.

Letters of support should also now be sought and the process of bid submission adhered to. Be careful to check how the funding body want to receive the application (electronic and/or hard copy); whether they require ink signatures and from whom – the research lead, all team members, host organisation, etc. If they require hard copies, how many do they require, and so on. Having worked so hard to construct a high-quality bid it would be a shame to be rejected because of a technical error.

Common reasons for applications failing

- The research question is not strong enough.
- The research question does not fit the funder's remit, i.e. it is out of scope.
- The researchers do not demonstrate a good acquaintance with the existing body of knowledge.

- The lead applicant does not have all the appropriate partnerships in place.
- The application is poorly written and presented.
- The administrative instructions have not been followed accurately.
- The team has unrealistic aspirations.
- The applicants underestimate the time it will take to complete.
- Co-applicant signatures have not been secured.
- The finances were inaccurate or incomplete.

Summary

- There is an art to applying for funding for research; learn from feedback from panels and other researchers who have been successful.
- A good research idea can fail to get funded as the result of a weak application and poor communication.
- You are in competition for the money that is available and you must therefore make a compelling case for why your study should be awarded.
- The team and their previous research experience matters.
- Be sure to pick an appropriate funding stream so your project fits their remit.
- Do not underestimate how long a good application will take, allow plenty of time.
- There is a plethora of information on funders' websites. Make use of it.

Questions for Discussion

1. In regards to your own research idea

   a. What aspects of your research could not be changed under any circumstances, e.g. topic, population, setting, method, aims, hypothesis or question? (Deciding on this will help you narrow down funding options.)

   b. What aspects can be changed? (Ascertaining this will help broaden your search of appropriate funding streams.)

   c. Draft a timeline of the tasks that you need to accomplish before you are in a position to submit an application.

Further Reading

Aldous, C., Rheeder, P. and Esterhuizen, T. (2011) *Writing your First Clinical Research Proposal*. Johannesburg: Juta Academic.

Berry, D. (2010) *Gaining Funding for Research: A Guide for Academics and Institutions*. London and Milton Keynes: Open University Press.

Gitlin, L.N. and Lyons, K.J. (2008) *Successful Grant Writing Strategies for Health and Human Service Professionals* (3rd rev. edn). New York: Springer Publishing Co.

Hackshaw, A. (2010) *How to Write a Grant Application: for Health Professionals and Life Science Researchers*. Oxford: Wiley-Blackwell.

Ogden, T.E. and Goldberg, I.A. (2002) *Research Proposals: A Guide to Success* (3rd edn). San Diego, CA: Elsevier Science.

Punch, K.F. (2006) *Developing Effective Research Proposals* (2nd edn). London: SAGE.

Reis, J.B. and Leukefield, C. (1995) *Applying for Research Funding: Getting Started and Getting Funded*. London: SAGE.

References

Aldridge, J. and Derrington, A. (2012) *The Research Funding Toolkit: How to Plan and Write Successful Grant Applications*. London: SAGE.

Chung, K. and Shauver, M. (2008) 'Fundamental principles of bid writing success', *Journal of Hand Surgery*, 33A: 566–72.

Goodman, I. (2011) 'Grant development for large scale research proposals: an overview and case study', *Journal of Research Administration*, 42 (2): 78–86.

Hickson, M. (2008) *Research Handbook for Healthcare Professionals*. Oxford: Wiley-Blackwell.

Kraicer, J. (1997) *The Art of Grantsmanship*, available from www.unige.ch/collaborateurs/recherche/financement/5/theartofgrantmanship.pdf (accessed Dec. 2012).

Koppelman, G. and Holloway, J. (2012) 'Successful grant writing', *Paediatric Respiratory Review*, 13: 63–6.

Kuruvilla, S., Mays, N., Pleasant, A. and Walt, G. (2006) 'Describing the impact of health research: a research impact framework', *BMC Health Services Research*, 6: 134.

National Institute for Health Research's (NIHR) (2012) commissioned call 2/133,September2012 http://www.phr.nihr.ac.uk/fundingopportunities/pdfs/12_133_older_age_more_active.pdf (last accessed March 2013).

5

BUDGET AND FUNDING

Roz Sorrie and Andy Barton*

Helen Hancock and Helen Close**

Learning Objectives

- Be able to define and describe the various categories of costs associated with non-commercial research in the NHS
- Be able to attribute the different costs associated with delivering a research project so that the relevant costs are included in the grant application and a plan is in place to ensure other non-grant related study activities are financially accounted for
- Be able to identify and implement practical steps to managing the budget for your study
- Demonstrate an understanding of the remit and requirements of grant funders to enable you to identify potential sources of funding for your study, and give yourself the best chance of success in obtaining funding

---

*Budget

**Funding

Introduction

The Department of Health in the UK recognises that research is a core activity in health care settings, having a value in terms of driving forward evidence-based practice and innovation. However, health care providers are usually on a very restricted budget, and any research activities that involve health service resources, e.g. equipment, treatments, staff, premises, etc., should not divert these resources from the delivery of normal services to patients. It is therefore important that the cost of research activities is attributed and calculated accurately to ensure there is no detrimental financial impact on service delivery. The calculation of the cost of research conducted in the National Health Service (NHS) in the UK has become increasingly rigorous since the mid-1990s. The Culyer Report in 1994 led to widespread acknowledgement that, although research in hospitals was to be encouraged, its cost to the service was, at best, unclear. Today, advice on how research costs are to be calculated is based on guidance published in 1997 by the Department of Health (HSG(97)32) and although it has been refined as ARCO (2005) and AcoRD (2012), the basic principles of that guidance survive. (Department of Health guidance provides the key reference material for all aspects of attributing costs to NHS research projects.) Even with these documents however, the calculation of the costs of a research project remains complex and it is important to seek expert guidance as early as possible when designing your study. Furthermore, Research and Development financial arrangements are constantly evolving so it is important to ensure that the advice you receive reflects the latest guidance. Often, a non-commercial study, i.e. research whose objectives are not the protection of a commercial institution's interests (Schimetta et al., 2005), will involve one NHS trust (or more if multi-centred) and at least one medical school or other university department. Each participating organisation will wish to assure itself that all of their costs are covered by the award before they allow the application to be submitted. However, whether they are a university or NHS trust, they will be keen for an application to succeed and thus should be willing to provide advice. You must consult the finance departments of any academic and health care partners early to allow time for the appropriate budgetary authorities to give their approval.

Costing a study

You will normally have produced an outline protocol for your proposed study before drafting your initial budget, which will become more detailed as the application develops. The most pragmatic approach to ascertaining costs is to identify all activities that need to be undertaken during the project to ensure the timely delivery of outcomes. This entails breaking the study down into constituent parts and asking the following questions:

- What? Quantify what is being done, e.g. number of tests/investigations, time taken to perform a procedure, etc.
- Who? Who will be undertaking these activities, e.g. members of the research team, healthcare professionals who are not part of the grant-funded research team, etc?

- Why? State the purpose of the activity. Is it solely for research purposes or is the activity related to patient care whilst they are in your study and also, potentially, once the research is finished?

- Where? Which setting are the activities taking place in?

At the time of writing, there is no national template in existence to support the costing of non-commercial studies, although there has been a great deal of discussion about the requirement for this type of tool in order to facilitate the costing exercise. NIHR is keen to address this and an Attribution Capture and Activity Template is being developed as part of a pilot pre-application support service initiative to support investigators during 2014.

Attribution of costs

Gone are the days where a research grant would cover the costs associated with a project entirely. Today a health services research project is funded from a variety of sources, and the costs associated with delivering a study need to be attributed correctly. This is an important, if complex and time-consuming activity, and requires a thorough understanding and appreciation of the health care organisations which are to host the research, together with a detailed knowledge of the research activities that are going to be involved. Most major grant awarding bodies require a comprehensive financial breakdown of all costs involved in delivering the study. Current guidance identifies three categories of costs:

1. *Research costs* are the expenditure for the research activity itself. These costs will end when the research finishes and relate to activities that are being undertaken to answer the research question. These are paid for from the research grant and will cover:

- Research staff costs such as applicants' time, research associates, statistical advice and support. These costs are normally expressed in terms of the proportion of time the individual spends on the study for the lifetime of that study, e.g. if you were to spend 4 hours per week on the study over the 18 months the study will take, based on a 37.5 hour working week, this would equate to 0.1 full time equivalent of your salary for 18 months in your budget.

- Tests or intervention(s), required to help answer the research question that are not part of usual care. These could include devices, tests and investigations stipulated in the protocol, as well as the staff time needed to undertake them, e.g. technician time, nurses' time, etc.

- Equipment for the research project, e.g. laptop computers, specialist laboratory equipment, tape recorders, statistical software, etc.

- Meetings, e.g. site initiation visits, steering committee meetings, conferences, etc.

- Travel and subsistence for researchers.

- Participant payments – to cover expenses such as travel, car-parking, recompense for time, etc.

- Patient and public involvement – including payment, training, travel, etc.

- Additional study-related costs – sponsorship fee, trial registration fee, Research and Development Office fee, audit and monitoring, study archival, dissemination of results, etc.

2. *Treatment costs* are the expenditure associated with the usual care (which is often current best practice for that condition) and the cost of the care under investigation. Therefore treatment costs includes all types of patient services, including diagnostic, preventive, rehabilitative-care and continuing-care services, e.g. medicines, devices, therapies, etc. Depending on your research design, if you have a control group, your study may also involve participants receiving usual care. For example, a randomised controlled trial evaluating the clinical effectiveness of a new medicine may involve randomising participants to either an arm where usual care is provided, or an arm where the new medicine under investigation is being provided. In this example, usual care is provided as part of the research protocol, i.e. it is an arm of the study, and therefore the costs of the usual care is the responsibility of the health care organisation as part of its normal service delivery. Where the patient care provided is either an experimental treatment or a new service which differs from usual care, the difference between the treatment costs for your research project and the costs of the usual care (if any), is called Excess Treatment Costs. This is the cost that would be introduced as a result of your research if you obtained positive findings and the health care providers wanted to implement your results in clinical practice after the research had stopped. For example, you may be testing a new drug which costs £10 per day, against an old drug, which is currently usual care, at £5 per day. Therefore the excess treatment cost is £5 per day. However this is where health economics comes in (please see Chapter 9), as although it may sound expensive, the costs are balanced against the benefit (or quality of life) it gives. Excess treatment costs are paid for by your hosting trust through the usual commissioning process, and they need to agree to cover both the treatment costs and the excess treatment costs if your research is funded. In order for them to agree to do so, depending on the level of additional funding required, they may ask you to provide a business case, which may require further discussion and agreement with the commissioning organisation. There may be some situations where the excess treatment costs are huge, and in these cases your study may qualify for subvention support to help pay for them from the Department of Health.

3. *Support costs* are the additional patient care costs associated with the research which would end once the study finishes, even if the patient care involved in the study continued to be provided. Examples of support costs could be the identification of potential participants by the clinical care team; obtaining informed consent from patients; additional tests or investigations where the results are provided to the clinical care team to ensure patient safety and clinical management whilst the patient takes part in the research; supplying and administering the medicine being studied. Support costs may be paid for by the hosting trust or, if funded by the National Institute for Health Services Research (NIHR) in England, or a recognised non-commercial partner your research will be eligible for inclusion on the NIHR portfolio, and thus these support costs will be paid for by their Clinical Research Networks.

Subtle, but distinct, differences between the same activities in different types of study can alter the attribution of the costs, depending on the role of the individual responsible for undertaking the activity and what the purpose of the activity is, for example, if your trust employs a pharmacist who supports clinical trials and will be responsible for repackaging the trial drugs (so the placebo and the new medication look the same) this does not incur service support costs. However, if the trust does not employ a pharmacist to support trials in this way, they may require service support costs in the form of a 'per patient fee' to cover the costs of staff in the pharmacy department (please see the case study for another example).

Case study

A researcher is hoping to conduct a qualitative focus group study (please see Chapter 7: 'Qualitative Data Collection') to ascertain the experience of being first diagnosed with polycystic ovary syndrome. As this involves newly diagnosed patients, she needs to recruit participants via primary care and general practitioners (GPs). Due to the estimated number of newly diagnosed women within a single practice, and from that, the percentage of women who will consent, she calculates that she will need to recruit from three practices, using one of two different approaches:

Option 1: She will identify a local Collaborator, a GP, at each site who, as part of the patient's clinical care team, is able to provide information about the study to potential participants. If the patient is interested in taking part, they will be then directed to contact the researcher directly. A member of the research team then arranges to obtain consent from each participant and take some demographic data. The time of the 3x GP Local Collaborators to identify potential participants is categorised as a Support Cost. The researcher's time to obtain consent is already covered by the grant award and is therefore categorised as a research cost.

Option 2: The 3x GP Local Collaborators will identify potential participants, obtain their consent to take part in the study and also collect the demographic data. Once patient consent and demographic data has been obtained, the researcher can then contact the patient directly to arrange the date and time of the focus group. In this scenario, the GPs should be reimbursed for their time to identify potential participants with whom to discuss the study, provide participant information and then obtain consent and collect demographic data from those who wish to take part. Therefore these are all categorised as support costs.

Project budgets

The lead applicant for a grant will be primarily concerned with the need to ensure that the costs of the main research team, including co-applicants and other research staff, are covered by the research costs covered by the funders. To ensure the research team has the appropriate expertise to conduct the research in a timely way, salaries may take up the bulk of the award. Your award will also need to cover other research costs and, unless you have budgeted appropriately for these, it can result in practical difficulties in setting up and running the study, as additional sources of funding, beyond the original grant award, may be required. Therefore you need to have drafted an inclusive budget, which not only covers the necessary staff, but also the required research costs. If after doing this, the research award you would like to apply for is not enough, you will either need to find and apply for a larger award, scale your project back or split the project into smaller, individual projects and apply for funds for each smaller project, for example, instead of conducting a mixed-methods project funded by one award, you may wish to complete the qualitative project first with one award, followed by the quantitative project with a separate award.

Indirect costs (overheads)

Your budget should also contain information about indirect costs, also known as overheads. Overheads are normally non-specific cost estimates that are not otherwise included under the research costs and are applicable to grant applications that involve Higher Education Institute (HEI) staff. Overheads are intended to ensure that the indirect costs to support research such as through the provision of consumables, office facilities, etc., as well as support departments, such as Estates, Finance, Human Resources, etc. are also reflected in the grant application. Many funding organisations declare a maximum percentage that will be paid for indirect costs incurred by HEIs. HEIs use their own protocol for calculating overheads (known as Full Economic Costing, or FEC). If you are based in a university, or any of your co-applicants are, you should engage in an early discussion with the relevant financial accountants who can advise you on the appropriate level of indirect costs that should be included in the grant application. NHS organisations are no longer expected to claim indirect costs from a research grant as most will be in receipt of extra funding to support research activities (currently known as Research Capability Funding).

Case study

A gastroenterologist is developing a grant proposal for a randomised controlled trial to compare the clinical and cost effectiveness of two types of bariatric surgical interventions for obesity. One intervention is more invasive and more costly than the other but is anecdotally associated with better outcomes for patients. The study will be run in six different sites, including the site where the gastroenterologist is based. Depending on the particular trust, either one, or the other, or both surgical interventions are offered as usual care. In the gastroenterologist's own trust, both interventions are offered, therefore both arms of the trial should be considered a treatment cost as the trust would normally take responsibility for bearing the cost of either intervention, regardless of the trial. However in trusts where the more expensive intervention is not offered, the costs associated with its provision due to the trial are categorised as excess treatment costs. In trusts where the least expensive intervention is not routinely offered, this intervention remains as a treatment cost, as it is less costly to provide than the other intervention. Two of the six sites do not routinely provide the most expensive intervention. Therefore the gastroenterologist negotiates the excess treatment costs at these two sites and has produced a business case highlighting the hypothesised improved outcomes for patients and potential resultant cost savings.

Budget management

A successful grant application marks not only the start of the research project, but the need for the chief investigator to begin actively managing the budget, which will involve ensuring that salaries are paid and that any payments to participating sites are made, including any treatment costs and service support costs. An award can typically last for two to three years, but may involve longer periods of time, depending on the terms of the grant. A robust approach to budget management provides an audit trail that can be used to demonstrate that study finances are being fully utilised in feedback reports to the grant-awarding organisation. All funders require regular interim reports which describe progress against targets and an outline of solutions to any delays in achieving them. Some funding bodies release funding on a yearly basis, dependent on successful progress in the preceding year as evidenced in the interim reports. A final report is normally submitted after the study has finished, which is reviewed and approved by the funding body; these are often also required by ethics committees and governance bodies. All outputs resulting from NIHR-funded research must be approved prior to the final publication. For many studies, budget management will be uneventful; for some, however, some contingency planning will be required as the following common pitfalls demonstrate.

Delays and extensions to studies

Delays to starting the research can occur periodically, usually concerned with organisational or study personnel matters. Starting the study at a later date than planned will impact on both the study delivery and on the budget, which may then start to register slippage. It is important to ensure that the grant-awarding organisation is kept fully informed of any delays and key milestones and deadlines are renegotiated if possible. If the study is not progressing as planned, the chief investigator may have to consider extending the study life beyond the original end date. This decision will have to be made taking into account the available funds and whether these will be sufficient to cover the extra costs incurred. Again, it is recommended that discussion takes place with the grant sponsor as occasionally these organisations will act favourably in agreeing to provide some short-term additional funding.

Recruitment problems

As the study gets under way, problems with participant recruitment can become apparent at an early stage, when it is clear that the recruitment target is not being achieved. One option is for the chief investigator to approach clinicians at other sites to enlist their support in delivering the study. Whilst this may benefit overall recruitment, it may have unplanned consequences for the budget management, particularly if there is no funding to cover the research costs of the new sites. The chief investigator may have to either use existing monies, thus stretching the budget, or rely on the additional sites having sufficient research infrastructure in place to absorb the additional costs. Of course, individual sites may decline to take part if they feel that the study is financially onerous. The other option is to extend the length of the trial, however, as noted above, this has its own financial considerations.

Changes to study personnel

Study personnel can change as the study progresses owing to career changes, maternity leave, health reasons and so forth. These changes are challenging to manage and will affect the budget. Taking an appropriate course of action as soon as the change is noted is advisable. In terms of budget management, this may mean some slippage is incurred against posts, for example, if a staff member leaves and the recruitment of a new post holder takes time. This slippage will mean that there is a little more funding available in the budget that can be set aside and used to offset other areas that may be overspent. The chief investigator also needs to be mindful that, owing to employment legislation, staff who are absent due to health reasons or on maternity leave will still require some or all of their salary paid for a period of time. This means that there is less flexibility in the budget to pay for the time of other staff to cover the workload of these individuals and consideration will need to be given to how the work will get done and how additional staff will be funded.

Funding

Unless you are funded for your research by private sector organisations, such as by pharmaceutical companies, you will need to compete for the scarce resources offered by charities or the government. The Organisation for Economic Co-operation and Development has estimated that approximately a third of all research is conducted by universities and the government, whilst the remainder is carried out by private industries. But there is funding for research out there. In 2010–11 the NIHR, through which the Department of Health supports and facilitates research in the NHS in the UK, awarded approximately £210.5 million (NIHR Annual Report 2011), whilst the National Institutes of Health in the USA awarded over $30.9 billion (USD), and the National Health and Medical Research Council in Australia awarded approximately $800 million (AUS). Aside from grants offered by these organisations, there are other funders such as the Medical Research Council (MRC) in the UK, which in 2010–11 awarded almost £400 million in research grants and training awards, whilst the Economic and Social Research Council (ESRC) awarded £200 million, and the Biotechnology and Biological Sciences Research Council (BBSRC) almost £390 million (2011 annual report for each). Elsewhere medical, research and social care charities make hundreds of millions of pounds available each year for research via funding competitions (for more on this see Berry, 2012: chs 3 and 4).

Searching for funding

In order to find the most appropriate research award, you need to develop and refine your research question and methodology, as different sponsors have different award remits. For example, charity awards are usually focused on research examining a particular disease or illness, whereas NIHR funding is for applied health research, and the MRC is for lab-based or methodological work, such as the MRC Methodology Research Programme which will fund the development of research methods in disciplines underpinning health research including: biomedical, behavioural and social science, experimental medicine, randomised trials, cohorts and other research designs investigating health, health care, health services and health policy, with no defined upper monetary limit, and four calls per year. You may also need funding for other research-related activities such as forming collaborations, or convening conferences; and there are different, smaller funds specifically for these types of activities, which are often awarded by associations or charities. For example, the European Association of Social Psychology (EASP) gives postgraduate and postdoctoral scholarships of up to 800 to pay for visits to departments elsewhere in the world in order to conduct research, complete ongoing projects or undergo training in a particular methodology or technology. The EASP will also support attendance to meetings, conferences or summer schools (currently an annual award with a December deadline).

Your health care organisation or university may have staff employed who can help you to find appropriate funding sources. If you wish to conduct your own funding search you can find funding programmes through journals in your discipline such as the *British Medical Journal*, or a generic research journal such as *Research Fortnight*, which give details of available research awards in all areas (as well as health). *Research Fortnight* also has an excellent search engine for funding: www.researchprofessional.com (accessed Dec. 2012), as does Europe Pubmed Central: http://europepmc.org/GrantLookup/ (accessed Jan. 2013).

Once you have identified a potential funder, look carefully at the variety of awards they support. Some may have specific remits associated with each award. For example, the NIHR Research for Patient Benefit (RfPB) Programme supports research which will have demonstrable effect on the health or health care of patients within three to five years and currently funds projects of up to £350,000 and of 36 months duration. Having some information about the amount of funding you will need, and the time it will take, is therefore helpful in these early stages.

If you need to conduct a pilot or feasibility study prior to a main award application, some funders will support this type of work, such as the RfPB. You could also enquire at your place of work, as often research departments have small 'pump-priming' awards. These pump-priming awards are also useful for your first project as chief investigator. You can also search for small awards, often organised by charities such as Starter Grants for Clinical Lecturers (Academy of Medical Sciences), which offer awards of up to £30,000 to enable clinical lecturers some money and freedom in order to pursue research. Another way in which you can pursue research is with the support of a fellowship award. Various funders have fellowships ranging from PhD stipends to postdoctoral awards and beyond. Both the MRC and NIHR offer fellowships, as do the Wellcome Trust who offer a variety of fellowships, including a career re-entry one for postdoctoral scientists who have had a break from their scientific career for at least two years. Fellowships vary in length, and monetary amount, but often pay the applicant's salary, costs of the research and any training required.

Your final consideration when choosing a funding stream is the frequency and timing of submission deadlines. As discussed in Chapter 4: 'Developing an Effective Research Proposal', you may need a year to develop and write an application from scratch. Sometimes meeting short deadlines is unavoidable with the commissioned calls which, in general, have quite short turnaround times. However, for researcher-led awards, they are often rolling with yearly calls, for example, RfPB is three times per year. It is advisable that you take your time and aim for a subsequent call rather than rush it as often funders will ask for the history of the application, including whether it is a resubmission and, if so, how it differs from the original application. They may also ask whether or not the application is being considered by another funder as some programmes do not allow dual submission.

Unsuccessful research applications are common. For example, the MRC in 2011–12 received 1095 applications for their awards, of which 280 (26%) were funded. Failure can be difficult to accept when you have submitted what you thought was a good and worthy application. However, this process is part of being a researcher and most, if not all, academics, including professors, will have had applications rejected. If it is rejected, you can use any feedback from the funder to revise and resubmit if appropriate. You will have also gained experience of the application procedure, including the approvals process, as well as writing a research grant, drafting Gantt charts and budgets, and developing a patient involvement strategy.

Commercially sponsored and funded studies

Although the above section is regarding competitive publicly funded awards, there are commercially sponsored and funded (industry) studies, which should be fully funded by the industry and should have no financial impact on the site hosting the research. The NIHR has developed an industry costing model and template for commercial studies. Pharmaceutical companies are encouraged to use this in negotiation with individual sites, prior to commencement of the research. The investigator will need to draft a budget including staff time, tests and investigations, pharmacy costs and other procedures that will be involved in the study. These are then entered into the costing template, which will then calculate overall costs, normally expressed as a fee per patient recruited into the trial. Once the budget for the study has been finalised, this will be made explicit in a Clinical Trial Agreement which is signed off by all parties (sponsor, participating site and any party with delegated sponsor responsibilities). Commercially funded studies also include an element of funding to enable research capacity to be built at the site, such as investment in research nurse posts and other study-related personnel, with the aim of establishing a strong track record in delivering industry studies at the site.

Summary

- Drafting a budget is a complex task and you must allow plenty of time for this, and to collect the approvals necessary for submission.
- Appropriate attribution of the costs involved in delivering a study is important.
- Funding bodies ask for a very clear and detailed account of the study budget; this plan should provide the blueprint for managing the budget through the life of the study.
- The budget needs to be actively managed, to ensure that all funding is being utilised as described in the grant application.
- Wherever possible, the study should be delivered within the identified budget and timescale.
- There are a plethora of awards by various funders. To find one suitable for your project, you need to be aware of your topic, and a ballpark figure of what you need, and what you need it for.
- Funding applications being rejected are the norm. Do not let it dishearten you; instead focus on the experience you have gained, and the peers you have collaborated with, to utilise in the future.

Questions for Discussion

1. As a university-employed researcher, if you are involved in developing a grant proposal, who are the key stakeholders you would need to engage with to discuss and agree the finances that need to be included in the grant application for your project you will conduct within a hospital?
2. An NHS organisation participating in your study does not provide one of the treatments in the study protocol as routine care. How would you set about convincing this site that it should fund these Excess Treatment Costs?
3. What key factors do you need to establish, in order for you to search for appropriate funding?

Further Reading

Berry, D. (2010) *Gaining Funding for Research: A Guide for Academics and Institutions.* Milton Keynes: Open University Press.

Crombie, I. and Florey, C. (1998) *The Pocket Guide to Grant Applications.* London: Wiley-Blackwell.

National Institute for Health Research (2010) *Clinical Research Networks and NHS Service Support: A Guide for Researchers.* London: NICE.

References

Arain, M., Campbell, M.J., Cooper, C.L. and Lancaster, G.A. (2010) 'What is a pilot or feasibility study? A review of current practice and editorial policy', *BMC Medical Research Methodology*, 10: 67.

Berry, D. (2010) *Gaining Funding for Research: A Guide for Academics and Institutions.* Milton Keynes: Open University Press.

Culyer, Anthony (1994) *Supporting Research and Development in the NHS.* London: HMSO.

Department of Health (2005) *Attributing Revenue Costs of Externally-Funded Non-Commercial Research in the NHS (ARCO).* London: Dept of Health.

Department of Health (2012) *Attributing the Costs of Health and Social Care Research and Development (AcoRD).* London: Dept of Health.

NHS Executive (1997) *Responsibilities for Meeting Patient Care Costs Associated with Research and Development in the NHS.* HSG (97) 32. London: NHS Executive.

Schimetta, W., Pölz, W., Haring, H.P., Baumgartner, H. and Aichner, F. (2005) 'When is a clinical study non-commercial?', *Wien Med Wochenschr*, 155 (9–10): 233–6.

Part II

GENERAL METHODOLOGIES

6

QUANTITATIVE DATA COLLECTION

Laura Gray and Katherine Payne

- Understand what quantitative research is and what type of questions it can answer
- Be familiar with the main designs used in quantitative studies and the benefits and limitations associated with these
- Appreciate some of the practical issues that must be considered when choosing a quantitative design methodology.

Introduction

One key question to ask when determining the most appropriate method for your research is whether it should use primarily a quantitative or qualitative methodological focus. One approach is not better or more robust than the other; rather, the two methods are used to answer different types of questions. In some instances, it might be more appropriate to answer a particular research question by using a combination of both quantitative and qualitative research paradigms, commonly termed 'mixed-methods' studies (please see Chapter 8). Qualitative methodologies aim to explore and understand people's beliefs, experiences, attitudes, behaviours and interactions through the use of methods such as interviews or focus groups, and thus usually generate non-numerical data from a small sample of participants for which statistical analysis is not normally appropriate. In contrast, quantitative methodologies are interested in collecting objectively measured data and counting/ quantifying the effect of one or more variables of interest. For example, in a study of pain, a quantitative study would attempt to measure the level of pain in a study sample, whereas a qualitative study would explore the experience of pain in the sample. Qualitative methodologies are described in detail in Chapter 7.

Quantitative research generates numerical data (or data which can be converted into numerical data) on which statistical analysis can be carried out in order to describe (quantify) the relationship between variables within a sample from a particular population. In a rigorous, valid study with a representative sample it is often deemed feasible to generalise the results seen to the larger population (please see Chapter 17: 'Sampling'). Therefore a key component of any quantitative methodology is the statistical analysis of the data collected and the interpretation of the results. So when deciding whether a quantitative method is appropriate for your research project, you need to think about how you might analyse the data in order to answer your research question. It is good practice to produce a statistical analysis plan before data is collected detailing the analysis to be carried out at the end of the study (please see Chapter 11: 'Clinical Trials').

Quantitative methods to inform clinical practice

One key objective of any piece of health services research is to provide evidence to aid decision-making. The 'evidence pyramid' is routinely used to grade the level of quality of studies when assessing the efficacy or effectiveness of treatments or services (please see Figure 6.1). An important factor to consider when you need the results from your quantitative study to inform decision-making is to ensure that your study generates evidence of a sufficient quality, which may mean obtaining a high level of evidence. As can be seen in Figure 6.1, systematic reviews are at the top of the evidence pyramid and, when assimilated into a meta-analysis, produce the highest level of evidence. Meta-analysis (quantitative) or meta-synthesis (qualitative) are methods to combine data from multiple studies using analysis to give an overall pooled result, thereby making the results more robust.

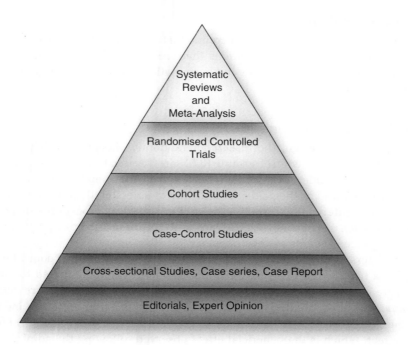

FIGURE 6.1   Evidence pyramid

Systematic reviews can incorporate either qualitative or quantitative studies depending on the nature of the research question of interest, and are an attempt to identify, appraise and synthesise all the empirical evidence that meets pre-specified eligibility criteria to answer a given research question. Researchers conducting systematic reviews use explicit methods aimed at minimising bias, in order to produce more reliable findings that can be used to inform decision-making (Higgins and Green, 2011). Quantitative systematic reviews and meta-analysis often form the basis of disease-specific guidelines or the development of services for patient populations, and are also important methods used by health economists when developing economic models to assess the relative cost-effectiveness of new interventions compared with current practice. The results of such economic models are now used routinely to inform decisions regarding health care resource allocations at a national level by bodies such as the National Institute for Health and Care Excellence (NICE) (please see Chapter 9: 'Health Economics' and Chapter 14: 'Systematic Reviews' for more in-depth discussions).

Quantitative methods in research

There are a number of different types of quantitative methods you can use for your research project. These can be categorised broadly into the following designs: experimental, observational or descriptive.

Experimental methods

In experimental studies it is the researcher that controls who is exposed, and to what. They are controlled investigations that are designed to be as objective and systematic as possible; this enables the examination of the probability of a causal relationship amongst variables.

Randomised controlled trials (RCTs)

In this experimental design, the researcher randomly allocates participants to an intervention group or a control group. RCTs are the next category down on the evidence pyramid under systematic reviews and meta-analysis/meta-synthesis. RCTs are often viewed as the gold standard way of assessing the efficacy and effectiveness of new interventions such as medicines, surgical procedures or complex interventions such as psychological therapies. RCTs are termed prospective studies because they record events as they happen.

Efficacy refers to how well the intervention works under optimal controlled conditions, i.e. a highly controlled research environment, when compared to placebo. Placebos are inert substances which contain no active ingredients that are delivered in the same way, for example, injection, tablet, etc., as the intervention being tested and are also designed to look the same. Placebos are used in order to control for the placebo effect, which is the beneficial effect observed following the administration of any 'treatment' (whether active or inactive) because of the patient's belief in the treatment. By using a placebo control, the researchers can also be blinded to which arm the participant is in to avoid observer expectancy effect, where researchers unconsciously influence the participant's responses, for example, by using eye contact, or tone of voice. As you can see, testing for efficacy does not replicate 'real life' and instead is an extremely controlled situation. Effectiveness on the other hand, is a measure of what you would expect to happen in real life and the comparator is current practice. For example, a trial of efficacy might have very strict inclusion criteria which limit the trial to those who are expected to achieve the maximum outcome, whereas a trial of effectiveness would be open to anyone who would potentially receive the treatment in routine care (Compher, 2010). Alternatively, some RCTs do not have a 'control' group *per se*, but compare two or more interventions to try and establish superiority of one over another, such as when comparing different regimens of the same medication.

Randomisation is a core advantage of the RCT design, ensuring that everyone in the study has an equal chance of being in either arm. It removes sources of selection bias, i.e. the systematic difference in the selection of study participants based on exposure to a risk factor or other predisposing characteristics, and ensures that both known and unknown factors which could affect outcome are evenly distributed between the arms. When deciding whether an RCT is the appropriate methodology to answer your research question, there are some ethical and practical issues to consider such as whether it is unethical to assess treatments which have the potential to be harmful (please see Chapter 15: 'Designing and Conducting an Ethical Research

Study'). Other treatments may be ethical to test but unfeasible, such as when an untested treatment has already become part of routine practice. This was the case with an RCT of counselling in general practice, where GPs were unwilling to randomise patients to not receive counselling even though its efficacy and effectiveness had not been proven (Fairhurst and Dowrick, 1996). RCTs also tend to be more time consuming and expensive than other designs. However after considering all of these facts, if you think that this type of quantitative method is still appropriate for your study, please see Chapter 11 which discusses RCTs in detail. The case study here shows an example of how to use an RCT to address a particular research question.

Case study

It is well documented that the prevalence, i.e. the proportion of cases of a particular condition in a population at a given point in time (please see Chapter 10: Epidemiology for further description) of type 2 diabetes mellitus (T2DM) is higher in women with polycystic ovary syndrome (PCOS) than those without (Moran et al., 2010). Additionally, there is evidence that following a Mediterranean diet might alleviate T2DM risk (Salas-Salvadó et al., 2011). The Mediterranean diet is generally considered to consist of a high concentration of 'good oils' (mono-saturated fatty acids), usually from olives and olive oil; a daily consumption of fruit, vegetables, whole grains and low-fat dairy; weekly consumption of fish, poultry, nuts and legumes; together with low red meat consumption and moderate alcohol intake.

Therefore a dietician would like to answer the research question: does following a Mediterranean diet prevent T2DM in women with PCOS? However they need to determine the most appropriate research design for answering it.

The first design the dietician considers is the RCT. Using an RCT to answer the research question would involve selecting a sample of women who have PCOS (the target population) and do not have T2DM (the study outcome). These women would then be randomised to either follow a Mediterranean diet or not for a given period of time (follow-up). The outcome would be the number of participants developing T2DM in each arm which could then be compared to see if less women in the diet arm go on to develop T2DM than in the control arm (please see Figure 6.2).

Although this sounds feasible, things to consider are, first, how the dietician would ensure that those in the Mediterranean diet arm follow the diet specified (or those in the control arm are prevented from beginning a similar diet of their own accord)? Tactics could be used for measuring these factors, such as asking participants to keep a diet diary. However this is not failsafe as participants may forget to complete it, or not want to keep the diary if they stop following the diet. Another consideration for the dietician is how long the follow-up period should be. The dietician may want women with newly diagnosed PCOS, otherwise there may already be prodromes of T2DM. Therefore as the disease may take many years to become clinically relevant, the trial may be very lengthy, and the longer the trial, the more the trial costs, and the higher the attrition rate (drop out) which can invalidate the results.

(Continued)

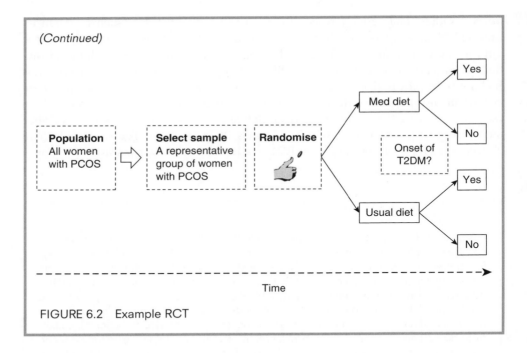

FIGURE 6.2   Example RCT

Observational methods

Cohort, cross-sectional and case-control designs are collectively referred to as observational methods, so-called because the researcher has no control over who is exposed to what.

Cohort studies

The level below RCTs in the evidence pyramid is the cohort study. The main advantage of cohort studies is that they allow researchers to investigate risk factors for which it would be unethical to randomise participants, for example, a researcher cannot allocate participants to a smoking or non-smoking group; they can only observe what happens to people who smoke. In a cohort study, a sample of people who do not have the outcome of interest are selected. The sample is then divided into two cohorts, those who have the risk factor (exposure) being investigated, and those who do not. The two groups are then observed for a period of time to see if they develop the outcome of interest. Cohort studies allow researchers to calculate both incidence and relative risk. Incidence is a measure of the risk of developing a new condition within a specified period of time, whilst relative risk is a measure of an event occurring in one cohort (the exposed) compared to another (the unexposed). A relative risk of 1 means that there is no difference between the cohorts, greater than 1 means that the exposure increases the probability of developing the outcome, and less than one means the exposure lowers the probability of the event occurring. For example, your research question could be: does smoking cause pancreatic cancer? Here your outcome of interest would be pancreatic cancer, with the exposure being smoking. Therefore your two cohorts would be smokers and non-smokers who you will observe over a specified period of time to see if there is any difference in the numbers developing pancreatic cancer between the two cohorts. Once the study has been completed, you would then be able to calculate the relative risk of developing pancreatic cancer in the smoking group compared to the non-smoking group. Once the two cohorts have been established you can assess more than one outcome. For example, as well as looking at pancreatic cancer, data on other types of cancer or mortality could also be assessed (for further description please see Chapter 10: 'Epidemiology').

The main disadvantage of cohort studies is that they often require long periods of follow-up which leads to potential drop out which can bias the sample (attrition bias). To account for this, cohort studies are generally quite large, and combined with the long follow-up time this means that they are expensive to conduct. Another major disadvantage is that the two cohorts might differ in other important factors over and above the exposure of interest and what you are actually measuring is a confounding variable. For example, a study of mortality and diabetes showed that 40% of patients with type 2 diabetes compared with 29% of patients with type 1 diabetes died (Gatling et al., 1989; Julious and Mullee, 1994). However, type 2 diabetes usually develops later in life than type 1 diabetes. When age was taken into account in the analysis the reverse was found and fewer patients with type 2 diabetes compared to those with type 1 diabetes died. Therefore age is confounding the relationship between diabetes type and mortality (Figure 6.3). In any study there are usually an infinite number of possible confounders. The only way to eliminate confounding is to use a RCT design where people are randomly allocated to group and therefore any confounders should be present in equal numbers randomly across both groups.

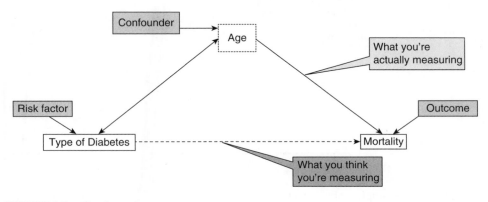

FIGURE 6.3   Confounders

The case study shows an example of how to use a cohort study to address a particular research question.

Case study

Using a cohort design to assess the dietician's research question would involve selecting a group of women who have PCOS (population) and do not have T2DM (outcome). These women would be split into two cohorts – those who follow a Mediterranean diet (exposure) and those who do not. They would then be followed up over a specified period of time, after which the number of women developing T2DM in each cohort would be compared (see Figure 6.4). Some of the issues in the cohort study are the same as those which may occur in the RCT, namely, will the participant's diet change over time? Also what is the length of follow-up, and how will this affect recruitment and retention? There are confounders that may be present in this cohort study such as are those who are following the Mediterranean diet different in other ways than just their diet to those who are not following the diet, e.g. different lifestyles, socio-economic status, etc.? Of major concern for the dietician is that having low vitamin D (which is naturally obtained through sunlight) is related to insulin resistance and diabetes. It is probable that the women who follow a Mediterranean diet are more likely to live in a sunny climate and therefore may have the preventative measure of a steady supply of vitamin D which would then be a confounder.

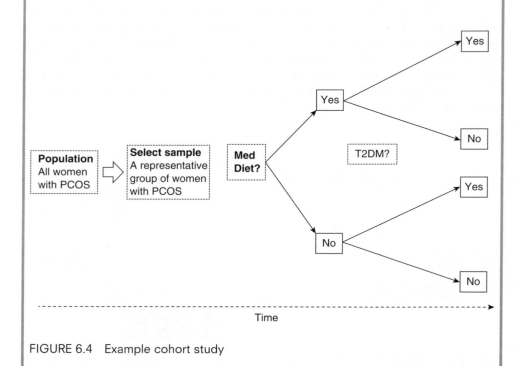

FIGURE 6.4   Example cohort study

Case-control studies

Following on from the cohort studies in the evidence pyramid are the case-control studies. Case-control studies identify people for inclusion based on the outcome of interest and then look back for possible related risk factors/exposures. For example, if you wanted to look at the association between psychosis and smoking cannabis you could find a group of people who had developed psychosis (the cases) and a group who had not (the controls), usually matched in some way to ensure comparability (usually by age and sex as a minimum). Then you would gather from them information about their previous cannabis smoking which would allow you to calculate the prevalence of this risk factor within each group. However, because these studies are retrospective (data collected regarding the past), it is not possible to calculate disease incidence.

As cases are included based on their outcome status, case-control studies are appropriate for rare diseases, such as leukaemia, because an unrealistically large sample size would be needed to ascertain relative risk in a rare disease using a cohort study design. Also, because cases are included based upon their outcome status, it is possible to measure multiple risk factors for a single outcome, in contrast to cohort studies which can measure multiple outcomes for one risk factor. For example, from your participants with psychosis, you could also collect data regarding other drugs previously taken. Another benefit of case-control studies is that, because they are retrospective, when compared to cohort studies, case-control studies tend to be quicker and cheaper to complete as you are not expecting participants to stay in your study to follow them up for any length of time, which also results in low attrition. The main disadvantage of this study design is that they rely on people's memories so it is subject to recall bias, which is when memory affects the data provided, and thus prone to error, which may leave it difficult to measure the exact amount of an exposure to a risk factor participants have had in the past. Another problem with the design, which is shared with cross-sectional studies (please see next section), is that being retrospective it can be difficult to ascertain the direction of causality. Temporality of exposure is the timing of when the person was exposed to the disease or risk factor, in relation to the outcome, i.e. the outcome has to come after the risk factor. For example, was the psychosis triggered by the cannabis smoking, or was the cannabis smoking a form of self-medication for prodromal symptoms? For further discussion regarding temporality please see Chapter 10: 'Epidemiology'.

The case study shows an example of how to use a case-control study to address a particular research question.

Case study

Using a case-control design, our study would identify a group of women with PCOS and then divide them into those that have T2DM (cases) and those who do not (controls). They would all be asked about their diet over a defined period of time in the past, probably helped with the use of food frequency questionnaires. The number of

(Continued)

(Continued)

women following a Mediterranean diet within each group would then be compared (please see Figure 6.5).

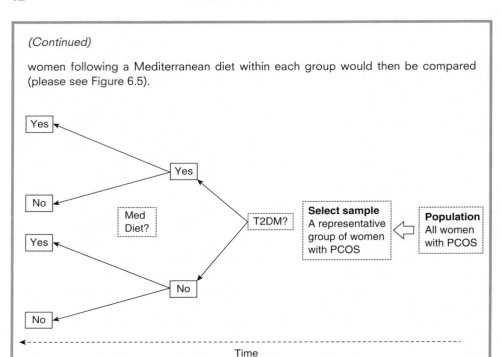

Time

FIGURE 6.5   Example case control study

However as the diet must be adhered to over a long period of time for it to make a difference to the outcome, the dietician is worried about the participants' ability to recall food intake as long ago as a year. Another concern is that participants with T2DM may overestimate or underestimate their intake of unhealthy foods due to the influence of having that disease. The dietician also has concerns regarding the sample. Due to funding, they need to collect the data in the UK; however they believe that following a Mediterranean diet would be rare in this population, which might have a dramatic negative impact on recruitment.

The selection of cases and controls is an important consideration when designing a case-control study, as the cases should be a representative sample of all patients with the disease of interest to avoid sampling bias, i.e. some members of a population are less likely to be included than others leading to a biased sample. Avoiding all sampling bias in a study is generally not feasible for two reasons; first, some people who have the disease may be undiagnosed or misdiagnosed. Secondly, it may only be feasible to collect data from a specific geographical locality (please see Chapter 17: 'Sampling'). Once a group of cases has been recruited it can be difficult to select a group of controls who are similar to the cases apart from their outcome status. Controls should be selected from the same population as the cases otherwise the study may be affected by selection bias. However, using a similar sampling procedure as the one used with the cases, such as attending the same outpatient department, or recruiting a sample from the same locality, may help. It may also help to have more than one control group recruited by different ways, e.g. outpatients, colleges, etc. Then if your analysis shows a significant difference in one of your outcome measures, your conclusion will be more robust if it remains significant between the cases and a number of differently recruited control groups (Mann, 2003).

Usually one control is selected for each case but it is possible to have more than one control per case to increase statistical power. Being able to increase statistical power in this way can be useful when the outcome of interest is uncommon. For example, in a cross-sectional study (please see next section) where the outcome of interest has a prevalence of 1%, you would need to study 10,000 people to obtain 100 cases. In a case-control study you would instead select these 100 cases and then select 100 (or more) controls, resulting in a considerably smaller total study population of only 200. It has been demonstrated, however, that increasing the number of controls to more than three to four per case does not yield further gains in statistical power or efficiency (Taylor, 1986).

Cross-sectional studies

The last group of quantitative methods towards the bottom of the evidence pyramid are the cross-sectional studies. As the name suggests, cross-sectional studies involve participants at a single time point and are used for two main reasons, first to assess prevalence, for example, a cross-sectional study ascertaining the prevalence of chronic pain in Australia, interviewed a random sample of adults by telephone. From the 17,543 interviews completed, chronic pain had a reported prevalence of 17.1% in males and 20.0% in females (Blyth et al., 2001). Secondly, cross-sectional studies can look for associations between variables, by assessing participants at one time point when data on exposure to risk factors and outcomes of interest are collected.

The main advantage of the cross-sectional study design is in its simplicity. Participants are only contacted once and are not selected based on their exposure or outcome (in contrast to cohort and case-control studies). Therefore these designs do not work well for rare diseases as even if a very large sample was obtained, there would still be relatively few participants identified with the disease of interest (Mann, 2003). The data collected can be used to assess multiple hypotheses and therefore these studies are relatively cheap and quick to carry out. This simplicity also leads to a number of disadvantages though, as mentioned above, it can be difficult to determine temporality due to both the outcome and exposure being measured at the same time point and not knowing which came first. A cross-sectional study carried out in Finland, for example, assessed depression and insulin resistance and found a positive association (more depression with more insulin resistance). However, this association cannot tell us whether depression causes insulin resistance or vice versa or whether the relationship is due to a confounder (Timonen et al., 2005).

A key logistical issue with cross-sectional designs is the impact of the response rate. If a study has a low response rate the results may be biased if there are important, quantifiable differences between responders and non-responders. In a study of the prevalence of undiagnosed T2DM in Leicester, UK, only 22% of those who were invited to be screened attended. Those who attended were older than those who did not and were more likely to be female. Therefore the results from this study had to be interpreted with caution as they reflected the population recruited rather than the population in general (Webb et al., 2011). The case study shows an example of how to use a cross-sectional study to address a particular research question.

Case study

A cross-sectional study could collect data at a single time point from a sample of women with PCOS. This sample would then be questioned to see if they also have T2DM (outcome of interest) and questioned about their diet to see if they follow a Mediterranean diet or not (exposure) (see Figure 6.6). Analysis would be able to tell the dietician whether following this diet is associated with diabetes with a negative correlation, i.e. the more you follow the Mediterranean diet the less likely you are to develop T2DM. The dietician might need a very large sample size if they chose a cross-sectional method, as the prevalence of the combinations of PCOS, T2DM and the diet might be low. One way around this would be to recruit women with PCOS who follow a Mediterranean diet and then compare the number with T2DM and without.

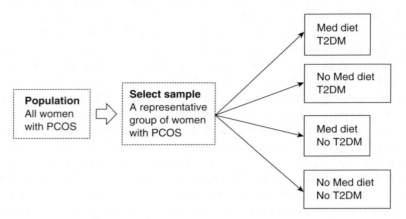

FIGURE 6.6   Example cross sectional study

The way the dietician could collect this data is through using surveys (please see Chapter 12: 'Surveys'). By conducting the research with mail, telephone or online surveys, the dietician could reach a large sample from a large geographical area which may help increase the numbers. However, issues that the dietician needs to consider before choosing this method are: whether the surveys would give an accurate reflection of the participants' actual food intake, given that following a healthy diet is desirable and therefore subject to prestige bias. The survey may be prone to sampling bias also. Because they are being asked about their diet, the probability is that women will respond who are interested in diet or healthy living. This may prove useful in identifying more people who follow the Mediterranean diet, though you may get less respondents with a unhealthy diet, and because obesity is linked with T2DM, you may get less respondents with this also.

Descriptive methods

Descriptive methods do not aim to compare groups to establish a causal relationship, but aim instead to describe a sample in order to make inferences about the rest of the population. The method used in the majority of descriptive studies is surveys, which consist of a structured set of questions that are used to systematically describe a situation, such as current practice for managing people with T2DM, or to measure attitudes and behaviours in a standardised way (Rubenfeld, 2004). Surveys can either be designed with bespoke questions that have been generated to address a particular set of research questions, or be validated and already in existence for standardised outcome measures, such as anxiety or exercise scales, or for measuring values or preferences for health economic analysis (Brazier et al., 2007) (see Chapter 9: 'Health Economics'). Another benefit with a survey is that you can use the same survey at a later time point with the same respondents. This might be useful if you were trying to examine the effectiveness of an intervention and need to compare baseline data, i.e. data collected before the programme begins, with post-intervention data. If you were seeking to determine whether art therapy is an effective intervention for treating depression, you could compare baseline data with post-intervention data using the same validated depression scale so the outcomes are directly comparable. However, although surveys can provide a cheap and simple way of gathering information, there are some important potential limitations, such as sampling bias due to a poor response rate, or instrument bias which occurs when the way a question is asked affects the response given. For example, question wording might influence the way the respondents answer, or complex vocabulary might make the questions difficult to interpret. (For a more in-depth discussion of surveys, please see Chapter 12.)

Summary

- Quantitative designs use numerical data to answer research questions.
- Quantitative methods can be categorised into experimental, observational or descriptive designs, each having specific benefits and limitations which need to be considered before choosing a particular design.

- Experimental methods are when the researcher controls who is exposed and to what. This method includes the randomised controlled trial.
- Observational methods are when the researcher has no control over exposure and includes cohort, case-control and cross-sectional designs.
- Descriptive methods do not attempt to compare groups to infer a causal relationship, but rather collect data with which to describe a sample. Surveys are the main method for descriptive studies.

Questions for Discussion

1. What are the advantages and disadvantages of using a prospective observational study compared with an RCT to evaluate the effectiveness of a new diagnostic test?
2. For an RCT of a new medicine, how would you ensure the results were useful for a decision-maker who wanted to develop a drug formulary in their hospital?
3. In what circumstances would a quantitative design be used to explore why young mothers choose not to breastfeed?

Further Reading

Balnaves, M. (2001) *Introduction to Quantitative Research Methods: An Investigative Approach.* London: SAGE.
Vogt, W.P. (2011) *SAGE Quantitative Research Methods* (4 vols). London: SAGE.

References

Azziz, R., Woods, K.S., Reyna, R., Key, T.J., Knochenhauer, E.S. and Yildiz, B. (2004) 'The prevalence and features of polycystic ovary syndrome in an unselected population', *Journal of Clinical Endocrinology and Metabolism,* 89 (6): 2745–9.
Blyth, F.M., March, L.M., Brnabic, A.J., Jorm, L.R., Williamson, M. and Cousins, M.J. (2001) 'Chronic pain in Australia: a prevalence study', *Pain,* 89 (2–3): 127–34.
Brazier, J., Ratcliffe, J., Tsuchiya, A. and Salomon, J. (2007) *Measuring and Valuing Health Benefits for Economic Evaluation.* Oxford: Oxford University Press.
Compher, C. (2010) 'Efficacy vs effectiveness', *Journal of Parenteral and Enteral Nutrition,* 34(6): 598–9.
Fairhurst, K. and Dowrick, C. (1996) 'Problems with recruitment in a randomized controlled trial of counselling in general practice: causes and implications', *Journal of Health Service Research Policy,* 1(2): 77–80.
Gatling, W., Mullee, M.A. and Hill, R. (1989) 'The general characteristics of a community based population', *Practical Diabetes,* 15: 104–7.
Higgins, J.P.T. and Green, S. (eds) (2011) *Cochrane Handbook for Systematic Reviews of Interventions Version 5.1.0.* The Cochrane Collaboration: www.cochrane-handbook.org (accessed Oct. 2012).

Julious, S.A. and Mullee, M.A. (1994) 'Confounding and Simpson's paradox', *British Medical Journal*, 309: 1480.

Legro, R.S., Kunselman, A.R., Dodson, W.C. and Dunaif, A. (1999) 'Prevalence and predictors of risk for type 2 diabetis mellitus and impaired glucose tolerance in polycystic ovary syndrome: a prospective, controlled study in 254 affected women', *Journal of Clinical Endocrinology and Metabolism*, 84 (1): 165–9.

Mann, C.J. (2003) 'Observational research methods: research design II. Cohort, cross sectional, and case-control studies', *Emergency Medicine*, 20: 54–60.

Moran, L.J., Misso, M.L., Wild, R.A. and Norman, R.J. (2010) 'Impaired glucose tolerance, type 2 diabetes and metabolic syndrome in polycystic ovary syndrome: a systematic review and meta-analysis', *Human Reproduction Update*, 16 (4): 347.

Rubenfeld, G.D. (2004) 'Surveys: an introduction', *Respiratory Care*, 49 (10): 1181–5.

Salas-Salvadó, J., Bulló, M., Babio, N., Martínez-González, M.A., Ibarrola, N., Basora, J., Estruch, R., Covas, M.I., Corella, D., Arós, F., Ruiz-Gutiérrez, V. and Ros, E. (2011) 'Reduction in the incidence of type 2 diabetes with the Mediterranean diet: results of the PREDIMED-Reus nutrition intervention randomized trial', *Diabetes Care*, 34 (1): 14–19.

Taylor, J.M. (1986) 'Choosing the number of controls in a matched case-control study, some sample size, power and efficiency considerations,' *Stat Med*. Jan–Feb. 5(1): 29–36.

Timonen, M., Laakso, M., Jokelainen, J., Rajala, U., Meyer-Rochow, V.B. and Keinänen-Kiukaanniemi, S. (2005) 'Insulin resistance and depression: cross sectional study', *British Medical Journal*, 330: 17–18.

Webb, D.R., Gray, L.J., Khunti, K., Srinivasan, B., Taub, N., Campbell, S., Barnett, J., Farooqi, A., Echouffo-Tcheuqui, J.B., Griffin, S.J., Wareham, N.J. and Davies, M.J. (2011) 'Screening for diabetes using an oral glucose tolerance test within a western multi-ethnic population identifies modifiable cardiovascular risk: the ADDITION-Leicester study', *Diabetologia*, 54 (9): 2237–46.

7

QUALITATIVE DATA COLLECTION

Jonathan Ives and Sarah Damery

- Understand what qualitative research is
- Gain a theoretical understanding of how interviews, focus groups and participant observation function as methods for collecting qualitative data
- Appreciate some of the advantages and disadvantages of these methods
- Appreciate some of the practical issues that must be considered when choosing a qualitative data collection method

Introduction

Qualitative research can furnish us with rich data that provide insight into human behaviour, and are concerned with documenting and understanding people's experiences, beliefs, values, motivations, perspectives and desires. Historically, qualitative research has been viewed with some scepticism by the medical community. This was largely due to an unreasonable comparison to quantitative research, with complaints about small sample sizes, lack of generalisability, reproducibility and statistical power. Over time however, qualitative methodology has gained popularity and established itself as an important group of methods in health research, both as a stand-alone approach, and for complementing quantitative research. Any direct comparison with quantitative methods is inappropriate because qualitative research is concerned with answering very different kinds of questions. As such, qualitative research should never try to mimic or compete with quantitative research paradigms, as the data cannot be reduced to something that can be merely counted.

If you decide that a qualitative methodology is appropriate for your study, it is important that you not only have an understanding of the data collection method you will use, but also how you intend to analyse the data you collect (please see Chapter 20: 'Qualitative Analysis'). Data collection and analysis are intimately connected, and cannot be considered separately or thought about linearly. The analytic approach you decide to take will influence the way you collect your data and, similarly, the way you collect your data will affect the kind of analysis you can conduct; therefore both need to be considered *prior* to data collection.

Data collection and analysis combine to form a methodology when both are driven by an overarching theoretical framework or philosophy about the nature and status of knowledge (epistemology). You may be tempted to think that you have no such theoretical or philosophical commitments but chances are you do; you just may not be conscious of it. Even asking certain kinds of questions makes assumptions about the way the world works and the way we acquire knowledge about the world. Your choice of methods for data collection and analysis will be influenced by the theoretical and philosophical assumptions you have made, often without giving them a moment's thought. Good qualitative research makes explicit those assumptions, justifies them and makes them coherent within a theoretically informed methodology, for example, ethnography, grounded theory, etc. Theoretical and methodological sensitivity come with time, practice and experience, and develops alongside one's practical understanding of data collection and analysis. Given this, we would recommend that, as you begin to explore the practical aspects of qualitative methodology, you also refer to more theoretically orientated texts (please refer to Howell, 2013; Crotty, 2009; and Cheal, 2005 in the Further Reading section of this chapter).

Case study

This case study is based on Dowswell et al.'s (2011) qualitative study which explored men's experience of erectile dysfunction after surgery for colorectal cancer.

It was decided that qualitative methods were appropriate because the study wanted to access rich, in-depth data regarding men's attitudes and experiences. This is potentially a very sensitive topic. Men may not feel comfortable talking about erectile dysfunction, as it can be experienced as a challenge to one's masculinity, and sense of masculine identity. It may, therefore, be very difficult to access this data.

Study objectives

- Describe the experiences of men with erectile dysfunction after surgery for colorectal cancer.
- Ascertain what information about erectile dysfunction the men felt they needed, and how they felt the currently provided information might be improved.

Interviews

An interview is, broadly speaking, a dialogue between you and your participant(s), in which you attempt to elicit information that will help you answer your research question(s). Burgess describes a qualitative interview as a 'conversation with a purpose' (1982: 102), and what your 'purpose' is will dictate how you go about having that 'conversation'. There are a variety of approaches to qualitative interviewing that will suit a variety of purposes.

A qualitative interview is an appropriate method of data collection when you require in-depth data about a participant's thoughts, feelings, experiences or reported behaviours. Interviews allow us to obtain data that is focused on what is important to the participant, and which can be clarified through careful questioning and probing, i.e. asking a follow-up question for further clarification or more detail. Often, the aim of qualitative research is to understand the experiences of others from their own perspectives, and Jones notes that to do this 'we would do well to ask them ... and to ask them in such a way that they can tell us in their own terms' (1985: 46). An interview allows us to do just that by providing the space and opportunity for participants to talk, using their own vocabulary, about what they find significant and important. The extent to which the interview is dictated by the agenda of the participant or the interviewer will be dependent upon the questions driving the research. The real strength of an interview, however, is that it gives us flexibility during the research encounter, which allows us to be both proactive to obtain the data we need, and also reactive to the data we get.

It is important to recognise that although we might describe an interview as a 'conversation', conducting an interview is by no means as straightforward as that suggests. Qualitative interviewing is a skill, requiring practice and constant reflection on one's own performance. Roulston et al. (2003) conducted an interview study exploring the difficulties experienced by novice researchers carrying out qualitative interviews. Four main themes emerged from this study: (1) difficulty dealing with unexpected participant behaviours; (2) difficulty recognising and managing one's own beliefs and prejudices; (3) difficulty in constructing and delivering questions; and (4) difficulty handling sensitive topics. It must also be remembered that an interview can only capture retrospective accounts, so data generated by an interview are based on participants' recollections of past events (Taylor, 2005).

Choosing your interview method

Your choice of what kind of interview to conduct will be dictated by the aims of your research and what kind of data you wish to generate, as well as any practical factors that might constrain the choices available to you, such as time or financial limitations.

Face-to-face interviews

This is the traditional and most recognisable form of interview, where the researcher and participant sit together and have a 'conversation'. This kind of interview is particularly suited to research where it is important to develop a personal rapport with participants, such as when exploring sensitive topics. Developing personal rapport may encourage the participant to give you access to their personal and private accounts, which they would not ordinarily make public. Additional insight into the data can be obtained by observing and responding to non-verbal communication. Similarly, if the interview is conducted in the participant's own environment this can provide contextual insight for the analysis (when relevant). Practical factors to consider when choosing this kind of interview are:

- The time and financial cost of travelling to and from interview sites.
- Cost of recording equipment.
- Personal safety. You may be travelling to different sites, perhaps even to participants' own homes. How will you ensure your safety? Consider developing a safety protocol, and make certain that someone always knows where you are.
- Data storage and recording equipment. Can you carry equipment around safely and comfortably, and how will you securely transport and store the recording? Consider how you will store any non-anonymous data.

Telephone interviews

Whilst telephone interviews might lack the personal touch that enables personal rapport to develop, they are often easier to arrange than a face-to-face interview and do not have the time or cost implications of travel. Many researchers are concerned that the loss of non-verbal communication (body language) and contextual (social/ geographical) data undermine the quality of the findings. As such, telephone interviews are often considered the second-best option, to be employed only when a face-to-face interview is not possible for practical reasons. Novick (2008) has claimed that these concerns merely reflect a bias against telephone interviewing, which is not supported by evidence. She argues that telephone interviews might, in fact, encourage participants to disclose information more freely, as they are not subject to the interpersonal stresses of a face-to-face encounter. Practical factors to consider when choosing this method are:

- Do all your potential participants have access to a telephone, with the cognitive and physical abilities to use it?
- Do you have the facility to record the conversion over the telephone?
- Cost of the telephone calls and recording equipment.

Novel interview methods

An alternative to telephone interviewing is video interviewing using the internet (please see Chapter 14: 'The Internet as a Research Medium'), which some may feel combines the beneficial features of face-to-face and telephone interviews. One might also consider the use of techniques like photo voice/photo elicitation, which have been found to be effective in encouraging people to talk about sensitive and emotive subjects. This method involves asking participants to take photographs that illustrate the way they feel about an issue, and then using those photographs to generate discussion (Sandhu et al., 2013; Drew et al., 2010; Frith and Harcourt, 2007).

Conducting an interview

Once you have chosen your interview method you need to decide how to carry it out. This demands careful thought about how your interview will be structured. As a general guide, there are three forms of interview structure: open, structured and semi-structured.

An open interview involves the researcher introducing the research topic using a very open question, and then allowing the interview to follow its natural course. This kind of interview generates entirely participant-led data and is designed to allow the conversational agenda to be dictated by the participant. You, as a researcher, would respond to your participant, exploring items of interest by asking additional questions, but every question you ask is formulated in response to something the participant says and is not defined in advance. Accordingly, open (sometimes called 'unstructured') interviews tend to be unique, and never follow the same pattern twice. This kind of interview is often associated with exploratory research that uses grounded theory (for more detail please see Chapter 20: 'Qualitative Analysis') or ethnographic methodology.

A structured interview involves the use of an interview schedule, with predefined questions that are not deviated from. The interview schedule may incorporate a set of pre-defined probes that allow the researcher to ask for clarification, but in a structured interview the researcher does not think up new questions or follow new lines of thought that are not covered in the schedule. The advantage of a structured interview is that each participant is asked identical questions in an identical order. This standardisation helps improve reproducibility, and ensures that only data pertinent to the research question are obtained. It is open for debate whether or not a structured interview is genuinely a 'qualitative' method, as it does not allow for the kind of exploration that is characteristic of a qualitative approach. However, if the questions are sufficiently open, a structured interview can generate discursive responses which can be analysed qualitatively. Structured interviews, because they are limited in the extent to which they can explore new areas, are more suited to research that asks very specific questions about specific topics, or where there is a specific hypothesis to be examined.

A semi-structured interview sits somewhere between structured and open interviews. This kind of interview usually has a few key questions or topics that the researcher will cover during the interview, but the researcher is free to respond to the participant flexibly to explore unanticipated topics. However, it is perhaps unhelpful to think of interviews as being either structured or not, and it is worth bearing in mind Britten's warning that:

> [although] qualitative interviews are often described as being unstructured in order to contrast them with [structured] interview[s], the term 'unstructured' is misleading as no interview is completely devoid of structure: if it were, there would be no guarantee that the data gathered would be appropriate to the research question. (1995: 251)

It may, therefore, be more useful to think about structure in interviews as a continuum, with interviews being more or less structured according to the bespoke needs of your research.

How many interviews, and how long?

One common view is that you should continue to interview participants until you reach the point where you are getting no new data, i.e. data saturation (when the information obtained in subsequent interviews is repetitive and contains no new ideas). This view is closely associated with grounded theory. It is difficult to predict, however, when nothing new will come up in the next interview, and working to saturation is particularly challenging in the health care context, where research governance normally requires researchers to state in advance how many participants they will be accessing. In addition, the number of interviews you can conduct will be constrained by your timeframe and other resources. Our view is that you should conduct as many interviews as you can within the budget and time you have, but be prepared to stop interviewing if you find that you are getting no new information in consecutive interviews.

Although the length of an interview should be 'as long as it needs to be to get the data you need', this is also largely impractical. As a general rule, an in-depth interview might last anything from 45 minutes to 2 hours, depending on the topic. The less structured the interview, the harder it is to predict how long you will need. In practice, much will depend on variables you cannot control, for example, how talkative your participant is, how interesting the data are, etc. When planning your project, you should consider how much time you have, how much time you think you will need (conduct a pilot or two and time them) and then build in some flexibility.

Case study

Interviews would be appropriate for this research project and, given the sensitive nature of the topic, a one-to-one interview may provide an environment in which participants feel sufficiently comfortable to talk frankly and openly about their experiences. Although the interview could be conducted in a number of ways, the advantage of a face-to-face interview is that it may allow rapport to be developed more readily, although a telephone interview may provide sufficient social distance for some men to talk more openly. This is a difficult decision because all participants are likely react differently to diverse kinds of interview encounter, which cannot be predicted in advance.

Careful thought needs to be given to who will conduct the interview, particularly the age and sex of the interviewer. Will men feel comfortable talking about erectile dysfunction to a male researcher, of any age, who may make them feel 'less masculine' by comparison, therefore inhibiting disclosure? Alternatively, the participants may feel embarrassed talking to a female about their sex lives. The potential for embarrassment may be lessened if the female interviewer is older, or of a similar age to the participants, who can demonstrate sufficient life experience to handle sensitive discussions?

Where to conduct the interview is an important question. A comfortable location is vital, and this might suggest the participant's own home is an appropriate venue. However, the presence of other people must be considered and the need for a private space in the home must be emphasised. Alternatively, some participants may prefer a more neutral setting which has no personal association for them. The researcher's own office may be appropriate, but it risks emphasising the power differential and sets up the interviewer as the expert in their own environment. A public space may feel safe, but the conversation may be overheard and background noise may interfere with the recording. A good alternative may therefore be a neutral, private room.

How the interview is structured will depend on how focused the research questions are. In this case, the research is looking to explore experiences and obtain specific information about support needs. This suggests that the interview needs some structure to ensure that relevant data are obtained, but too much structure may inhibit the exploratory aims. A semi-structured interview would be appropriate, with general open questions asking about participants' experiences and support needs, whilst allowing scope for probing and exploring participants' answers.

Focus groups

A focus group is a data collection method that brings together a group of people to discuss a specific topic, with the aim of generating data through discussion. It is, in essence, a collective conversation aiming to 'describe and understand meanings and interpretations of a select group of people to gain understanding of a specific issue from the perspective of the participants of the group' (Liamputtong, 2011: 30).

Focus groups are an ideal tool for exploring people's experiences, opinions, beliefs and concerns, giving the researcher unique insight into the many different forms of communication that may not be evident in other research settings (Kitzinger, 2005). Focus groups can give the researcher access to the ways in which groups of people interact within a 'permissive environment ... that encourages participants to share perceptions and points of view, without pressuring participants to vote or reach a consensus' (Krueger and Casey, 2000: 4). Whilst consensus is one possible outcome of a focus group, another outcome may be difference and disagreement. The key point is that a focus group *exposes the process* of reaching consensus, or of discovering difference and disagreement, and through careful analysis, allows the researcher to gain insight into the topic studied.

The strength of a focus group, and that which sets it apart from the interview, is that if conducted properly it should require minimal interference from the researcher. Rather than being a conversation between the participant and researcher, a focus group is a conversation between participants, in which participants quiz and probe one another and determine the course of the conversation themselves, with the researcher acting as a facilitator of the discussion. This guards against the research agenda being dictated by the researcher, and therefore makes focus groups particularly suitable where the research questions are open and exploratory. They may be less suitable for extremely sensitive topics, which participants may not want to discuss in front of others. In the context of health research, focus groups are typically used to explore patients' experience of service use (possibly because of their history as a market research tool), although they are increasingly and frequently used to explore patient experience of illness (Schulze and Angermeyer, 2003; Dowswell et al., 2011); as well as staff attitudes and experiences (Hanratty et al., 2002; Ives et al., 2009).

Conducting a focus group

Once you have decided that a focus group is appropriate for collecting the data that will answer your research question, there are a number of practical and theoretical issues to consider.

Number of groups

When deciding how many groups to run, you will have to consider both your overarching methodology and your practical circumstances. Some methodologies will require theoretical sampling or theoretical saturation (please see Chapter 20:

'Qualitative Analysis', for further description), which means that you cannot specify in advance how many groups you will need to run. Alternatively, your project may be resource limited, and you may have to work out how many groups you have time for or can afford. Whilst focus groups are often thought to be time and cost efficient because they gather a lot of data from many people concurrently, they can be costly and time consuming for other reasons, for example, time to organise, paying for a venue and catering, participant expenses, etc. Transcription is also more time consuming and costly compared to one-to-one interviews. In addition, there is more chance of a focus group being cancelled at the last minute because it requires a critical mass of participants and cannot be run if too many people withdraw.

Composition of groups

Assuming that you have used a purposive sampling strategy that has identified potential participants (please see Chapter 17: 'Sampling' for further description), you then need to decide how to form them into groups. There are three key considerations when thinking about group composition. First, you need to consider what kinds of homogeneity or heterogeneity would produce the best environment for getting the data you need, for example, sex, age, profession, ethnicity, etc. Second, you need to consider whether the participants in your groups should know each other. For example, if you are gathering data on the experience of negotiating hospital power structures, it may not be appropriate to have consultant doctors in the same focus group as junior doctors from the same hospital, as this may inhibit the more junior staff from expressing their opinions. Alternatively, this formation might be appropriate if you are interested in looking at the way that people at different career stages talk about power in the workplace. Third, you need to consider how many people to have in each group. This is not set in stone but, as a rule of thumb, six to eight appears to be a common choice amongst qualitative researchers (Morgan, 1997). The group needs to have enough members so that a genuine group discussion can take place, but not so many that individuals cannot be heard. These factors, together with consideration of the interplay between your research questions and the kind of environment you need to create to facilitate participant disclosure, will dictate the composition of your group.

Structure and facilitation

A focus group is usually structured through the use of a topic guide, which introduces the various topics of interest and promotes discussion. A topic guide may be simply an *aide-memoire* for the facilitator to make sure that s/he does not forget the key topics of discussion, or it may be something more elaborate, such as a vignette, i.e. a description of a particular kind of experience; or photos that participants are asked to look at and discuss. Whether it is a list of open questions, photos, drawings or vignettes (to name but a few possibilities), the purpose of the topic guide is to generate discussion around the topic of interest.

The role of the facilitator (also referred to as the 'moderator') is to ensure that the group remains focused on the topic of interest, whilst allowing the direction and content of the conversation to be dictated by the participants. The facilitator must dictate the topic, but not the content of the discussion, by exerting 'mild, unobtrusive control' (Nyamathi and Schuler, 1990: 1286). Effective facilitation is a skill, and it requires practice to maintain control of a discussion without influencing precisely what is discussed. As a facilitator, you may have to respond to the discussion to ask for more detail, change the direction/topic, get the discussion going, or close the discussion down. Krueger and Casey suggest that thinking about different categories of question is helpful: 'opening' (to get people talking); 'introductory' (to get people thinking about your topic); 'transition' (to move the conversation towards the key study questions); 'key' (the questions that drive the study); and 'ending' (questions to close the discussion) (2000: 44–6).

Case study

Focus groups may be an appropriate method of data collection for this topic. It is possible that men may feel empowered to talk about their own experiences if they are in a positive and supportive environment, comprising other men who understand and share their experience. The advantage of conducting a focus group here is that there may be more scope for a genuinely participant-led discussion, with participants dictating where the discussion goes. However, despite a shared experience, participants may not feel comfortable talking to a group of strangers about an intimate aspect of their lives. Additionally, the data obtained from a focus group would not comprise the rich personal stories that interviews would yield, but a negotiated discussion of shared experiences instead. This may be very useful in meeting the second objective that looks at information requirements, but less useful in meeting the first.

Participants for group composition would be men over 60 who have erectile dysfunction, and therefore homogeneous in terms of age, sex and experience. It is unlikely to be possible to convene a group of participants who already know each other, and may not be desirable to do so. Therefore the group would be comprised of strangers.

Structuring the discussion could be done in a variety of ways. In this case, a simple topic guide comprising open questions might work well. Vignettes may be less effective here because the project wants to access personal experiences rather than generic comments, and would risk alienating those participants who do not recognise that experience as their own.

Participant observation

Participant observation is a method of collecting qualitative data that involves the researcher physically entering the field of study to experience and observe it directly. This data collection method is particularly useful for studying groups and structures, and understanding how people negotiate and construct culture (Sharkey and Larson, 2005). You might consider using participant observation if your research question is focused around institutional practice and power, or where you suspect there may be discrepancies between reported and actual behaviour. Whilst participant observation is closely associated with ethnographic methodology, it is important to note that the two are not synonymous. Ethnography is not limited to participant observation and may involve other data collection methods, including interviews (Marshall and Koenig, 2010) and diaries (Zimmerman and Wieder, 1977; Elliot, 1997). Hammersley and Atkinson characterise ethnographic participant observation as '...the ethnographer participating, overtly or covertly, in people's daily lives for an extended period of time, watching what happens, listening to what is said, asking questions – in fact, collecting whatever data are available to throw light on the issues that are the focus of the research' (1995: 1). It should be noted that there are particular ethical issues involved in covert participant observation, which require substantial justification and careful consideration (please see Li, 2008, and Johnson, 1992, in the Further Reading section of this chapter).

The data collected from participant observation is usually in the form of field notes that record observations, experiences, reflections and interpretations. The researcher's role is to record their experiences and observations as accurately as possible so that this written record can be subjected to analysis. It is important to remember, when planning how to record your data, that there is no single and 'best' way of capturing what you have observed and experienced. As Emerson et al., note:

> ... there is no one 'natural' or 'correct' way to write about what one observes. Rather, because descriptions involve issues of perception and interpretation, different descriptions of 'the same' situations and events are possible. (2011: 5)

Given this, the relationship between data and analysis is more complex for participant observation than for other qualitative methods as the data have already passed through the interpretative 'lens' of the researcher, and there is no independent data set, for example, interview transcript, etc., that can be scrutinised. It is important, therefore, that the observer is clear on what kind of data is being sought, and to what end, as this will influence the way data is collected and interpreted *in situ*. Allen (2010) describes a continuum of participant observation with the 'detached observer' at one end concerned with attempting to develop dispassionate descriptions of the field, and 'full participation' at the other, which attempts to describe the experience of being part of the field. Where you sit along this spectrum will be determined by your overarching methodology, theoretical orientation and research questions. It will influence how you write up your data and analysis, and will affect the extent to which your field notes are *part of* the analysis or *subject to* analysis.

Participant observation is a skill that needs to be practised and honed. Bernard (1988) suggests that key skills for participant observation are: learning the language of the people studied (including technical/insider language); building explicit aware-ness of what might initially appear minor details; building your memory in order to remember what you have observed; maintaining some level of naivety so that you do not take anything for granted; and developing writing skills so that you can communicate your findings effectively and clearly. One's first time in the field is always going to be challenging, and good reflexive practice will be key to your development as a participant observer.

Challenges in participant observation

One of the most significant challenges when conducting participant observation is the 'observer effect'. Broadly speaking, this is the notion that people will act differently when they know they are being observed. This can lead to the researcher observing a performance that is especially created for them rather than normal activity. The aim of the observer is to become part of the background, so that other people in the field do not think of the researcher as a stranger who is observing them, but as a normal part of the environment. This is one of the reasons why participant observation takes place over an extended period of time (usually many months), as it gives the researcher an opportunity to blend in and become part of the community. Another challenge, which may be particularly acute in a health care setting, is that of negotiating an appropriate role. A health care worker who is entering the field as an observer will have a specific skill set that they might be able to employ, such as nursing skills. A researcher in this situation can experience tension from being torn between maintaining distance as an observer and wanting to get involved, help or even take charge of a situation (Koch, 2006). The extent to which either remaining detached, or getting involved, is a problem will depend on where you sit along the participant-observer spectrum outlined above.

Case study

It is very unlikely that participant observation could yield useful data on this topic. First, it is not clear what could actually be observed. Observation would require the researcher to live intimately with the participant and observe/participate in the process and experience. This is unlikely to be considered ethical, or consented to by participants, and is unlikely to be something a researcher would feel comfortable doing. Whilst it may have the potential to yield valuable data that is not filtered through the participant's perceptions and memory of events, the obstacles to using this method outweigh any possible advantages.

Participant observation might be possible and appropriate if the project changed its focus to look at the ways in which men engaged with medical professionals about the condition. A researcher could embed themselves in a clinic that could allow valuable data to be collected about the way clinicians and patients interact regarding this topic. This could then be used to develop and inform health care service delivery. To do this, one would have to first consider the ethical and practical implications of observing clinical interactions. Permission would have to be sought from both clinicians and patients. One would also have to consider the length of time one would need to spend in the field, and this would require research into the number of cases that present in a given time period.

Summary

- There are a range of qualitative data collection methods available, each with different strengths and weaknesses. Careful consideration should always be given to which method will best help you answer your particular research question(s).

- Your method for data analysis must always be considered alongside your choice of data collection method. Data collection and analysis cannot be treated as entirely distinct processes.

- All qualitative methods present significant challenges to even the most experienced researcher and require practice, skill, and constant reflection.

Questions for Discussion

1. For a study exploring why young mothers choose not to breastfeed, what practical and theoretical factors would need to be considered when deciding between using focus groups and face-to-face interviews?

2. If you were planning a participant observation study of neonatal intensive care units, what kind of difficulties/obstacles could you expect to encounter?

3. For each of the three methods outlined in the chapter, i.e. interviews, focus groups and participant observation, to what extent is it possible and/or desirable to ensure that you, as the researcher, do not influence the data that is being collected?

Further Reading

Cheal, D. (2005) *Dimensions of Sociological Theory*. New York: Palgrave Macmillan.

Crotty, M. (2009) *The Foundations of Social Research*. St Leonards: SAGE.

DeWalt, K. and DeWalt, B. (2011) *Participant Observation: A Guide for Fieldworkers*. Maryland: AltaMirra Press.

Holloway, I. (ed.) (2005) *Qualitative Research in Health Care*. Maidenhead: Open University Press.

Howell, K. (2013) *An Introduction to the Philosophy of Methodology*. London: SAGE.

Johnson, M. (1992) 'A silent conspiracy? Some ethical issues of participant observation in nursing research', *International Journal of Nursing Studies*, 29 (2): 213–23.

Krueger, R. and Casey, M. (1990) *Focus Groups: A Practical Guide for Applied Research*. London: SAGE.

Li, J. (2008) 'Ethical challenges in participant observation: a reflection on ethnographic fieldwork', *Qualitative Report*, 13 (1): 100–15.

Liamputtong, P. (2011) *Focus Group Methodology: Principles and Practice*. London: SAGE.

Silverman, D. (2004) *Doing Qualitative Research: A Practical Handbook*. Trowbridge: SAGE.

Taylor, M.C. (2005) 'Interviewing', in I. Holloway (ed.), *Qualitative Research in Health Care*. Maidenhead: Open University Press.

References

Allen, D. (2010) 'Fieldwork and participant observation', in I. Bourgeault, R. Dingwall and R. de Vries (eds), The *SAGE Handbook of Qualitative Methods in Health Research.* London: SAGE.

Bernard, H.R. (1988) *Research Methods in Cultural Anthropology.* Newbury Park, CA: SAGE.

Britten, N. (1995) 'Qualitative research: qualitative interviews in medical research', *British Medical Journal*, 311: 251–3.

Burgess, R. (ed.) (1982) *Field Research: A Sourcebook and Field Manual.* London: Allen & Unwin.

Dowswell, G., Ismail, T., Greenfield, S., Clifford, S., Hancock, B. and Wilson, S. (2011) 'Men's experience of erectile dysfunction after treatment for colorectal cancer: qualitative interview study', *British Medical Journal*, 343: d5824.

Drew, S.E., Duncan, R.E. and Sawyer, S.M. (2010) 'Visual storytelling: a beneficial but challenging method for health research with young people', *Qualitative Health Research*, 20: 1677–88.

Elliot, H. (1997) 'The use of diaries in sociological research on health experience', *Sociological Research Online*, 2(2).

Emmerson, R., Fretz, R. and Shaw, L. (2011) *Writing Ethnographic Fieldnotes* (2nd edn). Chicago: University of Chicago Press.

Frith, H. and Harcourt, D. (2007) 'Using photographs to capture women's experiences of chemotherapy: reflecting on the method', *Qualitative Health Research,* 17: 1340–50.

Hammersley, M. and Atkinson, P. (1995) *Ethnography: Principles in Practice.* London: Routledge.

Hanratty, B., Hibbert, D., Mair, F., May, C., Ward, C., Capewell, S., Litva, A. and Corcoran, G. (2002) 'Doctors' perceptions of palliative care for heart failure: focus group study', *British Medical Journal,* 325: 581.

Ives, J., Greenfield, S., Parry, J., Draper, H., Christine, G., Petts, J., Sorrel, T. and Wilson, S. (2009) 'Healthcare workers' attitudes to working during pandemic influenza: a qualitative study', *BMC Public Health*, 9: 56.

Jones, S. (1985) 'Depth interviewing', in R. Walker (ed.), *Applied Qualitative Research.* Aldershot: Gower.

Kitzinger, J. (2005) 'Focus group research', in I. Holloway (ed.), *Qualitative Research in Health Care.* Maidenhead: Open University Press.

Koch, T. (2006) 'Establishing rigour in qualitative research: the decision trail', *Journal of Advanced Nursing,* 53 (1): 91–103.

Krueger, R. and Casey, M. (2000) *Focus Groups: A Practical Guide for Applied Research* (3rd edn). London: SAGE.

Liamputtong, P. (2011) *Focus Group Methodology: Principles and Practice.* London: SAGE.

Marshall, P. and Koenig, B. (2010) 'Ethnographic methods', in J. Sugarman and D. Sulmasy (eds) *Methods in Medical Ethics.* Washington, DC: Georgetown University Press.

Morgan, D. (1997) *Focus Groups as Qualitative Research.* London: SAGE.

Novick, G. (2008) 'Is there a bias against telephone interviews in qualitative research?', *Research in Nursing and Health*, 31: 391–8.

Nyamathi, A. and Schuler, P. (1990) 'Focus group interview: a research technique for informed nursing practice', *Journal of Advanced Nursing,* 15: 1281–8.

Roulston, K., deMarrais, K. and Lewis, J. (2003) 'Learning to interview in the social sciences', *Qualitative Enquiry,* 9: 643–68.

Sandhu A., Ives J., Birchwood, M. and Upthegrove, R. (2013) 'The subjective experience and phenomenology of depression following first episode psychosis: a qualitative study using photo-elicitation', *Journal of Affective Disorders* (in press).

Schulze, B. and Angermeyer, M. (2003) 'Subjective experience of stigma: a focus group study of schizophrenic patients, their relatives and mental health professionals', *Social Science and Medicine*, 56 (2): 299–312.

Sharkey, S. and Larson, J. (2005) 'Ethnographic exploration: participation and meaning in everyday life', in I. Holloway (ed.), *Qualitative Research in Health Care*. Maidenhead: Open University Press.

Taylor, M.C. (2005) 'Interviewing', in I. Holloway (ed.), *Qualitative Research in Health Care*. Maidenhead: Open University Press.

Zimmerman, D. and Wieder, D. (1977) 'The diary: diary interview method', *Journal of Contemporary Ethnography*, 5 (4): 479–98.

8

MIXED METHODS

Doreen Tembo

- Understand what mixed methods are and when using them might be appropriate
- Know what the benefits and drawbacks with using mixed-methods are
- Be able to consider important factors when designing a mixed methods study, including prioritisation, pacing and points of interface
- To distinguish between dynamic approaches and typologies

Introduction

Mixed methods refers to adopting more than one method within a single research project. This could be through combining both qualitative and quantitative approaches to each stage of the project, for example, defining the research question, data collecting, etc. or different approaches at different stages of the project, for example, using a focus group followed by a structured survey. Therefore, it involves working with and analysing different types of data. Quantitative and qualitative methodologies have previously been presented as two distinct paradigms of enquiry routed in opposing theoretical traditions (Chapters 6 and 7). Because mixed methods build upon these two approaches, it is important that you have a prior awareness of both.

The core characteristics of mixed-methods research (based on Creswell and Plano Clark, 2011) are that it:

- collects and analyses persuasively and rigorously both qualitative and quantitative data;
- mixes, integrates or links the two forms of data, either by having one build on the other (sequential), or embedding one in the other (concurrent);
- can give priority to one form of data, or to both forms of data equally;
- combines the approaches into a specific research design, i.e. a mixed-method design, which determines the protocol for conducting the study.

Although this chapter adopts these core characteristics as the governing definition of mixed methods, other definitions for mixed methods exist. For example, while mixed methods commonly refers to the use of both quantitative and qualitative methods within the same study, some authors also consider the mixing of methods from the same paradigm as mixed methods, i.e. utilising more than one qualitative method within the same study, for example, focus group and observation; or more than one type of quantitative method in a study, for example, structured survey and objective outcome measurement (see Morse and Niehaus, 2009). However, the term multimethod, as defined by Tashakkori and Teddlie, (2003), rather than mixed methods, is often used by authors when the methods employed in a study originate from the same research paradigm (see Andrew and Halcomb, 2009; or Johnson et al., 2007).

Green (2007: 20) describes mixed methods as 'multiple ways of seeing and hearing multiple ways of making sense of the world'. Therefore, if employed appropriately, a mixed-methods approach can provide a better understanding to a research question than single approaches alone, and can offer validation for your results, a form of *triangulation* if you like, where the premise is that no single research method ever solves the problem of opposing explanations (Patton, 1999). Thus the weakness of one method is counterbalanced by the strength of the other (Hugentobler et al., 1992), such as a qualitative method adding depth and richness to the data obtained by a quantitative method. For example, in your trial of a new diet pill, your participants are not losing the weight that you hypothesised they would in the weekly weigh-ins, however you do not know why. Is it because the pill is truly not working, or is there a confounder, such as the participant not adhering to the recommended diet? This information could be ascertained through a series of interviews which would help you to determine any influencing factors.

When two methods are mixed, the validity criterion for judging the worth of inferences drawn from mixed-method research is referred to as 'legitimation' (Johnson and Onwuegbuzie, 2004). It is thus important to ensure legitimation is met in your study and that you ground your work in credible theory and background literature. Critical appraisal tools for mixed methods studies, such as the

TABLE 8.1　Reasons for carrying out mixed-methods designs (Bryman, 2012)

Triangulation or greater validity	Quantitative and qualitative research is combined to triangulate findings in order to be mutually corroborated.
Offset	Both quantitative and qualitative research methods have their own strengths and weaknesses so that combining them offsets their weaknesses and draws upon their strengths.
Completeness	A more comprehensive conclusion can be drawn if both quantitative and qualitative research methods are employed.
Process	Quantitative research provides an account of structures in social life, qualitative research provides a sense of process.
Different research question	Quantitative and qualitative research each answer different research questions.
Explanation	Each research method is used to explain findings generated by the other.
Unexpected results	Quantitative and qualitative research can be combined to understand surprising results.
Instrument development	Qualitative research is used to develop questionnaire and scale items.
Sampling	One approach is used to facilitate the sampling of participants.
Credibility	Employing both approaches enhances the integrity of the findings.
Context	The qualitative research provides contextual understanding coupled with generalisable, externally valid findings uncovered through a survey.
Illustration	Using qualitative data to illustrate quantitative findings.
Improving the usefulness of findings	Combining the two approaches will be more useful to practitioners and others.
Confirm and discover	Using qualitative data to generate hypothesis and using quantitative research to test them within a single project.
Diversity of views	Uncovering relationships between variables through quantitative research while revealing associated meanings from participants through qualitative research.
Building upon quantitative/qualitative findings	Making more of either quantitative or qualitative findings.

Health Care Practice R&D Unit's evaluation tool for mixed-methods studies (Long et al., 2002), or Tashakkori and Teddlie's evaluation criteria framework (2003) can assist you in assessing the quality of mixed-methods research. One thing to consider about any piece of mixed-methods research, however, is whether there is a clear rationale for carrying out a mixed-method study as opposed to using just a single method, as they tend to be more resource intensive in terms of research funds and time. Table 8.1 presents the main reasons that researchers give for carrying out mixed-methods studies.

When to use a mixed-method design

As with all research, choosing the appropriate method is top down and led by the question you wish to answer with your project (please see Chapter 1: 'Asking the Right Question'). Questions that address different social levels may require the use of different methods for each of the levels studied, i.e. micro (individual, partner and family) may require qualitative methods, whilst meso (community) and macro (policy) would probably require quantitative methods due to the sheer size of the population. Therefore your research question will determine whether more than one method is required to comprehensively answer all aspects posed by it. Such research questions tend to be complex in nature and may often seek to both explain and understand the phenomena being studied (please see the case study).

Case study

Stewart et al. (2008) used mixed methods in a project which looked at reducing health inequalities by examining the impact of socioeconomic status on social exclusion and its relationship to health from the perspectives of both low- and high-income participants. They used a sequential mixed-method design in three phases, a qualitative project, followed by a quantitative project, concluding in another qualitative project. The qualitative method chosen for phase I were interviews which ascertained the key features of social exclusion which were influenced by the participant's socioeconomic status, and how these factors related to their health. Responses from these interviews were then used to develop a survey (quantitative phase II). After phase II was complete, the survey data were used to develop questions for two focus groups consisting of policy-makers to discuss the findings from phases I and II (qualitative phase III).

They found that the qualitative and quantitative data corroborated each other and showed the same pattern of the effect of socioeconomic status on social exclusion and health. The qualitative data added richness and understanding to the quantitative findings, such as feeling like you were included in society giving a sense of emotional, social and physical well-being. In turn, the quantitative data helped to generalise their findings to a wider population of vulnerable people.

Conducting a mixed-methods study

Once it has been established that mixed methods are required to fully address a research question, it is essential that the right research team is assembled. As methods are used from different paradigms, each requiring their own form of analysis, expertise is needed in the team to ensure there is rigour throughout the project regardless of which method is being employed, i.e. one member with qualitative and another with quantitative expertise. If you are conducting your mixed-methods project alone, either due to it being a dissertation, or unfunded, see if you can access some qualitative and quantitative methodology training. Once you have the appropriate expertise for the project, the next stage is designing the research.

Types of mixed-methods designs

Sometimes all components have equal weight, or importance, regardless of whether they are quantitative or qualitative, as would be the case for triangulation. However, sometimes a secondary method is utilised that does not directly relate to answering the research question *per se*, but rather adds detail or information, such as utilising a second method to enhance a certain part of the study. In such cases, the secondary method is referred to as being *embedded* or *nested* in the primary method. For example, if you were carrying out a quantitative project to look at learning a new task, although your main outcome is the length of time to learn the task (quantitative), you may also want to make field notes through observations (such as noting any off-task behaviour) which will add understanding to your overall results, and thus enabling you to refine the task or the instructions related to learning the task. Or it may be that your study is predominantly a qualitative study with a nested quantitative study. For example, you may be interviewing participants about the acceptability and usefulness of a new intervention to stop smoking. Your main study is a series of interviews; however you may also wish to collect carbon monoxide readings at the same time. An embedded design is particularly useful when you have limited time or resources (please see Figure 8.1 for an illustration in which the capital letters denote the primary research method, whilst lower case letters denote the secondary method).

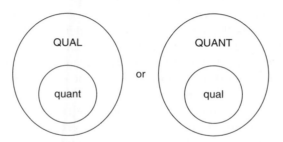

FIGURE 8.1   Concurrent nested study design

As you may be able to tell, there are various permutations in regards to whether one method has dominance, and whether you use the methods concurrently or sequentially, and if sequential, which method you use first. In sequential studies the analysis of the first, primary method is conducted to inform the secondary method of data collection, which differentiates it from the nested designs where data are collected concurrently and analysed at the end. Your research question will determine whether a project is predominantly quantitatively or qualitatively driven or whether there is an equal focus on both methods.

When choosing your research design, guidance can be taken regarding which design may be appropriate from similar previous studies, i.e. a typology-based approach, which you will have identified through your literature search (please see Chapter 2: 'Finding the Evidence to Support your Research Question') or you might decide to develop a design unique to your project, i.e. a dynamic approach.

Dynamic approaches

To help organise the different methods used, it is useful to distinguish the different components of research which make up the project (see Morse and Niehaus, 2009). The components may be qualitative or quantitative and will include all of the steps from posing the question the component will answer, through to collecting and analysing the data and ultimately interpreting results according to the paradigm of that component. Once you have distinguished which different components your research project requires to fulfil its objectives, you then need to prioritise them.

Prioritisation (or weighting) will be given to the component that is best suited to answering the primary part of the research question, i.e. the *core component*. The components that answer secondary questions are the *supplemental components* (see Creswell and Plano Clark, 2011: 65). Where a quantitative method is a core component and qualitative method is the supplementary component, the design is called a *quantitative priority design* (such as in the previous diet pill example). Where the opposite is true, i.e. the core component is a qualitative method and the supplementary component is a quantitative method, this is called a *qualitative priority design* (such as the previous smoking example). The focus of the project therefore primarily centres on the core component and the supplementary component cannot stand alone as a separate project (Morse and Niehaus, 2009). The results from the supplemental component should always add strength to the narrative of the findings from the core component. When equal weight is given to both qualitative and quantitative components this design is called an *equal priority design*. While equal priority studies do exist, in a project usually one method will implicitly or explicitly be the core component while the other will be the supplementary component.

Once you have determined the prioritisation of the components you also need to think about the *pacing,* i.e. the timing of implementation, of the components. If your methods are being conducted concurrently, both the core and supplementary components will be carried out at the same time in the project, i.e. a nested design, as discussed earlier. Concurrent designs are best suited when your project has a broad research question, includes complex concepts or different participant populations, or has variables with different attributes or measurements (Morse and Niehaus, 2009). However, you may have sequential pacing in your project where the supplementary component is carried out before, or after, the core component, although some authors feel that, in sequential designs, the supplementary component should always follow the core component (Morse and Niehaus, 2009). In practice, however, many studies have a supplementary component that precedes the core component, such as using data from focus groups to inform the design of an intervention which is then tested for efficacy using a quantitative design. Sequential designs are either planned at the proposal stage or develop when it becomes evident that a need exists to address questions that have arisen during the project which require a different research method to answer them, i.e. an *emergent mixed-method design*. Emergent designs may delay the study if ethical approval or clearance from the funding body/ host organisation is required to run the additional component.

The last issue to consider when designing your mixed-methods project is determining the *interface*, i.e. the approach used to mix the results from the components, and the point at which this happens, i.e. the *point of interface* (Morse and Niehaus, 2009). The point of interface can take place at either an *interactive level*, i.e. the two components are interfaced before the final stage of interpretation, or an *independent level*, i.e. the components are kept separate until inferences are determined at the end of the study (Creswell and Plano Clark, 2011). If you intend to interface the components before the end of the study, perhaps to ensure that you do not require another supplemental component, there are three time points where interface can occur. These are: (i) design, for example, using the results from qualitative interviews and a quantitative objective outcome measure together to develop an intervention; (ii) data collection, for example, the earlier example regarding smoking, using interviews together with objective carbon monoxide readings; and (iii) data analysis, where the two components are merged by combining the two data sets and analysing the results of the combined data set. However, since the two methods yield different types of data, the supplemental component's data will need to be transformed into data that can be analysed by the analysis methods used for the core method. For example, if your core component was quantitative, the qualitative data set should be transposed into numeric variables that can then be merged with the quantitative data set, or you might choose to identify common content in both components and then compare, contrast or summarise this in a table or discussion.

Case study

As mentioned earlier, Stewart et al.'s (2008) sequential designed project had the objective of reducing health inequalities. To do this they conducted a mixed-methods study with a dynamic approach, in that it had a research design unique to that project. Phase I at the beginning of the study was a supplemental component using

(Continued)

(Continued)

qualitative methodology and consisted of a series of in-depth interviews. The data obtained from these interviews then informed the next supplementary component (phase II) which consisted of a quantitative survey consisting of items defined by the interviews. The results from these two phases were then used to inform the final, core component, which used another qualitative method, i.e. focus groups with policy-makers. Therefore this study was a qualitative priority design with interactive levels of interface. Their point of interface was at the design stage in that the data they obtained from the supplementary components informed the core component in phase III, i.e. qual→quant→QUAL.

Typology approach

You may prefer to use an existing typology which will already have predetermined prioritisations, pacing and interfaces however. Typologies are useful because they inform your research design so that you know how to conduct your study, and are especially useful if you have not conducted a mixed-methods project before (Tashakkori and Teddlie, 2003). The following examples are adapted from Creswell and Plano Clark (2011) however there are others, and you may find one more suitable for your own project via your literature search.

Explanatory sequential designs (QUANT → qual)   Here the quantitative core component is followed up by a supplementary qualitative component. This design is normally used when a qualitative component is being used to help interpret or contextualise the results of the earlier quantitative core component (please see Figure 8.2). The qualitative sample is normally identified from the quantitative sample to enable comparability. However choosing a qualitative sample from an already randomly selected quantitative sample may undermine its validity, because the participants approached for the qualitative data collection may not necessarily represent the target population. The interpretation/reporting of this type of study should summarise the results from both components and discuss how the qualitative component helped to explain the quantitative results.

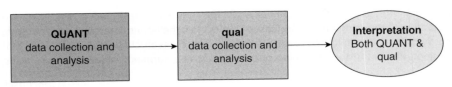

FIGURE 8.2   Explanatory sequential design (QUANT → qual)

Abidso et al. (2012) carried out an evaluation of a weight management programme first using a quantitative core component which consisted of the number of participants who completed the programme, the mean percentage weight loss and psychosocial measures. From the quantitative sample, they recruited people who were programme drop outs or completers for the following qualitative supplemental component which consisted of interviews. They also further broke down the sample of completers into those who had lost a lot of weight, and those who had not. This explanatory sequential design enabled them to not only assess the efficacy of the weight management programme, but to also explore the reasons why some people completed the course and some did not, and of those who did complete the course, why some people lost more weight than others. Therefore the added qualitative data were useful to further develop the programme.

Exploratory sequential designs (QUAL➔ quant) This design is when a qualitative core component precedes a supplementary quantitative component. The supplementary quantitative component can be used to generalise the exploratory findings from the qualitative core component to a larger, representative sample, or for the qualitative outcomes to be further tested and verified (please see Figure 8.3). When sampling for the quantitative component, the randomly selected sample should be from a group that is equivalent to the qualitative sample (see Morse and Niehaus, 2009). The interpretation or summarising of the results should report how the quantitative findings build on the qualitative findings.

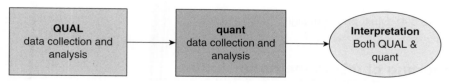

FIGURE 8.3   Exploratory sequential design (QUAL ➔ quant)

Plano Stoller et al. (2009) used an exploratory sequential design to investigate alcohol consumption decisions among non-abusing drinkers diagnosed with hepatitis C. The core qualitative component consisted of data generated from semi-structured interviews, electronic illness narratives, and internet-based discussions which enabled them to identify decision factors about drinking alcohol in this population. These decision factors were then used to design a survey, the supplementary quantitative component. The results from this survey then served to estimate the prevalence of drinking in this population, and the association of drinking behaviour with the decision factors as identified through the qualitative component.

Multiphase design

In most mixed-methods research each individual component will be answering a part of an overall research question. However, sometimes, the typology is guided by an overall programme of research which is composed of smaller individual studies with their own specific research questions, all evolving to answer the larger programme objective. This sequence of studies often mirrors the sequence that one might see in a basic mixed-method design, in that there is a research question for each of the studies, which builds upon the knowledge gained from earlier completed studies, but also contributes to the overall objective of the research program (Cresswell and Plano Clark, 2011). The results from each study can be published as each one in the programme comes to an end. It is only after the final study is complete, however, that the researcher can utilise mixed-method reporting to draw all of the programme data from all of the individual studies into one interpretation and discussion. The programme's objectives will determine the study designs used, including whether the studies within the programme are sequential or concurrent, and qualitative or quantitative. These programmes of research tend be large, funded studies which take place over many years (please see Figure 8.4).

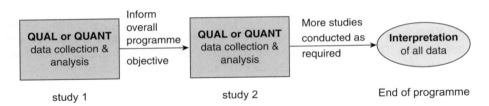

FIGURE 8.4   Multi-phase design

Reporting of mixed-methods studies

The final write-up will vary according the type of research design employed. However, in addition to following the normal procedures for writing up your findings, it is good practice to include the following things in your report:

- Include mixed methods as a keyword to enable others to find your work easily
- Name of the typology used (if applicable)
- Discuss the prioritisation, pacing, levels of interaction and points of interface
- Justify your choice of the research design
- For validation, provide reference to others that have used the same design
- Include a discussion on what was learned or achieved by using the mixed-methods approach you chose
- Limitations of your mixed-methods approach should be clearly outlined

Summary

- Ensure that your research question is one that merits a mixed-methods approach, with justification for each additional method used.
- The research question will determine the core method and supplementary methods.
- Ensure that each component has theoretical and methodological rigour.
- Give pacing of the components careful consideration.
- The analytical method of the core component will govern the analysis after interface.
- Results should report both the core and supplementary components. Supplementary findings should complement the findings from the core component and limitations should always be discussed.

Questions for discussion

1. Using a topic that you would like to study, identify and provide a justification for a research question that would merit the use of mixed methods.
2. Using your question developed in question 1, design a research project detailing prioritisation, pacing, the level of interaction and the point of interface, using either a dynamic or typology-based approach. Justify your choices along the way.
3. What do you perceive to be the advantages and disadvantages of your chosen design?

Further Reading

Bryman, A. (2012) *Social Research Methods* (4th edn). Oxford: Oxford University Press.

Creswell, J.W. and Plano Clark, V.L. (2011) *Designing and Conducting Mixed Methods Research* (2nd edn). Thousand Oaks, CA: SAGE.

Morse, J.M. and Niehaus, L. (2009) *Mixed Method Design: Principles and Procedures*. Walnut Creek, CA: Left Coast Press.

Saks, M. and Allsop, J. (2007) *Researching Health: Qualitative, Quantitative and Mixed Methods*. London: SAGE.

Tashakkori , A. and Teddlie, C. (eds) (2010) *Handbook of Mixed Methods in Social and Behavioural Research* (2nd edn). Thousand Oaks, CA: SAGE.

Teddlie, C., and Tashakkori A. (2009) *Foundations of Mixed Methods Research: Integrating Quantitative and Qualitative Approaches in the Social and Behavioural Sciences*. Thousand Oaks, CA: SAGE.

For developments in mixed-methods research see: *Journal of Mixed Methods Research*.

References

Abildso, C., Zizzi, S., Gilleland, D., Thomas, J. and Bonner, D. (2012) 'A mixed methods evaluation of a 12-week insurance-sponsored weight management program incorporating cognitive-behavioral counseling', *Journal of Mixed Methods Research*, 4 (4) 278–94.

Andrew, S. and Halcomb, E.J. (2009) *Introduction to Mixed Methods Research for Nursing and the Health Sciences*. Chichester, West Sussex: Blackwell.

Beck, C.T. and Gable, R.K. (2012) 'A mixed methods study of secondary traumatic stress in labor and delivery nurses', *Journal of Obstetric, Gynecologic, and Neonatal Nursing*, 41 (6): 747–60.

Branigan, E. (2003) 'But how can you prove it? Issues of rigour in action research', *Journal of the Home Economics Institute of Australia*, 10 (3): 37–8.

Bryman, A. (2012) *Social Research Methods* (4th edn). Oxford: Oxford University Press.

Creswell, J.W. and Plano Clark, V.L. (2011) *Designing and Conducting Mixed Methods Research* (2nd edn). Thousand Oaks, CA: SAGE.

Greene, J. C. (2007) *Mixed Methods in Social Inquiry*. San Francisco: Jossey-Bass.

Hesse-Biber, S. N. (2010) *Mixed Methods Research: Merging Theory with Practice*. New York: Guilford Press.

Hugentobler, M.K., Israel, B.A. and Schurman, S.J. (1992) 'An action research approach to workplace health: integrating methods', *Health, Education and Behavior*, 19 (1): 55–76.

Johnson, R.B. and Onwuegbuzie, A.J. (2004) 'Mixed methods research: a research paradigm whose time has come', *Educational Researcher*, 33 (7): 14–26.

Johnson, R.B., Onwuegbuzie, A.J. and Turner, L.A. (2007) 'Toward a definition of mixed methods research', *Journal of Mixed Methods Research*, 1 (2): 112–33.

Long, A.F., Godfrey, M., Randall, T., Brettle, A. and Grant, M.J. (2002) *HCPRDU Evaluation Tool for Mixed Methods Studies*. Leeds: University of Leeds, Nuffield Institute for Health: http://usir.salford.ac.uk/13070 (accessed Oct. 2012).

Morse, J.M. and Niehaus, L. (2009) *Mixed Method Design: Principles and Procedures*. Walnut Creek, CA: Left Coast Press.

Patton, M.Q. (1999) 'Enhancing the quality and credibility of qualitative analysis', *Health Services Research*, 34 (511): 1189–208.

Plano Stoller, E.P., Webster, N.J., Blixen, C.E., McCormick, R.A., Hund, A.J., Perzynski, A.T., Kanuch, S.W., Thomas, C.L., Kercher, K. and Dawson, N.V. (2009) 'Alcohol consumption decisions among nonabusing drinkers diagnosed with Hepatitis C: an exploratory sequential mixed methods study', *Journal of Mixed Methods Research*, 3 (1): 65–86.

Stewart, M., Makwarimba, E., Barnfather, A., Letourneau, N. and Neufeld, A. (2008) 'Researching reducing health disparities: mixed-methods approaches', *Social Science and Medicine*, 66 (6): 1406–17.

Tashakkori, A. and Teddlie, C. (2003) *Handbook of Mixed Methods in Social and Behavioral Research*. Thousand Oaks, CA: SAGE.

Teddlie, C. and Tashakkori A. (2009) *Foundations of Mixed Methods Research: Integrating Quantitative and Qualitative Approaches in the Social and Behavioural Sciences*. Thousand Oaks, CA: SAGE.

Part III

SPECIFIC METHODOLOGIES

9

HEALTH ECONOMICS

Matthew Jones and Casey Quinn

Learning Objectives

- To understand the importance of health economics, and the principles and methods of cost-effectiveness analysis
- To be aware of issues relating to the design and conduct of studies to support economic analysis
- To know how to select and measure appropriate health outcomes, resource use and cost data

Introduction

Expenditure on the health care sector is massive. In 2006, total spending on health care in the UK was £120bn, which represents 9.4% of the UK's gross domestic product (GDP) (Griffin, 2007). GDP is the market value of all products of a country, both goods and services, within a given period of time (usually a year), and is often used as an indicator of the country's standard of living. Health care expenditure is therefore a major consideration for government, as it is inextricably linked with the overall economic well-being of a country and its population, which is ultimately its workforce. Health economics emerged as a methodology due to a paper by Arrow in 1963, and has been developing in validity as a method, and in its importance to health service providers and policy-makers ever since. Health economics involves the use and development of economic methods in order to study the consumption of health care in relation to the population's health, illness and recovery. Health economics provides a framework in which we can assess how health care provision is associated with quality of life, and can help determine solutions to economic problems in health care (Morris et al., 2007). It also helps health care providers make informed decisions about how health care is funded, provided and distributed, with the ultimate aim of achieving the optimum allocation of resources, based upon the fact that resources to pay for health services are finite and constrained. This reflects the so-called economic problem: our wants and desires are limitless, but the resources to satisfy them are finite. Therefore, every choice and action comes with an opportunity cost, i.e. the loss of the next-most-preferred action. By paying for one thing you cannot pay for something else (Palmer and Raftery, 1999). For example, the National Institute for Health and Clinical Excellence (NICE) published a guideline on fertility treatment which recommended up to three cycles of *in vitro* fertilisation (IVF) (2004); although they did not recommend a drug for the treatment of bowel cancer (NICE, 2010). The media latched onto this fact with outrage. However, upon closer inspection, the bowel cancer drug is expensive – around £20,800 per patient to treat, with no significant benefits in either disease-free survival, or overall survival when compared with patients receiving standard chemotherapy and placebo (Allegra et al., 2012), whilst IVF is providing a future workforce.

Health, however, is not only a consumption good of which patients are the consumers, it is also an investment good, whereby providing health care can reduce work absenteeism or reduce the overall reliance on welfare in a country (Grossman, 1972). Therefore health economists need to balance cost against benefit and do so at both a macro level (large scale, economy as a whole) and a micro level (individual organisations, communities, etc.) In the previous example, investing in drugs to treat cancer can require an assessment on the macro level – overall budget impact of providing the new drug, wider societal benefit through reduced reliance on both formal and informal care and, potentially, increased economic output from patients returning to work – as well as the micro level which would include increased longevity and/or improved health-related quality of life, reduced out of pocket expenses for the patient and their family, etc.

> ## ⌐ Case study ⌐
>
> The government has approved for use a new drug (Treatinib) for colorectal cancer. Prof. Jones, chief executive of a health care organisation, realises that the cost of funding this drug for the eligible patients in her organisation is going to be about £1m per year. Prof. Jones's organisation does not have spare budget for prescribing Treatinib next year, but has £1m allocated to restore a local respite care centre that has been closed. In order to fund the use of Treatinib, the respite care centre would have to remain closed. Therefore to gain the benefits of treatment with Treatinib, Prof. Jones is going to lose the opportunity to gain the benefits that the respite care centre would have delivered, i.e. the opportunity cost. Prof. Jones's organisation has standing financial instructions that legally prevent them from incurring debt. Therefore, she has no choice in this matter: one beneficial use of the £1m must be sacrificed for the other – but which one? Treatinib may improve the lives of patients with colorectal cancer, and may even be effective enough for them to become well enough to rejoin the workforce. However, the welfare of the informal carers who will benefit from the respite care centre's support is also extremely important. Prof. Jones is aware that, from the 2001 census, 12% of the adult population in the UK were identified as carers, making an economic contribution of £119 billion per year (Carers UK, 2011). Therefore, there may be a direct economic gain from supporting them.

Economic evaluation

A useful tool for weighing the costs and benefits of a treatment or intervention is economic evaluation, which calculates true cost and benefit differences between alternatives, usually, a new intervention compared to current best practice. This is done by ignoring the costs and benefits that are the same between the alternatives, and only looking at the differences. For example, in the above case study, suppose Prof. Jones discovers that, although Treatinib is currently an intravenous drug, within the next six months there will be the alternative of buying it in tablet form. In this instance, if you were to conduct an economic analysis to compare the two methods of administration of Treatinib, although the benefits might remain the same between the alternatives, the cost will vary, as there will not only be the cost of the injecting paraphernalia with which to administer the intravenous drug, but there will also be the time of the health service professional who is injecting the patient, not to mention the patient taking time off work, driving to the doctor's surgery, etc.

Therefore economic evaluation helps us to make an informed decision about which option represents the 'best value for money' – remembering that 'best' will not always simply mean the 'most' value for money. In the case study, upon reading, Prof. Jones discovers that there is only a significant improvement in patients who are below the age of 50, and only for the first year of treatment with Treatinib, after which effectiveness tails off. Therefore the 'most value for money' could be to treat anyone indefinitely with colorectal cancer regardless of age with Treatinib

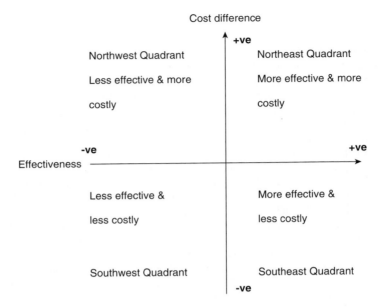

FIGURE 9.1   The cost-effectiveness plane

as there are benefits, just not significant ones. However the 'best value for money' would be to treat only patients 50 years of age or younger, for up to one year. Therefore economic evaluation's purpose is not to *make* the decision, but rather inform the decision-maker with the best possible information on which to base their decision. It is not always necessary to conduct an economic analysis, however. Sometimes it is clear that the treatment that is current best practice will dominate over new treatments, or that new treatments may dominate over current best practice.

A cost-effectiveness plane can be seen in Figure 9.1, with the horizontal axis dividing the plane according to the incremental effect (negative to the left and positive to the right), whereas the vertical axis divides the plane according to incremental cost (positive above, negative below). Therefore the plane is divided into four quadrants in which one can enter data regarding the costs and benefits of treatment A (the new intervention) compared to treatment B (current best practice).

Once all of the data points for treatment A have been plotted, it may become apparent that most of the data points fall into one of the quadrants. If they were clustered in the northwest quadrant this would mean that, for treatment A, the costs are high (as they are above the horizontal line) whilst the effects are low (as they are to the left of the vertical line) so treatment A is worse than treatment B in terms of both cost and benefit and therefore the new intervention should be excluded and current best practice maintained. If the cluster of data points falls in the southeast quadrant however, it is suggesting that treatment A is more effective and cheaper than treatment B and so should be implemented. These two quadrants show dominance of one treatment over the other and no analysis is required in these cases. If the data cluster were in one of the other two quadrants however, dominance is not clear as there is a trade-off between effectiveness and cost, with the northeast quadrant showing that the new intervention is more effective, but also more costly than current best practice, and the southwest quadrant showing that the new intervention is less effective than current best practice, but it is also less costly. In these instances an economic analysis will be required to determine: (i) whether the greater effectiveness is worth the greater cost (northeast quadrant); or (ii) whether the cost-savings are worth the loss of effectiveness (southwest quadrant).

There are three main subtypes of economic analysis to consider (Drummond et al., 2005).

Cost-benefit analysis (CBA)

This is the broadest form of economic analysis, as a given intervention can be compared easily with any other intervention – even across other sectors besides health care, such as when deciding whether to build a school, a hospital or a bridge. This is because both costs and outcomes are monetary measures and the analysis is based upon the comparison of the total of each inventory, i.e. all costs and benefits associated with one option are compared to those of another. However, calculating complete inventories of costs and benefits for all options is difficult. CBA also demands that outcomes are monetary, which poses technical, and often ethical and philosophical, challenges, such as assigning a monetary cost to human life.

Cost-effectiveness analysis (CEA)

Cost-effectiveness analysis is a method by which we can compare the cost of an intervention, relative to its effectiveness, against the cost and effectiveness of one or more alternative interventions. This is the most common form of economic evaluation. Costs are measured in monetary terms, but effectiveness is measured most often by a single natural unit, for example, bed-days, heart attacks avoided, life-years gained, etc. You can then calculate how much more costs you need for an improvement in effects.

The results are straightforward to interpret, but are not open to comparison with other CEAs because the outcome is incremental cost per outcome, and when the outcomes vary, comparison is impossible. This means that their costs must be measured consistently, and must reflect the same resource use from the same perspective. For example, the health service perspective which is most common (Johannesson, 1995) may choose to ignore National Institute for Care and Health Excellence (NICE) guidelines in the UK which advocate talking therapies for a variety of mental health conditions such as depression, in favour of cheaper options such as prescribing antidepressants, which may also have quicker effects in order for the patient to rejoin the workforce. This perspective may oppose the societal perspective which has society's welfare at heart and which, in this example, might give preference to talking therapies.

Perspective is also important in studies in which costs are not directly comparable. Talking therapies and antidepressants are comparable as they are treating the same thing and therefore the differences are incremental and costs can be those associated with items that are applicable to both, for example, cost of intervention, patient days off work, hospital admissions, etc. However in the case study, the two options are so different that the costs may not necessarily be comparable – days off work for carers versus increased life-years for patients with colorectal cancer. Thus, there needs to be a different type of analysis which instead of using a 'natural unit' uses an outcome that is generic enough to be applicable to a wide variety of clinical settings.

Cost-utility analysis (CUA)

In a cost-utility analysis, costs are measured in monetary terms but outcomes are utility-based, typically a combination of time and utility, i.e. patient satisfaction or preference, such as quality-adjusted life-years (QALYs) (Fanshel and Bush, 1970; Torrance and Feeny, 1989) or disability-adjusted life-years (DALYs) (Murray, 1994). Generic outcomes such as these encompass morbidity and mortality, and allow the comparison with other economic evaluations across the health care sector. Therefore this is one of the most used analysis types in health economics.

Quality-adjusted life-years

The quality-adjusted life-year (QALY) is a measure commonly used in health economics and is recommended by NICE (2013). QALYs not only takes into consideration the quantity of life lived, but also the quality, as it collects data on a large number of health-related factors such as mobility, pain and mood. QALYs calculate how many years and months of life are added by an intervention, and the quality of that life ranging from negative values below 0 (worst possible health) to 1 (the best possible health), whilst 0 is dead. Because the QALY collects data on so many health-related factors, it is generic enough to be used widely, and so disparate interventions can compared. There are a variety of validated scales with which to collect data suitable for calculating QALYs, such as the commonly used Short Form (36) Health Survey (SF-36) (Brazier et al., 2002).

Cost-effectiveness is ascertained by determining first, the incremental increase in life-years a given treatment will create; then, determining the health state(s) in which those life-years will be spent and the quality weight to give to those health states. Finally, the life-years are weighted accordingly to determined the incremental gain (or loss) in quality-adjusted life-years. Cost-effectiveness is then considered in terms of incremental cost per QALY.

Case study

A trial is being conducted to ascertain the efficacy of two medications to treat the human immunodeficiency virus (HIV), one of which is currently being prescribed. Alongside efficacy data, researchers collect data using the SF-36 in order to calculate QALYs so that they can conduct an economic evaluation. They discover that, if a patient continues receiving usual care, s/he will live for one year of extra life with a quality of life of 0.4 (0 is worst health and 1 is perfect health). If the patient receives the new medication s/he will live for 1.25 years of extra life with a quality of life of 0.6. In order to compare the medications the researchers calculate the QALY:

- Usual care: 1 (a year of extra life) × 0.4 (quality of life) = 0.4 QALY
- New medication: 1.25 (1 year, 3 months of extra life) × 0.6 (quality of life) = 0.75 QALY

By subtracting the QALY of the medication currently being subscribed from the new treatment QALY, i.e. 0.75 – 0.4 = 0.35, one determines the additional QALYs achieved per patient with the new treatment is 0.35.

Incremental cost-effectiveness

The primary outcome of an economic analysis will usually be a single statistic that captures the incremental costs and outcomes for one treatment compared to another. In health economics this is almost universally the incremental cost-effectiveness ratio (ICER) (Drummond et al., 2005). The ICER is defined as:

$$\text{ICER} = \frac{\text{Cost}_{\text{Treatment B}} - \text{Cost}_{\text{Treatment A}}}{\text{Outcome}_{\text{Treatment B}} - \text{Outcome}_{\text{Treatment A}}}$$

The ICER summarises the incremental difference in costs as a ratio of the incremental difference in outcomes. If this is above a pre-specified willingness to pay for those outcomes (established in the UK by NICE), the treatment will not be accepted. In the case study, the new treatment for HIV is £10,000, whilst the usual care is cheaper at £3,000, i.e. a difference of £7,000. Therefore to calculate the cost per QALY, this difference in costs is divided by the QALYs gained, i.e. £7,000 ÷ 0.35 = £20,000 per QALY. As a rule of thumb, a new drug with an ICER of below £20,000 per QALY should, in most circumstances, be approved. On the other hand, a new drug with an ICER of say £50,000 per QALY would almost certainly not be accepted (Devlin and Parkin, 2004), although implementation depends the decision-maker's willingness to pay, *and* on their willingness to accept the validity and robustness of the summary measure given. For example, an ICER of £33,000 per QALY with a high degree of uncertainty could mean rejection, while an ICER of £35,000 per QALY, but with a low degree of uncertainty, could be acceptable.

Measuring costs

When conducting cost-effectiveness analysis, 'costs' compared with 'effectiveness' are relatively more straightforward conceptually. Ideally, a research study would collect all resource use data which might differ between two treatment options. In reality however, some data are impractical to collect in detail, such as how many minutes are spent by different clinical staff following one method for stroke rehabilitation compared with another. This can result in a lack of robustness and generalisability of trial data and the results of incremental economic analyses which, in turn, limit the usefulness of these data and analyses for health care decision-making.

When costs are difficult to capture they may be determined instead via an economic model. However, models are based upon assumptions as well as data, and therefore modelling introduces more uncertainty into the data and analysis.

Regardless of whether intended analyses are of trial data only, or will incorporate economic models, there should exist a well-thought-out plan to ensure that all relevant costs (and outcomes) are included in the analysis. This may include primary as well as secondary data and analysis, and some assumptions. A taxonomy of these costs can be summarised as follows (Elliott and Payne, 2005).

Direct costs

These are the treatment costs directly associated with the disease or condition: (i) background treatment costs, for example, visits to a physician, blood tests, etc.; (ii) costs associated with the new intervention, for example, acquisition costs for a new drug, theatre time, labour costs, material costs for a new surgical procedure, etc.; and (iii) costs associated with the comparators. Focus on direct costs is usually associated with a health service provider perspective.

Indirect costs

These are only indirectly related to the illness or treatment, and usually fall outside of the perspective of the health care sector, but are considered within a societal perspective, for example, time off work due to illness or due to the treatment (attendance at clinics, adverse events), reduced productivity while at work, etc. They can be limited in scope to a patient and their family or carer(s), or broader in scope to include wider societal benefits.

Intangible costs

Intangible costs cannot be quantified or measured objectively, as they are factors that are not naturally monetary, but which do affect the patient (or their carers/ family members) directly, such as loss of quality of life (reduced QALYs), anxiety, pain, loss of function or capability. Which of these costs are collected during a study can depend on several considerations:

- The perspective of the analysis: to whom might the new intervention be cost-effective? Is it the provider only, the provider plus the patient, or society at large?

- The study: what resources are available for collecting very detailed resource utilisation?

- The treatment setting: how feasible is the relatively more labour-intensive micro-costing approach in which all resources used, e.g. surgical instruments, individual staff time, etc., are tracked and measured, multiplied by their unit costs and summed up at the end?

- The patients: does their health, frailty, expected survival, and so on, have an impact on what costs are relevant, e.g. long-terms costs, work absenteeism, etc.? Also what about the costs of managing adverse events or co-morbidities?

Careful consideration must be given to what costs are going to be relevant, and these may vary. Submissions to NICE, for example, typically have focused only on NHS and social services costs, i.e. the provider perspective, even when costs related to work absenteeism may be important (NICE, 2013). Alternatively, the same research funded by for example, Arthritis Research UK, would include work absenteeism, i.e. patient perspective, as this better reflects the experience of patients with arthritis.

Measuring outcomes

The measurement of outcomes is a more complicated problem than costs. While costs are essentially monetary, outcomes are often not. The type of analysis you intend to use will dictate the type of outcome data you collect. Outcome measures can be general, such as cases diagnosed or avoided if your purpose was to evaluate a screening programme together with the resulting lives saved or extended due to the programme. Alternatively, they can be clinical measures, for example, weight, cholesterol levels, etc. Clinical measurement data is often already being collected to calculate efficacy of the treatment. Not only the type of analysis but also the perspective taken will determine which type of outcome is relevant. In turn, the outcome chosen will dictate the extent to which direct, indirect and intangible costs are considered. In the UK, most publicly funded cost-effectiveness analysis, or economic modelling to support reimbursement by NICE, will need to include QALYs (NICE, 2013). For NICE this will mean including in the study an instrument that generates QALYs, such as the EQ-5D (EuroQol, 2012) or the SF-36 (Brazier et al., 2002).

Your study might not include a generic QALY generating instrument, but might instead include instruments that map onto these. In oncology, the EORTC QLQ-C30 and FACIT measures are often used (EORTC, 2012; FACIT.org, 2012). These instruments have the advantage of also containing symptom subscales. Health care providers may also demand some patient-reported outcomes measures to be used (Department of Health, 2009), which are broader instruments that better capture the functioning or capabilities of patients, such as the non-utility health-related quality of life (HRQol), or a symptom subscale from the EORTC or FACIT instruments which measures fatigue, pain, cognitive impairment, satisfaction and many more domains of quality of life.

Some careful, prior research should be conducted before an outcome measure, or instrument, is selected. This is to ensure that you take into consideration what the patients and payers most care about, what symptoms or adverse events of treatment are most prevalent, severe, etc. In general, thought must be given to symptoms, functioning, health status and health perception.

Discounting

Discounting is used to translate past and future costs or benefits into today's value (or value for any other indexed date), as studies often consider costs and outcomes for a period of more than one year. For example, a mammogram screening programme incurs costs at the time of the procedure. However, the benefits are fewer deaths, operations, etc., but these economic savings and benefits are a long way in the future. Discounting also allows common comparison between, for example, a treatment with greater short-term QALYs and a treatment with greater longer-term QALYs. The discount rate which you should use for economic modelling or cost-effectiveness analysis will be usually determined by your country's treasury department. However, whether using the same discount rate for costs and non-cost benefits is appropriate remains open to debate (Severens and Milne, 2004). Individuals are shown to have different time-preferences for health benefits – but these time-preferences also vary: across diseases, disease-severity and symptoms. For example, the perceived cost of smoking, loss of health and shorter life expectancy, are far in the future, whilst the perceived benefits of smoking (utility of smoking, preventing withdrawal) are immediate. To ensure that discounting is done appropriately, alternative rates should be explored when you conduct your analysis.

Case study

A multidisciplinary team of researchers has designed a study to assess the benefits of a new drug for rheumatoid arthritis. The natural endpoints are well understood: serum urate levels and flares, which are already being measured in the study to assess efficacy. However, these endpoints must also be translated into patient- and payer-relevant outcomes as they are also going to evaluate the drug's cost effectiveness. Therefore the team decide to use the following measures:

- A Quality of Life (QoL) scale. This is known to be relevant to the payer, but not patients or doctors, as it gives a score which measures the effect of the intervention, rather than a clinically useful outcome.
- An arthritis health status instrument which measures pain, mobility, emotional and social well-being, and global health. This will be more sensitive to changes in the disease and is relevant to the patient.
- Work absenteeism which is relevant to the patient and society in general.

Patients experiencing acute flares use health care resources, and these can be identified easily from patient records. Costing is therefore straightforward (the average cost of a flare can be used), but this crude measure will miss important differences: the drug is expected to reduce the severity of flare, as well as reducing the rate at which they occur. Micro-costing by formulating an inventory of all costs associated with the treatment, as might be collated for a cost-benefits analysis, is much harder to administer within the study due to the huge amount of data required, but would better reflect the true benefits of the new drug. The new drug also reduces mortality, which in turn, has implications on patient quality of life and lifetime earnings – but it will also mean drug costs persist over the long term. Therefore in the analysis, treatment costs and patient earnings will be discounted at 3.5%.

Design and conduct of an economic evaluation

Defining the question

Your question is the most important thing to determine (please see Chapter 1: 'Asking the Right Question'). This is a very important consideration, since the purpose of economic analysis is not to make the decision, but to allow the decision-maker to make an informed choice on the basis of the information provided. Therefore, if the wrong research question is answered, the analysis and results will not inform that decision as it will not be applicable. For an economic evaluation, it is important to remember that this does not need to be the same, and rarely is the same, as the clinical research question. To help you determine your health economic question, first consider what the objective is of the analysis. Is it to determine whether a new treatment is cost-effective, or whether an alternative treatment regimen is cost-effective? Or is it to show that a new regimen achieves similar benefits, but at a lower cost than current best practice? Or perhaps it is to demonstrate an improved safety profile? Second, think about who provides the care, and who funds the care, or are they the same? The final consideration is what you are going to compare the new treatment with? For example, many new drugs are evaluated against a placebo, but the decision-maker would be more interested in whether the drug is more effective when compared to the current best practice. Choosing an inappropriate comparator, such as placebo, will mean that the analysis can only be done indirectly, such as using current best practice data from a published source. This poses methodological challenges.

Choosing the perspective

As mentioned previously, the perspective is one of the most important parts of the evaluation to ascertain. It determines which costs and benefits are going to be appropriate and useful to measure. The narrower the perspective, the fewer costs and benefits needed to be collected. For example, a pharmaceutical company wishing to evaluate a drug would choose a provider perspective, and would only collect costs relating to themselves and outcomes relating directly to the treatment. A hospital, on the other hand, might consider a broader perspective, perhaps collecting costs associated with multiple factors within the hospital and out-comes relating to the treatment. A public perspective is perhaps the broadest in common use, taking into account the costs and outcomes associated with the provider, patients and carers, but not everyone, as in the societal perspective. When choosing the perspective of the analysis, a balance must be made between what costs and benefits are needed for the decision-makers, but also what can practically be measured.

Identifying and measuring the relevant costs and benefits

Only once the perspective has been determined can the appropriate costs and out-comes to be collected be ascertained. Costs and outcomes should be relevant to patients, disease and treatment setting and also directly relevant to the research question. You also need to choose the most appropriate way to answer it, taking into account the method most commonly used or accepted for doing a similar analysis, or economic model development as ascertained in your literature search (please see Chapter 2: 'Finding the Evidence to Support your Research Question').

Analysis

Like any other piece of research, consideration must always be given to the transparency, generalisability, reproducibility and validity of your results and data by performing univariate and multivariate sensitivity analyses (NICE, 2013), as well as probabilistic analyses of uncertainty. These analyses are important because all of the data in a model, assuming as is usually the case that cost and outcomes must be modelled, i.e. predicted beyond the duration of the study, will reflect an assumption. These assumptions should be analysed to ensure robustness.

Writing up

As an incremental economic analysis is often part of a trial, the clinical write-up regarding efficacy is usually regarded amongst the trial team as the main publication. However, any economic benefit will also need to be established for research to have impact at the policy or commissioning levels. The write-up of the economic analysis for the final report of a study is different to a journal article; likewise, a paper written for an economic, or health-economic, journal is going to be profoundly different to a paper written for a clinical journal, even when it is the same analysis being presented.

A report written for the funders of a primarily health-economic study should be a lot more detailed. There is often no word limit and much more detail of the study and analysis can be included. However, if the economic analysis is secondary, par-ticularly in clinical studies, the analysis must be written up in far fewer words, even though the economic analysis will have been no less complex. Therefore communi-cating the conduct and results of the economic work package within a study can be challenging.

For a journal publication, the first consideration is to determine who your audience is. Trial-based economic studies can often have been limited by the study, which will mean they are not likely to be accepted in an economics or methodological journal, which will require higher standards for the data and methods. Therefore, if the main purpose of your study is to affect change in treatment, a disease-specific clinical journal may be identified as the best outlet. If you decide to publish your economic analysis in a disease-specific journal, simple language should always be employed as much as possible, not complicated, methods-specific lexicon or jargon (Cochrane, 2005; Varian, 1994). Equations are best avoided, and keep graphs simple. The most important consideration here is the reader. The reader, presumably a peer, will only act upon your results if they can understand and accept them.

Unlike other quantitative studies, the results from your economic analysis might not be able to be reproduced elsewhere or in general practice, due to assumptions that have been made along the way, such assumptions about resource use, the costs of those resources, plus assumptions about how the clinical benefit translate into, say, QALYs – plus, after all of that, how each of these carries forth into the future, well beyond the observation period of the study. To aid the critical appraisal and reproduction of your work, state any assumptions you made and refer to a critical appraisal tool to ensure that you include all of the necessary information for an appraisal (e.g. Centre for Reviews and Dissemination, 2009; Drummond et al., 1997; McCabe and Dixon, 2000; McGhan et al., 2009; Sculpher and Mercey, 1998) (please see Chapter 3: 'Critical Appraisal').

Summary

- Economic evaluation demonstrates the effectiveness of interventions compared to their costs, giving decision-makers the information they need to determine whether the interventions are cost-effective.

- The most important things to consider when planning an economic evaluation is: what is the question to be answered; who is to be informed; and what perspective is being chosen? Only after considering these factors can a suitable method be chosen and relevant costs and outcomes be identified.

- When planning, conducting and writing the report, always consider whether your analysis/model is valid, transparent and generalisable.

Questions for Discussion

1. In 2012, after a review of the UK NHS's Pharmaceutical Price Regulation Scheme which controls drug prices in the UK, the Office of Fair Trading (OFT) recommended a move to Value-Based Pricing. In 2014 NICE will switch to this system, which rewards manufacturers according to the demonstrated benefit of

their drug. In particular, the new criteria will broaden the scope of 'benefit', to include societal benefits such as work productivity and impact on carers. Think of scenarios where this change of policy could lead to significantly higher prices. Can you think of scenarios in which the new policy might lead to lower prices?

2. Soft tissue sarcoma, i.e. a cancer that develops in connective tissue, is usually asymptomatic until it is relatively advanced. Suppose you are designing a clinical study to examine the benefit of treating patients with a new medication, which is reasonably effective but has several adverse events associated with it. You are deciding which scale to use for your economic evaluation, either a generic preference measure which collects data regarding mobility, self-care, usual activities, pain/discomfort and anxiety/depression, or a more sensitive instrument designed to measure QoL in patients with cancer, that has a greater number of questions and several symptom subscales. Which one would you decide and give your reasons why?

3. You are planning a clinical study to assess the benefit of a smoking cessation programme in prenatal care. Your study follows the smoking behaviour of women through their pregnancy and for six months' post-natally. What further long-term economic benefits of the smoking cessation programme might you expect to uncover?

Further Reading

Boardman, A.E. (2006) *Cost-Benefit Analysis: Concepts and Practice*. Englewood Cliffs, NJ: Prentice Hall.

Brazier, J., Ratcliffe, J., Salomon, J.A. and Tsuchiya, A. (2007) *Measuring and Valuing Health Benefits for Economic Evaluation*. Oxford: Oxford University Press.

Briggs, A.H., Claxton, K. and Sculpher, M.J. (2006) *Decision Modelling for Health Economic Evaluation*. Oxford: Oxford University Press.

Drummond, M.F., Sculpher, M.J., Torrance, G.W., O'Brien, B.J. and Stoddart, G.L. (2005) *Methods for the Economic Evaluation of Health Care Programmes*. New York: Oxford University Press.

Elliott, R. and Payne, K. (2005) *Essentials of Economic Evaluation in Healthcare*. London: Pharmaceutical Press.

Glick, H.A., Doshi, J.A., Sonnad, S.S. and Polsky, D. (2007) *Economic Evaluation in Clinical Trials*. New York: Oxford University Press.

Institute for Quality and Efficiency in Health Care (2012) *IQWiG's work procedures (Methods)*. Cologne: https://www.iqwig.de/en/methods/methods_papers/general_methods.3020.html (accessed Nov. 2012).

International Society for Pharmaeconomics and Outcomes Research (2012) *ISPOR Good Practices for Outcomes Research Index*. Lawrenceville: www.ispor.org/workpaper/practices_index.asp (accessed Nov. 2012).

James, M. and Stokes, E. (2006) *Harnessing Information for Health Economics Analysis*. London: Radcliffe.

McIntosh, E., Clarke, P., Frew, E. and Louviere, J. (2010) *Applied Methods of Cost-Benefit Analysis in Health Care*. Oxford: Oxford University Press.

Morris, S., Devlin, N. and Parkin, D. (2007) *Economic Analysis in Health Care*. Chichester: John Wiley & Sons.

National Institute for Health and Clinical Excellence (2008) *Guide to the Methods of Technology Appraisal*. London: www.nice.org.uk/media/B52/A7/TAMethodsGuideUpdatedJune2008.pdf (accessed Nov. 2012).

National Institute for Health and Clinical Excellence (2012) *NICE Decision Support Unit (DSU): Technical Support Documents*. London: http://www.nicedsu.org.uk/Technical-Support-Documents%281985314%29.htm (accessed Nov. 2012).

Pharmaceutical Benefits Advisory Committee (2012) *PBAC Guidelines*. Canberra: www.pbs.gov.au/info/industry/listing/elements/pbac-guidelines (accessed Nov. 2012).

World Health Organisation (2003) *WHO Guide to Cost-Effectiveness Analysis*. Geneva: www.who.int/choice/publications/p_2003_generalised_cea.pdf (accessed Nov. 2012).

References

Allegra, C.J., Yothers, G., O'Connell, M.J., Sharif, S., Petrelli, N.J., Lopa, S.H. and Wolmark, N. (2012) 'Bevacizumab in stage ii–iii colon cancer: 5-year update of the National Surgical Adjuvant Breast and Bowel Project C-08 trial', *Journal of Clinical Oncology*, 31 (3): 1–7.

Arrow, K. (1963) 'Uncertainty and the welfare economics of medical care', *American Economic Review*, 53 (5): 941–73.

Brazier, J., Roberts, J. and Deverill, M. (2002) 'The estimation of a preference-based measure of health from the SF-36', *Journal of Health Economics*, 21: 271–92.

Carers UK (2011) *Valuing Carers 2011*: www.carersuk.org/professionals/resources (accessed Nov. 2012).

Centre for Reviews and Dissemination (2009) *Systematic Reviews: CRD's Guidance for Undertaking Reviews in Health Care*. York: http://www.york.ac.uk/inst/crd/SysRev/!SSL!/WebHelp/SysRev3.htm (accessed Sept. 2012).

Cochrane, J.H. (2005) *Writing Tips for Ph.D. Students*. Chicago: http://faculty.chicagobooth.edu/john.cochrane/research/papers/phd_paper_writing.pdf (accessed Nov. 2012).

Department of Health (2009) *Guidance on the Routine Collection of Patient Reported Outcome Measures (PROMs)*. London: http://webarchive.nationalarchives.gov.uk/20130107105354/http://www.dh.gov.uk/en/Publicationsandstatistics/Publications/PublicationsPolicyAndGuidance/DH_092647 (accessed Nov. 2012).

Devlin, N. and Parkin, D. (2004) 'Does NICE have a cost–effectiveness threshold and what other factors influence its decisions? A binary choice analysis', *Health Economics*, 13: 437–52.

Drummond, M.F., Richardson, W.S., O'Brien, B.J., Levine, M. and Heyland, D. (1997) 'Users' guides to the medical literature. XIII. How to use an article on economic analysis of clinical practice. A. Are the results of the study valid? Evidence-Based Medicine Working Group', *JAMA*, 277: 1552–7.

Drummond, M.F., Sculpher, M.J., Torrance, G.W., O'Brien, B.J. and Stoddart, G.L. (2005) *Methods for the Economic Evaluation of Health Care Programmes*. New York: Oxford University Press.

Elliott, R. and Payne, K. (2005) *Essentials of Economic Evaluation in Healthcare*. London: Pharmaceutical Press.

EORTC. 2012. *EORTC QLQ-C30*. Brussels: http://groups.eortc.be/qol/eortc-qlq-c30 (accessed Nov. 2012).

EuroQol (2012) *EQ-5D*: www.euroqol.org/home.html (accessed Nov. 2012).

facit.org. (2012) *FACIT*. Elmhurst: www.facit.org/FACITOrg (accessed Nov. 2012).

Fanshel, S. and Bush, J.W. (1970). 'A health-status index and its application to health-services outcomes', *Operations Research*, 18, 1021–66.

Griffin, A. (2007) 'UK nears european average in proportion of GDP spent on health care', *British Medical Journal*, 334: 442.1.

Grossman, M. (1972) 'On the concept of health capital and the demand for health', *Journal of Political Economy*, 80 (2): 223–55.

Johannesson, M. (1995) 'A note on the depreciation of the societal perspective in economic evaluation of health care', *Health Policy*, 33: 59–66.

McCabe, C. and Dixon, S. (2000) 'Testing the validity of cost-effectiveness models', *Pharmacoeconomics*, 17: 501–13.

McGhan, W.F., Al, M., Doshi, J.A., Kamae, I., Marx, S.E. and Rindress, D. (2009) 'The ISPOR Good Practices for Quality Improvement of Cost–Effectiveness Research Task Force Report', *Value Health*, 12: 1086–99.

Morris, S., Devlin, N. and Parkin, D. (2007) *Economic Analysis in Health Care*. Chichester: John Wiley & Sons.

Murray, C.J. (1994) 'Quantifying the burden of disease: the technical basis for disability-adjusted life years', *Bulletin of the World Health Organization*, 72: 429–45.

National Institute for Health and Clinical Excellence (2004) *Fertility: Assessment and Treatment for People with Fertility Problems (CG11)*: www.nice.org.uk/guidance/index.jsp?action=byID&r=true&o=10936 (accessed Nov. 2012).

National Institute for Health and Care Excellence (2013) Guide to the methods of technology appraisal 2013. London: http://publications.nice.org.uk/guide-to-the-methods-of-technology-appraisal-2013-pmg9/the-reference-case

National Institute for Health and Clinical Excellence (2010) *Beacizumab for Treating Metastic Colorectal Cancer: Benefits for Some Patients; High Cost for the NHS*: www.nice.org.uk/newsroom/pressreleases/BevacizumabForTreatingMetastaticColorectalCancer.jsp?domedia=1&mid=400375CC-19B9-E0B5-D47397C25C5FC3B1 (accessed Nov. 2012).

Palmer, S. and Raftery, J. (1999) 'Opportunity cost', *British Medical Journal*, 318: 1551–2.

School of Health and Related Research (SCHARR) (2012) *SF-6D*. Sheffield: www.shef.ac.uk/scharr/sections/heds/mvh/sf-6d (accessed Nov. 2012).

Sculpher, M. and Mercey, D. (1998) 'How to assess an article on economic evaluation', *Sexually Transmitted Infections*, 74: 223–7.

Severens, J.L. and Milne, R.J. (2004) 'Discounting health outcomes in economic evaluation: the ongoing debate', *Value in Health*, 7: 397–401.

Torrance, G.W. and Feeny, D. (1989) 'Utilities and quality-adjusted life years', *International Journal of Technology Assessment in Health Care*, 5: 559–75.

Varian, H.R. (1994) *How to Build an Economic Model in Your Spare Time*. University of California, Berkeley: www.bus.lsu.edu/hill/writing/varian.pdf (accessed Nov. 2012).

10

EPIDEMIOLOGY

Puja Myles and Peter S Blair

Learning Objectives

- Recognise the scope and application of epidemiology in health services research
- Recognise the strengths and limitations of various epidemiological study designs
- Choose an appropriate epidemiological study design for your research question and context
- Be able to apply appropriate causal inference principles in interpreting epidemiological study findings

Introduction

Epidemiology studies the distribution (time, place and population), and determinants (physical, biological, social, cultural, economic and behavioural) of health-related states or events. This knowledge is then used to control the problem by allowing us to understand the cause, effect and distribution of diseases and therefore is the basis for public health, including informing policy decisions. Indeed, you have epidemiology to thank for the control of polio and typhoid and the total eradication of smallpox, which was directly responsible for 8–20% of all deaths in Europe in the 18th century (Bonanni, 1999). Epidemiological methods are used to identify epidemics, which occur when the number of new cases of disease exceeds that which is expected in a given population, and pandemics, which are essentially epidemics spread across a large geographical area, for example, the flu pandemic in 2009.

Epidemiologists can monitor increases in unfavourable events, for example, occurrence of disease, and by studying the associated factors can help us understand the potential causes or behaviour modification needed to reduce adverse outcomes. Factors may be related to the individual or to the environment and can be protective, such as breastfeeding which benefits a baby's immunity, or put people at risk, i.e. risk factors, such as smoking. Factors are sometimes called 'exposures' in epidemiology. Once the factors have been determined, advice can be given to reduce modifiable risk factors that are thought to be causally related to the disease, or both modifiable and non-modifiable risk factors can be used to define high-risk groups in order to design targeted public health or clinical interventions for high-risk individuals identified through screening programmes (Valanis, 1999). Once these programmes are in place, their success can be evaluated by comparing the reduction in disease incidence, prevalence or mortality, or improvement in overall health status. These comparisons can be carried out over time, i.e. before and after the intervention, or between groups of people who are in the programme or not.

Epidemiology also helps us understand the health event of interest in more detail, such as the identification of syndromes through the observation of clusters of signs and symptoms, and allows us to determine the natural history of a disease such as the stages in progression, and outcomes including recovery, complications and death (Valanis, 1999). Epidemiology can be used to establish patient characteristics and symptoms that are commonly associated with a given disease and its prognosis. This knowledge can aid clinicians in differential diagnosis and treatment planning. For example, we know that chronic obstructive pulmonary disease (COPD) affects mainly smokers in their forties, while asthma usually starts in childhood.

Epidemiological study designs

Chapter 6: 'Quantitative Data Collection' introduced the evidence pyramid and terms such as observational and experimental studies. Before considering individual epidemiological study designs in more detail, it is worth reviewing general terminology in relation to study designs.

Experimental designs

An experiment can be either 'randomised' where participants are randomly assigned to either treatment or to one or more control arms; or 'quasi-randomised', which is a method of allocating participants to different forms of care that is not truly random; for example, allocation by date of birth, medical record number, month of the year or the order in which participants are included in the study (alternation). Quasi-randomised poses a greater risk for selection bias when compared with randomised controlled trials with adequate allocation concealment. Non-randomised trials (quasi-experimental) are often used to evaluate health care interventions, such as cancer screening programmes or weight management programmes, when participants select, or are selected for, an arm of the trial. Non-randomised trials are sometimes used when it is difficult to achieve equipoise, i.e. the research should begin with a null hypothesis, not that one intervention will be greatly superior to the other, or where the assignment to the group has occurred due to a natural event.

Observational studies

Observational studies are ones where nature takes its course, the researcher has no control over who is exposed to what, and do not involve any intervention on the part of the investigator. In other words, the researcher adopts the role of a passive observer of health-related outcomes occurring in the study population. The epidemiological study designs that are 'observational' in nature are case-control, cohort, cross-sectional and ecological studies. Things can get slightly confusing when some quasi-experimental designs used in health care evaluations start looking very similar to cohort and case-control studies. Could a cohort design that compares the quality of life in a group of patients who receive a new cancer treatment when compared to current best practice without random assignment be classified as a quasi-experimental study? The distinction, if any, is subtle and Issel (2009) provides a useful clarification: observational studies such as case-control and cohort studies are used when the health outcome is 'bound' at the individual level. This means that there is no possibility of pre-test or baseline data before the intervention. Quasi-experimental designs on the other hand, would include pre-test or baseline data. Therefore the cancer programme project above would be a quasi-experimental study as you would collect baseline data.

Studying populations

Ecological studies investigate groups of people, communities or populations as a whole and therefore collect aggregated data (summary of all gathered data). Ecological studies are population-level studies that compare groups rather than individuals. They do this by assessing the relationship between summary population measures of exposure, for example, average household income, national gross domestic

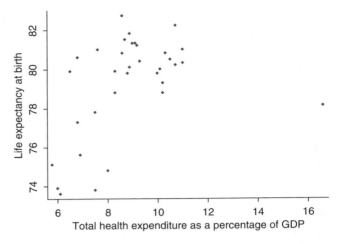

FIGURE 10.1   Scatterplot showing the correlation between total health expenditure and life expectancy at birth [Data source: *Health: Key Tables from Organisation for Economic Co-operation and Development*. DOI: 10.1787/20758480]

product, etc., and summary population measures of a disease/outcome, for example, average age of death for a region, prevalence of diabetes, etc. Ecological studies are one of the most cost-effective study designs to use and are quick to perform as they use routinely collected data. They are good for hypothesis generation and are often the first step in investigating potential associations between a risk factor and a disease. Though ecological studies are often positioned quite low in the evidence pyramid (the same level as cross-sectional studies, case reports and case series (see Figure 6.1, p. 85), they may be the most appropriate design for studying the effect of national policies on the population's health. The results of an ecological study can be presented graphically as scatterplots. The scatterplot in Figure 10.1 shows the relationship between total health expenditure and life expectancy at birth using data from 34 countries. You can see that, as the total health expenditure increases, life expectancy at birth increases.

A special type of ecological study is the time series analysis which involves multiple measurements of the outcome of interest over a period of time, thereby allowing trends to be detected. An interrupted time series is a particular type of analysis which involves measurements both before and after the introduction of an intervention and is useful for evaluating the impact of health and social policies on health-related outcomes in a specified population. A multiple time series on the other hand compares trends across multiple groups and allows for comparisons with a control group. For example, an interrupted time series study would involve comparing the mean number of asthma exacerbations in a region over time to see how changing levels of pollution are associated with asthma severity. A multiple time series study would compare the mean number of asthma exacerbations over time for more than one region. In this scenario, a multiple time series would be particularly useful if one of the regions had introduced a congestion policy that would impact on pollution and therefore could potentially have an impact on asthma severity. The other regions would then act as comparators or controls. It is important to note that an association observed between an exposure and an outcome at an aggregate level does not necessarily represent or reflect the association that exists at an individual level. This is known as the ecological fallacy, an example of which can be seen in the case study here. Both residual confounding, which is the distortion that remains after controlling for confounding in the design or analysis, and systematic measurement error, which is the non-random bias in measurement resulting in the mean of the measurements differing significantly from the true value, are also more likely to be problematic in ecological investigations as compared to other observational studies.

Case study

An ecological study by Zhang et al. (1999) showed that fish consumption was associated with lower rates of heart disease at a population level. However, on inspecting individual-level data you may find that the data on consumption of fish and heart rates come from two entirely different groups within that population. Therefore this association could be an ecological fallacy as we do not know whether it would remain true at an individual level. Indeed, there have been conflicting reports from individual-level epidemiological studies investigating the association between fish oil consumption and heart disease risk (Kris-Etherton et al., 2002).

Correlation

The term correlation refers to the linear relationship between the exposure and the outcome/disease and can be represented graphically using scatterplots or expressed as a correlation coefficient (presented as **r**) which measures the degree that two variables are linearly related. Correlation indicates the degree to which two variables increase or decrease together (positive correlation, **r** in the range 0 to +1), or go in opposite directions (negative correlation, **r** in the range 0 to -1), or appear to be unrelated to each other (**r** is 0 or close to 0). A perfect correlation is 1 either positive (Figure 10.2) or negative (Figure 10.3). The association between fish consumption and heart disease in the case study is an example of a negative correlation, i.e. eating more fish (y axis), means less heart disease (x axis). Whereas Figure 10.1 illustrates a positive correlation between total health expenditure and life expectancy at birth. A value of 0 on the other hand, indicates that there is no linear correlation at all between the two numbers (Figure 10.4), so the closer the **r** is to 0, the less certainty there is about the association. Therefore any **r** other than 0 will indicate an association, for example, a value of 0.89 would indicate a strong positive linear correlation, i.e. increasing exposure is associated with increasing outcome which is what you would see when the exposure is a risk factor. Conversely a value of -0.78 indicates a strong negative correlation, i.e. increasing exposure is associated with decreasing outcome, which is the pattern you would see when the exposure is a protective factor.

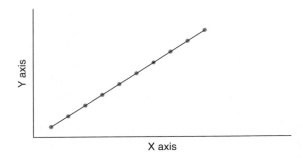

FIGURE 10.2   Perfect positive correlation **r** = +1

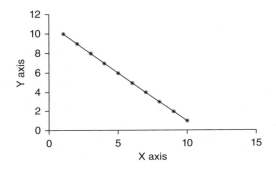

FIGURE 10.3   Perfect negative correlation **r** = −1

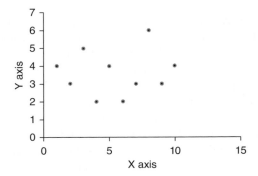

FIGURE 10.4   Zero linear correlation r = 0

Studying individuals

The research designs for studying individuals in epidemiology are: cross-sectional, case-control, cohort and RCTs. Cross-sectional studies can include either all persons in the population at the time of data collection or a representative sample of all such persons (Rothman et al., 2008) and can be either descriptive, such as measuring prevalence, or analytic, looking for associations between exposure and the outcome of interest. Case-control studies are analytical and aim to investigate the association between a given exposure and an outcome. Case-control studies start by identifying a group of people with the outcome of interest (cases) and another group of people without the outcome (controls). Data regarding the exposure of interest are then collected for both cases and controls; for example, people with asthma (cases) may be compared to people without asthma (controls) to study the relationship between cat ownership (exposure, which in this case is a risk factor as cats can exacerbate asthma due to allergens) and asthma (outcome). If on the other hand you were looking at the association between rural living and asthma, the exposure (living in the country) would potentially be a protective factor as a polluted urban environment could also exacerbate asthma. This association between the exposure and the outcome is represented using odds ratios.

Another research design which can be used in epidemiology is the cohort study. A cohort is a group of people with a common characteristic that is followed up over time. The aim of such studies may be to describe the experience of these cohorts including incidence of disease, survival, career achievements, educational outcomes, etc. An example of this type of cohort study is the 'Born in Bradford' study which recruited babies born to a population of all pregnant women attending a routine antenatal appointment at the Bradford Royal Infirmary, UK, between 2007 and 2010. The study successfully recruited a cohort of 13,500 babies who will be followed through into adulthood. Cohort studies may also be designed as comparative studies such that a cohort of 'exposed' people is compared to a cohort of 'unexposed' people. For example, a cohort of babies who have been breastfed could be compared to a cohort of babies that had not been breastfed and studied over a period of time to observe long-term health outcomes such as diabetes, cardiovascular disease and allergies. The incidence of these health outcomes in breastfed (exposed) and non-breastfed (unexposed) groups could then be compared. An advantage of using a cohort design is that you can be certain that the exposure preceded the disease or outcome, i.e. temporality. However, cohort studies can be very expensive and time consuming and may be affected by loss of study participants during follow-up, which can lead to attrition bias. It is possible to conduct a case-control study 'nested' within a cohort study for statistical efficiency. For instance, you could investigate potential risk factors for a rare outcome such as autism, typically diagnosed in mid-childhood, using cases and controls from a birth cohort, where the exposure could be a combined MMR vaccination to test Wakefield et al.'s theory (1998) as outlined in the case study in Chapter 3: Critical Appraisal. The advantage of a nested case-control study over the usual case-control study design is that once again you can be certain that the exposure occurred before the outcome.

Case study

An endocrinologist has noticed that there is a high rate of women in her care with diabetes who also have breast cancer. She would like to see if this is a true association and starts collaborating with an oncologist in her hospital to develop a research proposal.

To answer the question, they could choose a case-control study in which women with breast cancer (cases) and without breast cancer (controls) would be compared in terms of their exposure (whether they had diabetes or not). The limitation of this approach is that if they found a statistically significant association between diabetes and breast cancer, they would not be able to determine whether diabetes was present before the breast cancer or not. This problem would be averted if, instead, they conducted a cohort study in which they followed up women with or without diabetes (exposure) and compared the incidence of breast cancer (outcome) reported over a specified follow-up period in both groups. However, you would need to make sure that study participants in both the exposed and unexposed groups did not have breast cancer at the start of the study period.

Epidemiological measures

Prevalence

Prevalence is the frequency of an existing disease in a defined population at a particular point in time, and is a commonly used measure of disease burden. Prevalence is calculated by dividing the total number of cases of a disease by the total number of people in the population at a given point in time:

$$\text{Prevalence} = \frac{\text{Number of cases of a disease at a point in time}}{\text{Total number of people in the population at same point in time}}$$

Incidence

Incidence refers to the new cases of disease that occur in a population within a given time period and can be represented as incidence risk or incidence rates. The calculation for incidence risk assumes that the denominator population, which is the total population at risk, remains fixed over the entire research period, i.e. a closed cohort. If your study has a long follow-up period in which people may migrate in and out of the denominator population, for example, change age brackets, socioeconomic status, etc. this is called an open cohort.

$$\text{Incidence risk} = \frac{\text{Number of new cases of disease during a time period}}{\text{Total population initially at risk}}$$

If your study has an open cohort, incidence rates are used instead of incidence risk as it accounts for every person who migrates in and out of the denominator population by counting the 'time' they contributed to the study, for example, in a cohort study with a 10-year follow-up, a person who spent three years in the study would contribute three person-years, whilst someone who contributed six years, would contribute six person-years, and so on. Instead of adding up all of the people in the population at the start of the study, as you would in a closed cohort to calculate incidence risk, you would add up the person-years and use that as the denominator.

$$\text{Incidence rate} = \frac{\text{Number of new cases of disease during a time period}}{\text{Total person-years at risk}}$$

Risk ratios and odds ratios

A risk ratio is the measure of the risk of a certain event, such as a disease, happening in an exposed group compared to the risk of the event happening in an unexposed group. Therefore risk ratios are used to compare the prevalence or risk of a given disease in exposed versus unexposed groups.

$$\text{Risk ratio (RR)} = \frac{\text{Risk of disease in exposed group}}{\text{Risk of disease in unexposed group}}$$

An odds ratio on the other hand, compares the odds of exposure in people with the disease (cases) compared to the odds of exposure in people without the disease (controls). To calculate the odds of exposure for each group, simply divide the number of people with the exposure by the number of people without the exposure.

$$\text{Odds ratio (OR)} = \frac{\text{Odds of exposure in people with the disease}}{\text{Odds of exposure in people without the disease}}$$

When interpreting odds ratios and risk ratios a ratio of 1 means no difference in the odds or risk between the two groups. Therefore the exposure which is being studied is probably not associated with that disease. If you obtain a ratio <1 (less than 1) this means that cases are less likely to have been exposed (OR) or that the exposed group is less likely to have the disease (RR). You would be looking for a ratio <1 if your exposure was a protective factor. A ratio >1 (great than 1) means that cases are more likely to have been exposed (OR) or that the exposed group is more likely to have the disease (RR). Therefore the exposure is a risk factor. The finding would be significantly protective or a significant risk if the confidence interval, i.e. the range of values within which the true value lies, did not include the value 1 (please see Chapter 19: 'Quantitative Analysis' for a description of confidence intervals). In clinical studies the RR is often the statistic of greater interest and is a standard measure in biomedical research. The RR is easier to interpret, but it is not always possible to calculate the RR. The sampling method in case-control studies does not allow for the calculation of RR because you do not know the total exposed and unexposed populations at risk of developing the disease. In these instances, or when events are rare, the OR can be used to approximate the RR; however to do so the risks must be small (the rule of thumb is less than 10%).

Bias

Most of these research designs are open to bias and confounding. The design which is the least susceptible to these is the RCT, which is why this design is considered as one of the higher level designs in the evidence pyramid (please see Chapter 6: 'Quantitative Data Collection'). In epidemiology, bias refers to a systematic error in the collection, analysis or interpretation of data which can lead to an overestimation or underestimation of the association between an exposure and an outcome. Misclassification bias occurs when the disease (outcome) or exposure status is assigned inaccurately. Misclassification can be differential, where the errors in the measurements between groups are different. For example, diabetic cases may be more likely to correctly recall their dietary patterns than controls because diet is an important part of diabetes monitoring. Misclassification can also be non-differential, where the degree of measurement error is the same in both groups, such as when using an insensitive screening instrument which results in both cases and controls having a similar level of inaccuracy in assignment of exposure. Differential misclassification could either underestimate or overestimate the true association, but non-differential misclassification always leads to an underestimate of the true association. The differential accuracy of dietary pattern recall between diabetic cases and controls is due to recall bias, which is often because cases have more interest in, and awareness of, the possible contributory factors to their disease. Response bias, on the other hand, occurs because of differential reporting of exposures such as smoking or alcohol by cases, as a strategy to avoid blame for a 'self-inflicted' disease.

Minimising bias

Bias is best controlled for at the design stage. The randomisation process in RCTs breaks the association between the intervention and any confounding variables by balancing the distribution of known and unknown confounders between the comparison groups, but it is not always feasible or ethical to conduct an RCT. Therefore, strategies are employed to control for confounding, such as collecting data on potential confounders and then using statistical approaches such as multivariable modelling to adjust for them. For example, in the case study investigating the association between diabetes and breast cancer, the researchers may ask participants to keep a log of their exercise regime, or wear a pedometer, as previous evidence has shown that lack of physical activity is associated with both cancer and diabetes and therefore could be a confounder. However, it may not be possible to anticipate all possible confounders, so there may still be some degree of residual confounding in observational studies. However, the robustness of your project can be maintained through careful research design, such as minimising selection bias by considering a general population control group, or minimising response bias by using objective measures of exposure, or clinical records, rather than self-reported ones. To prevent attrition bias, you can put measures in place to achieve high response rates and low losses to follow-up, for example, maintaining a dialogue with the participants throughout the study, as seen in a cohort study with a follow-up of nine years, where birthday cards were sent to all child participants in each year of the study, thereby retaining 80% of the participants (Walker et al., 2011). For further discussion regarding retention please see Chapter 18: 'Recruitment and Retention'.

Causal inference

Most epidemiological studies aim to investigate the association between an exposure and an outcome. An observed statistical association may (or may not) represent a true causal relationship between the exposure and outcome under investigation because of factors like chance, bias or confounding. The Bradford Hill Criteria provide a framework to guide causal inference from epidemiological findings (Hill, 1965):

Strength: Strong associations (a large OR) are more likely to be causal.

Consistency: Similarity of findings across studies investigating the same association in different contexts indicates a causal relationship. It is worth noting though that study findings may differ because they are using different research methods or there is a variation in how outcomes or exposures are defined.

Temporality: The exposure must precede the outcome.

Specificity: The outcome, exposure and population need to be specific in order to exclude confounders which may be the reason for the association. This criterion is better suited to infectious diseases which can be attributed to a specific virus or bacteria but may be problematic when dealing with complex multifactorial health outcomes such as cardiovascular disease.

Biological gradient: This refers to a dose-response relationship between exposure and outcome. This criterion would not be applicable to threshold associations which is when exposure must exceed a given threshold limit before it triggers a disease outcome, e.g. exposure to sulphur dioxide becomes toxic at 10 particles per million or more. (National Institute for Occupational Safety and Health, 1981)

Plausibility: Biological plausibility would strengthen the argument for causal inference but its demonstration would depend on the scientific knowledge at any given time. For example, it is plausible that chewing tobacco could cause a cancerous lesion in the mouth based upon our prior knowledge of the association of tobacco and cancer.

Coherence: Could be seen as a corollary of the plausibility criterion: 'the interpretation of the data should not seriously conflict with the generally known facts on the natural history and biology of the disease' (Hill, 1965: 298)

Experiment: This criterion is about testing whether preventive action to remove or mitigate the exposure is effective in preventing or reducing the frequency of the outcome thus insinuating an association. This may be difficult or unethical to demonstrate in the case of complex, multi-factorial disease outcomes.

Analogy: Comparisons with similar exposures, similar biological pathways or similar outcomes may be employed to aid causal inference.

You will note that the Bradford Hill criteria are useful for causal inference but have some inherent limitations with regards to general applicability to all situations. In fact, Rothman et al. (2008) point out that the only necessary criterion for a causal relationship is temporality.

Reporting epidemiological research

The Strengthening of Reporting of Observational Studies in Epidemiology (STROBE) statement outlines good practice in writing up epidemiological research and includes a detailed checklist of items that should be reported for cohort, case-control and cross-sectional studies. A number of peer-reviewed academic journals require authors to follow the STROBE checklist when preparing manuscripts for submission (von Elm et al., 2008).

Summary

- Epidemiological methods can be used to investigate risk factors of disease, develop prognostic indices to aid clinical decision making, conduct health needs assessment for a population, disease surveillance and to evaluate the effectiveness of health care policies.

- Epidemiological studies include observational study designs such as cross-sectional, case-control, cohort and ecological studies as well as experimental designs such as randomised controlled trials.

- Potential bias and confounding can partially be dealt with at the design stage and controlled for in the analysis but a critical eye is still needed when interpreting the results.

- Epidemiological evidence of a statistical association cannot be assumed to represent a causal relationship between the exposure and outcome under investigation. A useful framework for causal inference is the Bradford Hill Criteria.

Questions for Discussion

1. You want to assess the impact of a national smoking ban on smoking prevalence. Which study design would you consider? Reflect on the pros and cons of your choice.

2. An occupational health physician has noticed an increasing number of cancer cases among workers in a chemicals manufacturing factory and is considering conducting an epidemiological investigation to test his hypothesis that one of the chemicals could be associated with the cancer. Which study designs could he use and what factors would determine his final choice?

3. Statins are prescribed to prevent heart disease in high-risk patients. A case-control study was conducted to investigate the association between statin use and myocardial infarction (heart attacks). The study found that statin use was actually associated with an increased risk of heart attack. How would you interpret this result (is this likely to be a true association)?

Further Reading

Bailey, L., Vardulaki, K., Langham J., and Chandramohan, D. (2005) *Introduction to Epidemiology*. Maidenhead: Open University Press.

Bhopal, R. (2008) *Concepts of Epidemiology: Integrating the Ideas, Theories, Principles and Methods of Epidemiology*. Oxford: Oxford University Press.

Elwood, M. (2007) *Critical Appraisal of Epidemiological Studies and Clinical Trials* (3rd edn). Oxford: Oxford University Press.

Koepsell, T.D. and Weiss, N.S. (2003) *Epidemiologic Methods: Studying the Occurrence of Illness*. Oxford: Oxford University Press.

Last, J.M. (2001) *A Dictionary of Epidemiology*. Oxford: Oxford University Press.

Savitz, D.A. (2003) *Interpreting Epidemiologic Evidence: Strategies for Study Design and Analysis*. Oxford: Oxford University Press.

Silva, S. and Fraga, S. (2012) 'Qualitative research in epidemiology', in N. Lumet (ed.), *Epidemiology: Current Perspectives on Research and Practice*: http://cdn.intechopen.com/pdfs/32600/InTech-Qualitative_research_in_epidemiology.pdf (accessed Dec. 2012).

References

Bonanni, P. (1999) 'Demographic impact of vaccination: a review', *Vaccine,* 17 (S3): S120–S125.

Chapman, T.F., Mannuzza, S., Klein, D.F. and Fyer, A.J. (1994) 'Effects of informant mental disorder on psychiatric family history data', *American Journal of Psychiatry,* 151 (4): 574–9.

Economic and Social Research Council (2010) *International Benchmarking Review of UK Sociology*, Economic and Social Research Council, British Sociological Association and Heads and Professors of Sociology Group: http://www.esrc.ac.uk/_images/Int_benchmarking_sociology_tcm8-4556.pdf (accessed Nov. 2012).

Gomez, M.B. and Muntaner, C. (2005) 'Urban redevelopment and neighbourhood health in East Baltimore, Maryland: the role of communitarian and institutional social capital', *Critical Public Health,* 15 (2): 83–102.

Green, J. and Thorogood, N. (2009) *Qualitative Methods for Health Research*. London: SAGE.

Hill, A.B. (1965) 'The environment and disease: association or causation?', *Proceedings of the Royal Society of Medicine,* 58: 295–300.

Issel, M.L. (2009) *Health Program Planning and Evaluation: A Practical Systematic Approach for Community Health* (2nd edn). Sudbury, MA: Jones & Bartlett.

Kris-Etherton, P.M., Harris, W.S. and Appel, L.J. (2002) 'Fish consumption, fish oil, omega-3 fatty acids, and cardiovascular disease', *Circulation*, 106: 2747–57.

Kromhout, D., Bosschieter, E.B. and de Lezenne Coulander, C. (1985) 'The inverse relation between fish consumption and 20-year mortality from coronary heart disease', *New England Journal of Medicine*, 9: 312 (19): 1205–9.

Lloyd, M. (2000) 'Analysis on the move: deconstructing troublesome health questions and troubling epidemiology', *Qualitative Health Research*, 10 (2): 149–63.

Muntaner, C., Eaton, W.W., Diala, C., Kessler, R.C. and Sorlie, P. (1998) 'Social class, assets, organizational control and the prevalence of common groups psychiatric disorders', *Social Science and Medicine*, 47: 243–53.

National Institute for Occupational Safety and Health (NIOSH) (1981) *Occupational Health Guidelines for Chemical Hazards*. London: DHHS (NIOSH) Publication No. 81–123.

Rothman, K.J., Greenland, S. and Lash, T.J. (2008) *Modern Epidemiology* (3rd edn). Philadelphia, PA: Lippincott Williams & Wilkins.

Shadish, W.R., Cook, T.D. and Campbell, D.T. (2002) *Experimental and Quasi-Experimental Designs for Generalised Causal Inference*. Belmont, CA: Wadsworth, Cengage Learning.

Valanis, B. (1999) *Epidemiology in Health Care* (3rd edn). Stamford, CT: Appleton & Lange.

von Elm, E., Altman, D.G., Egger, M., Pocock, S.J., Gøtzsche, P.C. and Vandenbroucke, J.P. (2007) 'The Strengthening the Reporting of Observational Studies in Epidemiology (STROBE) statement: guidelines for reporting observational studies', *PLoS Med.* 4: e296.

Stone, N.J. (1996) 'Fish consumption, fish oil, lipids and coronary heart disease', *Circulation,* 94: L2337–40.

Wakefield, A.J., Murch, S.H., Anthony, A., Linnell, J., Casson, D.M., Malik, M., Berelowitz, M., Dhillon, A.P., Thomson, M.A., Harvey, P., Valentine, A., Davies, S.E. and Walker-Smith, J.A. (1998) 'Ileal-lymphoid nodular hyperplasia, non-specific colitis, and pervasive developmental disorder in children' [retracted]. *The Lancet*, 28; 351 (9103) 351: 637–41.

Walker, D.-M., Marlow, N., Upstone, L., Gross, H., Hornbuckle, J., Vail, A., Wolke, D. and Thornton, J.G. (2011) 'The growth restriction intervention trial: long-term outcomes in a randomized trial of timing of delivery in fetal growth restriction', *AJOG*, 204 (34): e1–9.

Zhang, J., Sasaki, S., Amano, K. and Kesteloot, H. (1999) 'Fish consumption and mortality from all causes, ischemic heart disease, and stroke: an ecological study', *Preventative Medicine,* 28: 520–9.

11

CLINICAL TRIALS

Paul Silcocks and Adrian Gheorghe

- Describe what is meant by a clinical trial
- Understand the reasons for randomisation and the methods of treatment allocation
- Describe the characteristics, advantages, and disadvantages of main clinical trial designs
- Understand the principles underlying the choices of outcome variables and interventions
- Be aware of threats to the validity of trial conclusions
- Outline the principles of trial analysis and reporting

Introduction

A clinical trial is an experiment performed on humans with the aim of obtaining a convincing answer to a medical question. The medical question will refer to the effect of an intervention, for example, drug, surgery, public health programme, health service reorganisation, etc., on the outcome in a particular disease or condition that each participant has. Trials are not applicable for studies of prognostic factors or to evaluate diagnostic test performance (although trials can be done to compare outcomes using different diagnostic tests), and are unsuitable for interventions whose results will be obsolete by the time they are available due to the advent of a new medication, or policy. A single, high-quality clinical trial carries a lot of weight in the evidence pyramid (second only to a meta-analysis of several high-quality trials) for informing clinical practice and policy (please see Chapter 6: 'Quantitative Data Collection'). This is because other methods such as a single case report, or anecdotal evidence, may merely reflect the natural variation in the disease, whilst comparing outcomes of current and past patients, i.e. historical controls, is flawed because of the potential lack of comparability in terms of method of diagnosis, details of the intervention or outcome assessments. Clinical trials avoid this problem by using concurrent controls either in the form of parallel groups or by crossover of patients from one treatment to the other (see below). Single arm studies (without a control group) are also used in the early stages of drug development or for determining the feasibility of conducting a full-scale trial, but are not the basis to determine efficacy because a control group is lacking.

Building a trial team

If your research question is suitable for a trial, such as to determine the efficacy of a therapy, the first step is to build a multidisciplinary trial team who are responsible for the trial design, delivery, analysis, and reporting. A project team with the relevant expertise has been singled out as the major predictor of a trial's successful recruitment within its allocated budget (Swan et al., 2009). The chief investigator (CI) is the person who takes ultimate responsibility for the entire trial. As trials are primarily driven by answering clinically relevant questions, such as 'Is intervention X likely to be more beneficial for this patient population when compared with intervention Y?' the CI will usually be a clinician with advanced expertise in the subject. The CI is heavily involved in all stages of the research: (i) pre-trial, for example, designing the trial and applying for funding; (ii) in-trial, for example, motivating the trial team and overseeing the trial's progress; and (iii) post-trial, for example, dissemination of the trial's findings. In multicentre trials (where a trial is conducted concurrently in the same manner at various sites, usually to ensure the required size of the patient sample is met in a reasonable time), a principal investigator (PI) leads and takes responsibility for trial-related activities at each participating site. Ensuring efficient trial management is instrumental for successful delivery of outcomes (Farrell et al., 2010).

Therefore, appointing a dedicated trial manager to manage the day-to-day running of the trial is highly recommended. The responsibilities of trial managers include, but are not limited to: site selection; keeping to budget and monitoring recruitment (both are common problems in trials); ensuring efficient communication between sites; managing the flow and storage of trial documents; organising the activity of trial team members; and overseeing the data management which includes the creation of a secure, efficient environment for data storage (normally a database) and data entry into it. Key personnel directly involved in data entry are IT programmers, database managers and data assistants. The input of a trial statistician is vital both at the design stage, to ensure that the study questions can be reliably answered with the data collected, and at the analysis stage. If your trial aims to provide evidence to inform health policy by means of a built-in economic evaluation, it is also essential to involve a health economist at the trial design stage (please see Chapter 9: 'Health Economics'). Other useful team members could be members of the patient population you will be recruiting from (please see Chapter 16: 'Patient and Public Involvement'). A clinical trials unit (CTU) may provide most of the core expertise required for trial design and conduct, and may either host the entire trial or provide limited support, for example with the randomisation or the statistical analysis. For academic and NHS research, involvement of a registered CTU (UK Clinical Research Collaborative, 2012) is recommended for all trials and may be required by some funders, for which they will pay. Many trials units will require involvement prior to the funding application being submitted, thus early engagement with a CTU is strongly encouraged.

Trial committees

Although the overall responsibility for the conduct of a clinical trial rests with the sponsor and investigators, several other groups oversee different aspects of the trial. These may include:

- A trial steering committee (TSC) which ensures that the trial is conducted in line with good clinical practice (a quality standard for trials) on behalf of the funder and sponsor (National Institute for Health Research, 2012). The TSC should include an independent chair and independent members, one or two PIs and two or more patient representatives.

- A trial management group (TMG) which meets frequently to provide guidance on the day-to-day management of the study, and comprises key members of the trial team such as the chief investigator, trial manager and trial statistician.

- A data monitoring committee (DMC) oversees the accruing trial data and considers any new evidence that may impact on patient safety (European Medicines Agency, 2012; National Institute for Health Research, 2012) or outcomes. The DMC normally provides the sponsor and the TSC with recommendations on whether the trial should continue as planned or be terminated due to evidence of efficacy, futility or harm. A typical DMC comprises two or more clinicians and a statistician who are independent of the trial.

- Endpoint adjudication committees are for trials where patients or clinicians cannot be blinded to the intervention, such as when obviously different types of interventions are being evaluated, such as drugs versus radiotherapy, or when endpoints are particularly complex and require standardised interpretation (e.g. X ray images) to reduce variability. The committee, comprised of clinical experts who remain blinded to treatment allocation in order to minimise potential bias, adjudicate outcomes based on previously agreed criteria (European Medicines Agency, 2012).

Designing a clinical trial

Choosing your population

A rich body of evidence gathered from various therapeutic areas suggests that participants recruited in clinical trials are often not representative of the target population with the condition of interest (Costa et al., 2011; Cottin et al., 1999; Falagas et al., 2010; Hoel et al., 2009; Moore et al., 2000). A target population is the entire group that a researcher is interested in and about which they would like to draw conclusions, whereas the sample of participants actually studied may be very different. For example, women and the elderly are consistently excluded from cardiology trials (Gurwitz, 1992; Heiat et al., 2002) which may seriously limit the generalisability of their findings, i.e. they have poor external validity. Although patients within trials are bound to be unrepresentative to some extent (those who agree to randomisation are a self-selected group, and eligibility criteria aim to select patients who could benefit and exclude patients who may be harmed), the burden of proof is on researchers to demonstrate either that such differences are absent or are justified (please see Chapter 17: 'Sampling').

Determining outcomes

Study outcomes should be measured objectively but should also be relevant, such as carbon monoxide readings as an indication of smoking. If subjective outcomes are required, such as a quality of life measure, then appropriate validated tools suitable for the target population should be used. You may already have an idea of what efficacy means in the study, indicated by a pre-specified change to an outcome. The primary outcome (or primary endpoint) is the most important outcome in a trial and 'should be the variable capable of providing the most clinically relevant and convincing evidence directly related to the primary objective of the trial' (International Conference on Harmonisation, 1998: section 2.2.2:5). The choice of primary outcome should be informed by the views of key stakeholders (sponsor, funding bodies, patients, investigators and clinicians) and previous evidence. Ideally the primary outcome should be generally accepted as relevant and be suitable for a later meta-analysis. The COMET Initiative (Williamson et al., 2011) aims to address this issue by proposing a core set of outcomes that all trials in a field should adhere to.

The choice of primary outcome, the rationale for its selection and the planned statistical analysis must be pre-specified in the trial protocol and in grant applications, because it will form the basis of the power calculations and thus the sample size (please see Chapter 17: 'Sampling'). The primary outcome variable is measured on individual participants, for example, death, blood pressure, weight loss, etc., but these data are aggregated for the analysis. For instance, death applies to an individual; the risk of death (proportion dying) is an aggregate summary calculated for each trial arm. The aggregated primary outcome data for each arm can then be compared, i.e. the efficacy parameter (or effect measure), for example, the difference in risk, or the relative risk of death. Once the efficacy parameter has been chosen, the sample size calculation is based on a minimal clinically relevant effect, i.e. the smallest value of the efficacy parameter that will be 'worth knowing about'. Do not make the mistake of thinking that any improvement is worth having, because, other things being equal, trivial treatment effects will require truly enormous sample sizes. Try to find a consensus on a sensible value by discussion with other professionals and patients, but remember that how an effect is presented will alter perception. If survival changes from 90% to 94% this may not seem very much. Presented as a 40% reduction in death rate (from 10% to 6%) it can seem very different.

Generally, there should be only one primary outcome and it is advisable to stick to this principle. However, there may be occasions when two or more primary outcomes are required, i.e. co-primary outcomes. For example, if you were studying the effectiveness of a diet pill, you may want to have the primary outcomes of (i) the average percentage change weight loss, but also (ii) the percentage of participants achieving 5% or more weight loss from baseline to the end of the trial. The requirement for a successful result might then be expressed as 'all co-primary endpoints have to be significant' or 'either may be significant'. However, having more than one primary outcome raises concerns regarding multiple statistical testing and will also affect the power, so there will be a penalty in terms of sample size (Buzney and Kimball, 2008). When a single primary outcome cannot be selected (such as when the study's clinical question can only be meaningfully informed by a collection of variables), there is the option of combining multiple individual outcomes, for example, death, disabling stroke, heart attack, etc., into one composite outcome. This avoids the problems associated with multiple statistical testing, but in the absence of a consensus on what is a clinically important effect, the required sample size can be hard to estimate. Results based on a composite outcome may also be hard to interpret (Freemantle, 2003; Lauer and Topol, 2003; Montori et al., 2005), and care should be taken to report results from all component variables (Cordoba et al., 2010; Tyler et al., 2011).

Instead of having co-primary outcomes, or a composite outcome, it may be more appropriate to have one primary outcome, which is the best for answering the trial's main clinical question, and then some secondary (supportive) outcomes. These should also be pre-specified in the trial protocol and grant application. However, the trial will not be powered for these secondary outcomes and therefore their results should be interpreted cautiously. The probability of observing a statistically significant result by chance alone increases with the number of tests taken, i.e. type I error (please see Chapter 17: 'Sampling'), so the number of secondary outcomes and secondary analyses should be limited within reason. Similarly, subgroup analyses should also be pre-specified and ideally only undertaken when a significant result is observed for the primary outcome of interest (Freemantle, 2001). If your trial's results may influence policy, you may wish to assess not only clinical effectiveness, but cost-effectiveness too. If so, health-related quality of life and cost data should be pre-specified as secondary outcomes in the protocol (please see Chapter 9: 'Health Economics').

A surrogate outcome is a laboratory measure, or physical sign that provides a 'measurement of effect in situations where direct measurement of clinical effect is not feasible or practical' (International Conference on Harmonisation, 1998: section 2.2.6:7). For example, you may measure cholesterol as a surrogate outcome for mortality from heart disease which is your clinical endpoint of interest. Surrogate outcomes feature a number of advantages: the trial may be shorter, requiring smaller sample sizes, and therefore have fewer trial costs. However, surrogate endpoints have come under criticism due to lack of clinical relevance and reliability of predicting clinical benefit (Bucher et al., 1999; Gøtzsche et al., 1996) and are best avoided if a definitive clinically important result is needed.

Randomisation

This is an extremely important design factor to get right as poor randomisation procedures can introduce bias, and therefore will throw doubt on any conclusions you obtain. Randomly allocating participants ensures that patients are comparable at baseline with respect to variables that may affect the response, i.e. confounders, such as age or duration of illness, thus avoiding selection bias. Exact equality of distributions cannot be guaranteed except on average, so for any particular trial some chance inequality in distributions is to be expected. In addition to generating a random list of treatment assignments, the sequence of allocations also has to be concealed because otherwise patients could be 'steered' to one or the other arm. Such concealment can be more problematic than generating the list itself. The method for randomisation and sequence concealment needs to be specified in any ensuing publications (Moher et al., 2010) and using central randomisation independent of sites for sequence concealment, such as via a CTU, is generally regarded as the best.

Another method that reduces biased assessment due to phenomena such as expectancy effects from the patient or observer effects from the researcher is by blinding participants and/or those collecting the data to the treatment allocation, thus preventing both conscious and subconscious bias. A double blind trial is where neither the treating clinician nor the patients are aware of the treatment allocation. In a single blind trial, only the clinician is aware of the allocation. This terminology assumes that the clinician is also assessing outcome, but this is not always the case and it is therefore preferable to specify who is blinded. Achieving blinding may

TABLE 11.1   Sources of bias in RCTs

Source of bias	How it can arise	Solution
Selection	'Steering' patients towards one or other arm preferred by the clinician	Good randomisation procedure Blinding of researchers
Performance	Unequal provision of care (e.g. frequency of follow-up clinics) between the arms	Design of trial procedures Blinding of carers
Attrition	Different drop-out rates between the arms	Better trial procedures
Detection	Outcome requiring subjective assessments (e.g. pain scale, quality of life, etc.)	Blinding of assessors Multiple assessors used Standardised assessment tool

require extra complexity for some research questions. In psychotherapy for example, you may need the dummy intervention of a 'chat' to control for attention, whilst for surgical treatments 'sham' surgical incisions would have to be used (Cobb et al., 1959; Daniels et al., 2009; Dimond et al., 1960; Moseley et al., 2002). The use of controls like this is ethically contentious, but is most justifiable when the primary outcome is a subjective response and when the sham procedure is both convincing and has negligible risks. You may also need to use dummy medicines in a drug trial, as the two drugs you are comparing may differ in formulation (capsule vs pill), number of pills/dose, number of doses/day or duration of the treatment course. Dummy medications are thus created to augment the treatments so that they look the same and to ensure that patients in each arm take the same number of pills each day for the same duration. This adds to your trial costs, but if it is possible to do it, blinding is the most robust method for preventing bias, as can be seen in Table 11.1.

If you want to confirm that your randomisation is balanced, you may want to run some analyses during the data collecting period, although significance tests to compare baseline data are not recommended (Altman, 1985; Senn, 1994). This is because, if the randomisation process is working, some differences are expected due to chance. If baseline imbalance is detected which is not due to a breakdown in the randomisation process, then the effect can be allowed for in the statistical analysis. However there is no point in such adjustment except for variables known to strongly affect outcome (imbalance in variables not related to outcome is irrelevant).

Stratification and blocking

If there is reason to believe that different groups of participants may have different outcomes (such as mortality rates) you may want to stratify the trial, i.e. divide participants into groups defined by prognostic or demographic variables. The aim of stratification is to improve the comparability of the treatment arms, especially when trials are of small to moderate size, because with simple randomisation a chance imbalance of important prognostic or demographic variables may result in spurious treatment effects. For example, if by chance patients with advanced cancer tended to receive treatment B while less advanced cases tended to receive treatment A, then a crude comparison of B vs A could suggest treatment B was worse, even if the actual effects were the same. With stratification, B would be compared with A separately for more and less advanced cases and then the results averaged, thus giving a 'like with like' comparison. Stratification can either be part of the randomisation process (stratified randomisation), where a separate randomisation list is prepared for each stratum, or performed when the data are analysed (a post-stratified analysis), when a single randomisation list covers all patients at baseline with the strata being defined and analysed post-hoc. Only variables known to be strongly associated with your outcome should be candidates for stratification because the number of strata can easily become unmanageable. For example, with cancer stage as a prognostic variable (four categories) and sex as a demographic variable (two categories), there would be eight groups, or *strata,* needed to ensure that participants of both sexes in each of the four cancer stage categories are represented. Some combinations of sex and stage may be uncommon in practice and strata with only one treatment arm represented are wasted. In order to avoid this, the number of strata should be related to the size of the study (Silcocks, 2012). If in doubt it is better to omit a stratification variable, because it can always be controlled for later on in the statistical analysis (for discussion on stratified random sampling please see Chapter 17: 'Sampling').

Because the number of patients per stratum may be quite small, blocking is normally combined with stratified randomisation. Blocking ensures that there are equal numbers of participants from each arm, as each block contains a random order of arm allocation. A separate set of blocks is provided for each stratum and within strata blocks are completed in sequence (see case study). If the block order is too repetitive, treatment allocation can become predictable with the potential for bias, for example, for two treatments with an equal allocation the smallest block size is two. Thus it is easy to guess the next allocation if the block size and number of arms are known. Unpredictability can be strengthened by using larger block sizes such as four or six or a random mixture of these, for example, start with a block size of four and generate the first 24 allocations, then continue with a block size of six and generate a further 120 allocations and so on, and finally shuffling these blocks. However a block that is larger than the number of patients in a stratum is no better than simple randomisation so block sizes should not be too large.

There are alternatives to stratification and blocking to obtain balance in the trial, such as 'urn randomisation' where the probability of the next allocation within a particular stratum is tweaked after each treatment is assigned to favour the arm that is under-represented in that stratum. Minimisation is similar in that the probability of the next allocation is tweaked after each treatment. However, unlike urn randomisation, minimisation also takes into account the imbalance for other strata. Minimisation is useful if the number of strata is relatively large for the sample size, however it will not work well with very sparse data. Both urn randomisation and minimisation are dynamic allocation methods that create no randomisation list in advance, but allocate treatment instantaneously using computer software. This means that the sequence of allocations is concealed, but is also hard to audit and is vulnerable to software bugs or hardware malfunction. Therefore if you are going to use one of these methods, a back-up stratified randomisation list needs to be ready in reserve.

Case study

A researcher aims to equally allocate two treatments (A and B) in randomised blocks with a block size of four. First, he lists all the possible types of block according to the sequence of the two treatments:

Block type	Sequence of treatments
1	AABB
2	BBAA
3	ABAB
4	BABA
5	ABBA
6	BAAB

He then randomly orders the block numbers: e.g. 2, 3, 1, 5, 6 and 4 and lists the corresponding sequence of treatments (BBAAABABAABBABBABAABBABA). He repeats this process for more sequences of allocation until he has enough allocations for that stratum, the first of which is 'sex'. The process will be repeated for each of his strata in turn, such as cancer stages. Specialised software to perform this is used.

Trial designs

The design of the trial, or configuration, is dependent upon what you hope to get out of running the study and what questions you want it to answer. The most common configuration is the parallel group:

- Patients are randomised to one of two or more treatment arms.
- Each patient has only one of the treatments (although the treatment might consist of several components).
- Statistical analysis is straightforward (as fewer assumptions are needed).

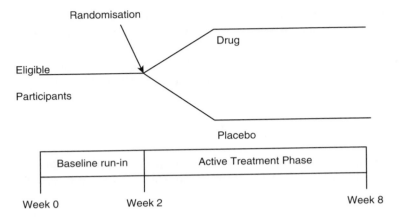

FIGURE 11.1   Parallel group design

The parallel group's essential features are shown in Figure 11.1 in which only two treatment arms are considered, although in theory any number of treatment arms can be used.

After obtaining consent from the participant, most trials will have a short interval before randomisation in which to take baseline measurements (run-in) and possibly establish 'good habits', for example, completing a symptom diary. After randomisation the treatments should start as soon as possible, and at the same time as each other, otherwise some participants may die, get worse or change their minds about taking part. If this happens more often in one arm, there is potential for bias if these patients are omitted from the analysis. If the outcome is measured at multiple times for each participant (usually baseline, at the end of the trial, and at specified time points during the trial) this is a repeated, or serial, measures design. How many measurements are taken, and when, should be determined by the hypothesised difference between the treatment arms. For example, if your trial is assessing a weight-loss drug, comparisons of serial measurements could identify the rate of initial weight loss, the time taken to stable weight, within-patient consistency of weight loss and so on (for more information please see Matthews et al., 1990).

The results from a trial usually take a long time to influence practice. Sequential designs, such as the parallel group, allow trials to stop earlier by taking repeated looks at the results as the trial progresses, i.e. interim analyses. This configuration is ethically justifiable as the results can be disseminated earlier and no more participants are needed than to give the answer. However these designs have a price: sample size, significance tests and confidence intervals are complicated by the combination of multiple comparisons; there is also the issue of dependence of progression to the next stage being dependent on the result of the previous one, so sophisticated software is needed. Also the results tend to be biased, and trials stopping early have been criticised for insufficient information on longer-term or rarer effects. Therefore trials such as these should not be undertaken lightly.

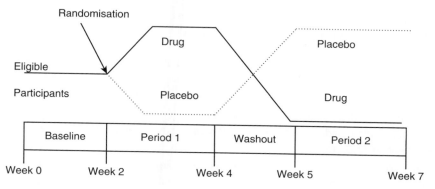

FIGURE 11.2   Cross over design

Another configuration to consider is the crossover where participants are randomised to treatment sequences, as can be seen in Figure 11.2:

- Each participant gets more than one treatment
- Responses are compared *within* participants
- The simplest is a 2×2 design, i.e. two treatments and two time periods

A crossover design has a number of advantages: The patient acts as their own control, which makes the design less susceptible to confounders; because within-patient variability is likely to be much less than between-patient variability, therefore more precise treatment comparisons can be made, so a smaller sample size is needed. The disadvantages of this design are its limited applicability. Only chronic, stable, reversible conditions, for example, high blood pressure, elevated blood sugar levels, asthma, etc., and interventions with quick and reversible effects are suitable (this excludes surgery, for instance). You also need to ensure that the washout period between treatments is adequate, as there is a possibility of carry-over if it is not. Even if there is an appropriate washout, it can make the duration of participant involvement unacceptably long, and the longer the duration the greater the risk of a period-effect due to seasonal or other time trends on response. In addition, it is harder to ascribe adverse events to a specific treatment, and participants may drop out after the first treatment. Data from such participants are usually excluded from analysis, and in general, a more complicated analysis is needed, especially in the presence of drop-outs, or if more than two treatments are involved. Single patient trials are a special kind of crossover design with just one participant, in which multiple periods on each treatment ensure precision in identifying the best treatment for a given individual (as opposed to identifying the best treatment for people in general). Otherwise, the techniques and limitations are like those of the crossover design.

In cluster-randomised trials whole groups (clusters) of individuals – rather than the individuals themselves – are randomised to treatments, in either parallel group or crossover configurations (for discussion of cluster sampling please see Chapter 17: 'Sampling'). These designs are applicable when:

- Inferences from the trial naturally apply at a group level. For example, if looking at the effect a hand-washing policy in hospitals has on cross-infection rates, it would be sensible to randomise hospitals to have the policy or not.
- The intervention has to be applied at a cluster level. For example, a trial to prevent malaria could randomly assign villages to have their local ponds sprayed with insecticide or not.
- There might be contamination from one treatment arm to the other, for example, when participants share information. This factor would be a problem in an unblinded trial of behavioural therapy for smoking for instance.
- It is administratively more convenient to cluster randomise than randomise individuals.

Another configuration is the factorial trial which evaluates two or more treatments simultaneously in the same participants. They are useful if the motivation is to study the separate and joint effects of treatments on a given disease, or to study unrelated conditions in the same sample. The simplest example of a factorial trial is a 2×2 design, with four arms (please see the case study which gives examples for the two distinct reasons for conducting a factorial trial).

Case study

A. The Physician's Health Study (Hennekens and Eberlein, 1985) aimed to answer two medically unrelated research questions: 'Does aspirin prevent myocardial infection?' and 'Does beta-carotene prevent cancer?' This was the first application of the 2×2 factorial design and, as it happened, the first large RCT conducted entirely by mail. A total of 22,071 US physicians were enrolled and randomised to one of the four arms, as in the allocation in Table 11.2.

TABLE 11.2   Treatment allocation in the Physicians' Health Study

Treatment	Aspirin placebo	Aspirin
ß carotene placebo	Arm 1: Beta-carotene placebo + aspirin placebo	Arm 2: Aspirin + beta-carotene placebo
ß carotene	Arm 3: Beta-carotene + aspirin Placebo	Arm 4: Aspirin + beta-carotene

The aspirin arm was stopped early due to evidence of significant benefit in reducing the risk of myocardial infarction, while beta-carotene eventually showed neither benefit nor harm.

B. The Medical Research Council's Thrombosis Prevention Trial (MRC General Practice Research Framework, 1998) aimed to answer one question about two treatments: 'Does either low-dose aspirin or low intensity oral anticoagulation with warfarin reduce the risk of ischemic heart disease?' A total of 5,499 UK patients were randomised to one of the four arms, as in the allocation in Table 11.3.

TABLE 11.3 Treatment allocation in the MRC Thrombosis Prevention Trial

Treatment	Aspirin placebo	Aspirin
Warfarin placebo	Arm 1: Warfarin placebo + Aspirin placebo	Arm 2: Aspirin + Warfarin placebo
Warfarin	Arm 3: Warfarin + Aspirin placebo	Arm 4: Aspirin + Warfarin

This is an example of a trial which demonstrated an interaction between two treatments as well as their individual efficacy. The results showed a beneficial effect for both aspirin and warfarin individually, but even more importantly, that a combination (Arm 4) was more efficacious than either of the two on their own.

Intervention(s)

The intervention and comparator for the trial will be influenced by new developments in your clinical area such as an emergence of a new drug or therapy. Policymakers are often interested in a trial's results, as not only does a trial determine efficacy, it can also determine resource allocation through its cost-effectiveness analyses (please see Chapter 9: 'Health Economics'). However the results will only be implemented in clinical practice when the intervention being evaluated in the clinical trial is compared to current best practice rather than placebo (Drummond et al., 2005).

Although the intervention that you study in one of the arms will often be a drug or a device, a skill-based intervention such as surgery or psychotherapy may also be tested. Drugs and devices are less open to variation, as they are uniform products. In contrast, for skill-based interventions, the level of expertise and background of the person delivering the intervention is a source of variation that is increased when a range of individuals deliver the treatment. This variation can be reduced by having specific requirements, for example, length of experience, qualification level, etc., and by bespoke training in the delivery of the intervention, documented in a trial-specific procedure manual. The extent to which this manual is adhered to is termed 'treatment fidelity'. Compliance is closely related to this, measuring the patient's contribution to treatment fidelity, for example, by taking medicines as directed, attendance at scheduled visits, etc. Compliance is only an issue for interventions that are taken over a period of time and will not affect one-off treatments such as surgery or a vaccination. Some apparently one-off interventions do require extended compliance however, such as the implantation of a medical device such as a pacemaker, which then needs follow-up treatments.

Number of arms

An inactive, placebo arm (suitably structured to ensure comparability) is needed if the aim is to show that an intervention works 'at all', i.e. efficacy. However, if an effective treatment already exists, the normal comparison would be against this existing treatment, i.e. effectiveness. A variation on this is to compare withdrawal of a standard treatment against its continuation; here the 'new' intervention is the absence of a treatment, such as a randomised study which looked at the discontinuation of long-term antipsychotic drugs in patients with dementia (Van Reekum et al., 2002). Some trials employ 'usual care' as the control arm, but this can cause problems because 'usual care' reflects a range of practice, both bad and good, a consequence of which is an underpowered trial unless this variability is allowed for by increasing the sample size. Therefore the fairest comparison should be against 'current best practice', but this may require some non-standard element of care, and it may be more difficult to recruit investigators or centres if a standardised current best practice protocol is felt to be inferior to local practice, or because it requires additional resources.

Sometimes rather than the standard two-arm trial, it is necessary to have three or more arms. For example, you may wish to run a three-armed trial comparing a drug both with placebo and against an alternative treatment (which could be current best practice so to inform policy). However the number of arms in your trial will affect your sample size calculation: the more arms you have, the more participants you will need for the same minimum significance between treatment effects. Your analysis strategy will also be affected: the use of global statistical tests, or multiple standard tests reflecting the number of arms, will mean that you will have less certainty in your results (because the analysis will result in wider confidence intervals, please see Chapter 19: 'Quantitative Analysis'). Thus, wherever possible, try to keep the number of arms low:

> For the best chance of a straightforward conclusion at the end of a study, use a straightforward design. A series of two-arm trials will not ask many questions but will provide answers to most of them (if sample sizes are adequate). (Green et al., 2012: 112)

Why trials fail

The main reason why trials fail is due to not collecting the proposed amount of data, which will impact heavily on the validity of the results. A major cause is under-recruitment which reduces power and widens confidence intervals. More than 50% of trials fail to recruit the proposed number of patients due to recruitment forecasts being far too optimistic. Telephone reminders, opt-out schemes (rather than opt-in) and open trial designs have been suggested as having potential benefit in addressing this issue (Treweek, 2010). There can also be difficulties in recruiting clinicians who will promote and conduct your trial. Getting health professionals involved in research is a challenge in itself and barriers to clinician recruitment and adherence to the trial protocol may be diminished by minimising the administrative burden of data collection, such as by using simple, electronic case report forms (Rendell et al., 2008). Evidence suggests that an effective strategy would be to conduct a qualitative study alongside the main trial in order to understand the difficulties that clinicians face with recruiting patients (Fletcher et al., 2012). Furthermore, if the shortfall in data is due to participant attrition, there may also be serious possibilities of bias if the attrition is related to outcome or side effects. Even if target recruitment is met, the proposed amount of data will be absent if there is extensive missing data (likely with burdensome assessments or poor-quality data management) and this poses more serious problems in analysis and interpretation than simple under-recruitment (please see Chapter 18: 'Recruitment and Retention'). The final reason why a trial may fail is due to going over budget. The length of the research, employment of administrative staff as well as the logistical effort involved in running a trial can all be very costly so ensure that you budget appropriately, and adhere strictly to your trial deadlines, as slippage in timings will affect the trial costs (please see Chapter 5: 'Budget and Funding').

The trial protocol

The trial protocol is a 'document that describes the objective(s), design, methodology, statistical considerations, and organization of a trial' (International Conference on Harmonisation, 1996: section 1.44:6). The protocol is written before the onset of the trial and fulfils a multitude of roles: it documents the investigators' decisions regarding the handling of participants and data; it presents the trial to funding and regulatory bodies (including ethics committees) when applying for grants and approvals; it demonstrates the trial's compliance with official regulations, norms and guidelines; and it acts as a reference document for trial conduct. Amendments to the protocol are allowed, subject to notification and approval from regulatory bodies. A list of standard protocol items to include has been developed by the Standard Protocol Items for Randomized Trials (SPIRIT) initiative (Chan et al., 2013) to help. Additional online resources are also available to assist the researcher with planning and writing a trial protocol (Treweek et al., 2006) such as www.practihc.org (accessed Oct. 2012).

Although your trial protocol will pre-specify an outline of your statistical analysis, covering the outcomes that will be analysed, the timing of the analyses, the main statistical methods, the statistical significance level, the selection procedure for trial participants who will be included in the analysis and procedures for handling missing data, it is modern practice for the full technical details of the analysis to go into a separate document, the Statistical Analysis Plan (SAP). The reasons for having such a plan are:

- It provides much more detail than is feasible or desirable in the statistical section of the protocol.
- It ensures that the methods followed by the statistician and/or statistical programmer are appropriate and meet the aims of the trial.
- By pre-specifying analyses and methods it minimises bias produced through the use of inappropriate post and ad hoc data dredging or 'chasing' the most favourable statistic.
- By explaining in detail what is required, it enables others to perform the actual analysis in the event of changes in personnel or other absence.

The golden rule is that all the analyses to be performed must be specified either in the protocol or in the SAP, prior to any analyses being conducted. This will indicate, for example, whether your primary analysis will be based on 'intention-to-treat' (ITT) or 'per-protocol' (PP). An ITT analysis compares outcomes between groups defined only by the initial treatment assignment. For example, you might have a trial of a new medication, but people tend to withdraw from the treatment because they feel more ill on the drug. It may be that the small proportion who do complete the trial treatment with no severe side effects, have outcomes better than the placebo arm, so if you just analysed such completers, you would have a positive result. ITT analysis would provide a more realistic estimate of the average effect by incorporating attrition (and other deviations from the protocol, such as non-compliance with the medication), therefore giving you a direct estimate of the practical value of a new medication. ITT is only possible however if patients who withdraw from trial treatment remain 'on trial' so that the outcome can still be assessed. A PP analysis uses data from patients to whom the trial protocol has been applied in full, for example, adhering to regime, having all outcome measures obtained, etc. This does indicate the treatment effect among those who take the treatment as specified, but the answer is also potentially biased as the resultant arms may differ in important ways. In the trial of a new medication from the earlier example, you would expect fewer participants to complete in the treatment arm due to the severe side effects than the control arm, and that the participants completing the trial treatment are atypical. Because ITT analyses preserve the initial randomisation and reflect what would happen in clinical practice, they are almost always preferred to PP and every effort should be ensured to make them possible.

Another consideration which must be pre-specified is how you will handle missing data because this introduces bias and reduces statistical power. Although missing data are inevitable in principle, particular efforts should be made to obtain complete data on outcome, stratification variables and covariates related to outcome. The trial protocol must include both methods for minimising the occurrence of missing data and indicate methods for handling missing data in the analysis. It is also important to investigate the reasons for which the data are missing in order to estimate the degree of bias likely to be incurred and to inform the methods for dealing with it (Douglas and Bland, 2007).

Summary

- Well-designed clinical trials aim to provide an unambiguous answer to a well-posed medical question.
- Clinical trial teams with appropriate membership are imperative.
- All stages of RCT conduct require integration of sound scientific, ethical, management and statistical principles to avoid bias, and to ensure validity.
- Clinical trials continue to develop methodologically, but adherence to guidelines on design provides a reliable frame of reference and ensures that current practice has the potential to reliably inform future developments.

Questions for Discussion

1. A randomised double-blind placebo-controlled crossover trial investigated the effect of alcohol consumption on hormone levels. Women were asked to drink a given measure of alcohol on one day and a placebo drink on the other, with the order being randomised. The outcome measure for each woman was the difference in the level of hormones (oestradiol and oestrone) in the blood for the alcohol and placebo days.

   a. Why was the order of the drinks randomised?

   b. What are the advantages and disadvantages of this design compared to a trial randomising women to an alcohol group and a placebo group?

2. You have developed a new pill that improves concentration. The effects from the pill are short-lived and participants need to take one per day for a continuous effect. Which trial configuration would you chose and why?

Further Reading

Green, S., Benedetti, J., Smith, A. and Crowley, J. (2012) *Clinical Trials in Oncology* (3rd edn). Boca Raton, FL: CRC Press.
Hackshaw, A. (2009) *A Concise Guide to Clinical Trials*. Chichester: Wiley-Blackwell.
Piantadosi, S. (2005) *Clinical Trials: A Methodologic Perspective* (2nd edn). Hoboken, NJ: John Wiley.

References

Altman, D.G. (1985) 'Comparability of randomised groups', *The Statistician*, 34: 125–36.
Bucher, H.C., Guyatt, G.H., Cook, D.J., Holbrook, A. and McAlister, F.A. (1999) 'Users' guides to the medical literature: XIX. Applying clinical trial results A; How to use an article measuring the effect of an intervention on surrogate end points', *Journal of the American Medical Association*, 282 (8): 771–8.

Buzney, E.A. and Kimball, A.B. (2008) 'A critical assessment of composite and coprimary endpoints: A complex problem', *Journal of the American Academy of Dermatology,* 59 (5): 890–6.

Calvert, M., Wood, J. and Freemantle, N. (2011) 'Designing "real-world" trials to meet the needs of health policy makers at marketing authorization', *Journal of Clinical Epidemiology,* 64 (7): 711–17.

Chan, A.W., Tetzlaff, J.M., Altman, D.G., Laupacis, A., Gøtzsche, P.C., Krleža-Jeri, K., Hróbjartsson, A., Mann, H., Dickersin, K., Berlin, J.A., Doré, C.J., Parulekar, W.R., Summerskill, W.S.M., Groves, T., Schulz, K.F., Sox, H.C., Rockhold, F.W., Rennie, D. and Moher, D. (2013) 'SPIRIT 2013 Statement: defining standard protocol items for clinical trials', *Annals of Internal Medicine,* 158 (3): 200–7.

Cobb, L.A., Thomas, G.I., Dillard, D.H., Merendino, K.A. and Bruce, R.A. (1959) 'An evaluation of internal-mammary-artery ligation by a double-blind technic', *New England Journal of Medicine,* 260 (22): 1115–18.

Cordoba, G., Schwartz, L., Woloshin, S., Bae, H. and Gøtzsche, P.C. (2010) 'Definition, reporting, and interpretation of composite outcomes in clinical trials: systematic review', *British Medical Journal,* 341: c3920.

Costa, D.J., Amouyal, M., Lambert, P., Ryan, D., Schunemann, H.J., Daures, J.P., Bousquet, J. and Bousquet, P.J. (2011) 'How representative are clinical study patients with allergic rhinitis in primary care?', *Journal of Allergy and Clinical Immunology,* 127 (4): 920–6.

Cottin, V., Arpin, D., Lasset, C., Cordier, J.F., Brune, J., Chauvin, F. and Trillet-Lenoir, V. (1999) 'Small-cell lung cancer: patients included in clinical trials are not representative of the patient population as a whole', *Annals of Oncology,* 10 (7): 809–15.

Daniels, J., Gray, R., Hills, R.K., Latthe, P., Buckley, L., Gupta, L., Selman, T., Adey, E., Xiong, T., Champaneria, R., Lilford, R., Kahn, K.S. and the LUNA Trial Collaboration (2009) 'Laparoscopic uterosacral nerve ablation for alleviating chronic pelvic pain: a randomized controlled trial', *Journal of the American Medical Association,* 302 (9): 955–61.

Dimond, E.G., Kittle, C.F. and Crockett, J.E. (1960) 'Comparison of internal mammary artery ligation and sham operation for angina pectoris', *American Journal of Cardiology,* 5 (4): 483–6.

Douglas, G.A. and Bland, J.M. (2007) 'Missing data', *British Medical Journal,* 334 (7590): 424.

Drummond, M.F., Sculpher, M.J., Torrance, G.W., O'Brien, B.J. and Stoddart, G.L. (2005) *Methods for the Economic Evaluation of Health Care Programmes.* Oxford: Oxford University Press.

EQUATOR Network (2012) *Library for Health Research Reporting:* http://www.ema.europa.eu/docs/en_GB/document_library/Scientific_guideline/2009/09/WC500002874.pdf (accessed Oct. 2012).

European Medicines Agency (2012) *Guideline on Data Monitoring Committees:* www.emea.europa.eu/docs/en_GB/document_library/Scientific_guideline/2009/09/WC500003635.pdf (accessed Oct. 2012).

Falagas, M.E., Vouloumanou, E.K., Sgouros, K., Athanasiou, S., Peppas, G. and Siempos, I. (2010) 'Patients included in randomised controlled trials do not represent those seen in clinical practice: focus on antimicrobial agents', *International Journal of Antimicrobial Agents,* 36 (1): 1–13.

Farrell, B., Kenyon, S. and Shakur, H. (2010) 'Managing clinical trials', *Trials,* 11 (1): 78.

Fletcher, B., Gheorghe, A., Moore, D., Wilson, S. and Damery, S. (2012) 'Improving the recruitment activity of clinicians in randomised controlled trials: a systematic review', *British Medical Journal Open,* 2(1).

Freemantle, N. (2001) 'Interpreting the results of secondary end points and subgroup analyses in clinical trials: should we lock the crazy aunt in the attic?', *British Medical Journal*, 322 (7292): 989–91.

Freemantle, N. (2003) 'Composite outcomes in randomized trials: greater precision but with greater uncertainty?', *Journal of the American Medical Association*, 289 (19): 2554–9.

Gøtzsche, P.C., Liberati, A., Torri, V. and Rossetti, L. (1996) 'Beware of surrogate outcome measures', *International Journal of the Technological Assessment of Health Care*, 12 (2): 238–46.

Green, S., Benedetti, J., Smith, A. and Crowley, J. (2012) *Clinical Trials in Oncology* (3rd edn). Boca Raton, FL: CRC Press.

Gurwitz, J.H., Col, N.F. and Avorn, J. (1992) 'The exclusion of the elderly and women from clinical trials in acute myocardial infarction', *Journal of the American Medical Association*, 268 (11): 1417–22.

Heiat, A., Gross, C.P. and Krumholz, H.M. (2002) 'Representation of the elderly, women, and minorities in heart failure clinical trials', *Archives of Internal Medicine*, 162 (15): 1682–8.

Hennekens, C.H. and Eberlein, K. (1985) 'A randomized trial of aspirin and beta-carotene among U.S. physicians', *Preventive Medicine*, 14: 165–8.

Hoel, A.W., Kayssi, A., Brahmanandam, S., Belkin, M., Conte, M.S. and Nguyen, L.L. (2009) 'Under-representation of women and ethnic minorities in vascular surgery randomized controlled trials', *Journal of Vascular Surgery*, 50 (2): 349–54.

International Conference on Harmonisation (1996) *ICH E6: Guideline for Good Clinical Practice*: www.ich.org/fileadmin/Public_Web_Site/ICH_Products/Guidelines/Efficacy/ E6_R1/Step4/E6_R1_Guideline.pdf (accessed Oct. 2012).

International Conference on Harmonisation (1998) *ICH E9: Statistical Principles for Clinical Trials*: www.ich.org/fileadmin/Public_Web_Site/ICH_Products/Guidelines/Efficacy/E9/ Step4/E9_Guideline.pdf (accessed Oct. 2012).

Lauer, M.S. and Topol, E. (2003) 'Clinical trials–multiple treatments, multiple end points, and multiple lessons', *Journal of the American Medical Association*, 289 (19): 2575–7.

Matthews, J.N., Altman, D.G., Campbell, M.J. and Royston, P. (1990) 'Analysis of serial measurements in medical research', *British Medical Journal*, 300 (6719): 230–5.

Medical Research Council's General Practice Research Framework (1998) 'Thrombosis prevention trial: randomised trial of low-intensity oral anticoagulation with warfarin and low-dose aspirin in the primary prevention of ischaemic heart disease in men at increased risk', *The Lancet*, 351 (9098): 233–41.

Moher, D., Hopewell, S., Schulz, K.F., Montori, V., Gotzsche, P.C., Devereaux, P.J., Elbourne, D., Egger, M. and Altman, D.G. (2010) 'CONSORT 2010 explanation and elaboration: updated guidelines for reporting parallel group randomised trials', *British Medical Journal*, 340: c869.

Montori, V.M., Permanyer-Miralda, G., Ferreira-Gonzales, I., Busse, J.W., Pacheco, V., Bryant, D., Alonso, J., Akl, E.A., Domingo-Salvany, A., Mills, E., Wu, P., Schunemann, H.J., Jaeschke, R. and Guyatt, G.H. (2005) 'Validity of composite end points in clinical trials', *British Medical Journal*, 330 (7491): 594–6.

Moore, D.A., Goodall, R.L., Ives, N.J., Hooker, M., Gazzard, B.G. and Easterbrook, P.J. (2000) 'How generalizable are the results of large randomized controlled trials of antiretroviral therapy?', *HIV Medicine*, 1 (3): 149–54.

Moseley, J.B., O'Malley, K., Petersen, N.J., Menke, T.J., Brody, B.A., Kuykendall, D.H., Hollingsworth, J.C., Ashton, C.M. and Wray, N.P. (2002) 'A controlled trial of arthroscopic surgery for osteoarthritis of the knee', *New England Journal of Medicine*, 347 (2): 81–8.

National Institute for Health Research (2012) *Efficacy and Mechanism Evaluation Programme: Data Monitoring and Ethics Committee*: www.eme.ac.uk/investigators/pdfs/DMECGuidelines.pdf (accessed Oct. 2012).

Rendell, J.M., Merritt, R.K. and Geddes, J. (2008) 'Incentives and disincentives to participation by clinicians in randomised controlled trials', *Cochrane Database of Systematic Reviews,* issue 2.

Schulz, K.F., Altman, D.G. and Moher, D. (2010) 'CONSORT 2010 statement: updated guidelines for reporting parallel group randomised trials', *British Medical Journal,* 340: c332.

Senn, S. (1994) 'Testing for baseline balance in clinical trials', *Stat Med,* 13 (17): 1715–26.

Silcocks, P. (2012) 'How many strata in an RCT? A flexible approach', *British Journal of Cancer,* 106 (7): 1259–61.

Sloan, J., Symonds, T., Vargas-Chanes, D. and Fridley, B. (2003) 'Practical guidelines for assessing the clinical significance of health-related quality of life changes within clinical trials', *Drug Information Journal,* 37 (1): 23–31.

Swan, J., Robertson, M. and Evans, S. (2009) *Managing Clinical Research in the UK: Evidence on the Challenges of Conducting Clinical Research Projects in the UK*: www.qmul.ac.uk/docs/research/65669.pdf (accessed Oct. 2012).

The Lancet (2010) 'Strengthening the credibility of clinical research', 375 (9722): 1225.

Treweek, S., McCormack, K., Abalos, E., Campbell, M., Ramsay, C. and Zwarenstein, M. (2006) 'The Trial Protocol Tool: the PRACTIHC software tool that supported the writing of protocols for pragmatic randomized controlled trials', *Journal of Clinical Epidemiology,* 59 (11): 1127–33.

Treweek, S., Pitkethly, M., Cook, J., Kjeldstrøm, M., Taskila, T., Johansen, M., Sullivan, F., Wilson, S., Jackson, C., Jones, R. and Mitchell, E. (2010) 'Strategies to improve recruitment to randomised controlled trials', *Cochrane Database of Systematic Reviews,* issue 4.

Tyler, K.M., Normand, S.L. and Horton, N.J. (2011) 'The use and abuse of multiple outcomes in randomized controlled depression trials', *Contemporary Clinical Trials,* 32 (2): 299–304.

UK Clinical Research Collaborative (2012) *UKCRC Registered Clinical Trials Units*: www.ukcrc-ctu.org.uk/ (accessed Oct. 2012).

Van Reekum, R., Clarke, D., Conn, D., Herrmann, N., Eryavec, G., Cohen, T. and Ostrander, L. (2002) 'A randomized, placebo-controlled trial of the discontinuation of long-term antipsychotics in dementia', *International Psychogeriatrics,* 14 (2): 197–210.

Williamson, P., Altman, D., Blazeby, J., Clarke, M. and Gargon, E. (2011) 'The COMET (core outcome measures in effectiveness trials) initiative', *Trials,* 12 (suppl. 1): A70.

12

SURVEYS

Roy Powell

- To understand the main purpose of a survey and know when to use the survey method
- To recognise the main sources of potential errors when applying the method and know how to minimise them
- To appreciate the main advantages and disadvantages of the different modes of data collection
- To appreciate some of the practical and ethical issues that must be considered when implementing the survey method

Introduction

Most readers will be very familiar with the idea of a survey. Surveys and the results that come from them, regularly feature in our personal and professional lives, for example, consumer satisfaction surveys, electoral voting intentions survey or a workplace staff survey. The survey is a method of collecting information, from a sample of individuals from the target population. This makes the survey a relatively efficient way to collect information. This is commonly achieved by researchers interviewing individuals (face-to-face, by telephone or on the internet), mailing out questionnaires to individuals for self-completion and return, or by inviting individuals to complete an online questionnaire. However although surveys are commonplace in health services research, they need thought to ensure that the survey method is appropriate to answer your research question. Once we have determined that a survey is appropriate, we then need to carry out the survey according to best practice. That is, to generate, analyse and report valid and reliable data and findings.

Surveys are commonly used to measure an individual's knowledge, attitudes, behaviour and preferences as well as collect factual information, such as age, sex or details of a particular health condition. They are also useful to collect longitudinal data at various time points. Surveys can be qualitative or quantitative. Which paradigm you choose will depend on your overall research questions and aims (please see Chapters 6: 'Quantitative Methodology'; and 7: 'Qualitative Data Collection'). Surveys could incorporate both paradigms, for example, a quantitative survey incorporating some open, qualitative questions, or if you were conducting a mixed-method study, you could combine a quantitative survey with other qualitative methods such as focus groups (please see Chapter 8: 'Mixed Methods').

A crucial element in planning a research study is to select a method that is appropriate to the research question being asked. The purpose of a survey is often to estimate some prevalence (or proportion), or a mean (or average) value. For example:

1. Have you ever been told by a doctor that you have psoriasis (skin condition)?

- Yes
- No

By calculating the total for 'Yes' you get and subtract from your total of 'No' answers you will obtain the prevalence of psoriasis in your sample.

2. How many times have you visited your family doctor in the last month?

This can be free text where they write the figure down. You can then add them up and divide by the number of respondents to obtain the mean number of family doctor visits per month.

Measures such as these can contribute towards many objectives often seen in health services research, for example:

- *To evaluate health services need.* An epidemiological survey study ascertained mental health prevalence, co-morbidity, disability and health service use (Andrews et al., 2001). Surveys such as these can help us to ensure appropriate health care provision, for now and the future.

- *To monitor trends.* The National Institute of Drug Abuse (National Institutes of Health, United States of America, http://www.drugabuse.gov, accessed Jan. 2013) conduct a yearly survey to measure drug use amongst school-aged children. Once again, this can help us identify health provision for now and the future, but also any issues of note such as a new type of drug being used.

- *To measure health outcomes.* Health outcomes are often measured before and after an intervention to determine its effect. For instance, Dworkin et al. (2009) used the McGill pain questionnaire in a study of a new analgesia.

- *To assess experiences of care.* The series of national inpatient surveys (DeCourcy et al., 2012) conducted in the National Health Service (NHS) in the UK have provided insights into patients' views on their experiences of hospital care for over 10 years.

- *To formulate and test hypotheses.* As illustration, Gartner et al. (2012) used survey data to test the 'hardening' hypothesis in smokers in Australia. According to this hypothesis, persons who continue to smoke cigarettes in the face of strong societal disapproval and discouragement will be more nicotine dependent and less likely to quit than those people who have already quit. Contrary to the theory, they found little evidence that the population of Australian smokers was hardening, as the prevalence of smoking continued to decline. These findings will help shape future public health strategies aimed at reducing smoking prevalence to near zero.

Advantages and disadvantages of survey study design

The advantages of the survey design largely relate to efficiency. Its efficiency lies in the use of appropriate statistical (typically random) sampling of the population of interest (please see Chapter 17: 'Sampling'). When combined with appropriately designed and tested data collection tools and methods, and analysed with appropriate statistical analysis techniques, the approach generates robust findings. These can then be generalised from the sample to the rest of the target population with calculable degrees of confidence. The survey study design is therefore relatively cost-effective when compared with other approaches.

The design is also flexible as it offers a range of methods for implementation according to sample characteristics and study requirements such as cost and time constraints. These include: (a) postal surveys – enabling sampling of a relatively large number of individuals across widely spread geographical areas; (b) face-to-face interviews – to collect data on more complex issues and improve response rates; and (c) online surveys, which could be self-completed, or 'face-to-face' using software such as Skype. The final advantage of using surveys is that they generally pose few ethical problems, particularly postal questionnaires, as they are not intrusive and they can be completed anonymously.

There are several disadvantages of the survey method. The first is due to the possibility of selective or low response rates, only those within the sample who have particularly strong views or feelings on the survey topic respond, for example. This can give misleading results if you do not consider this possibility or take steps to check the generalisability of the data. Secondly, studies have shown that respondents may under or overestimate in their replies. This is common in health-behaviour-related surveys regarding topics such as alcohol or tobacco consumption, healthy eating or participation in physical exercise. Thirdly, the representativeness of a sample is predicated on having a complete and accurate sampling frame; if this is not available or possible, then the generalisability of the findings is dubious. Finally, interview surveys require skilled and experienced interviewers to help minimise potential bias and leading questions that would invalidate the findings.

Error in surveys

The disadvantages of surveys mainly relate to potential sources of error that arise within the method, although most, if not all, methods of research will be open to some kind of error. Error in surveys comprises two elements: (i) sampling error, and (ii) non-sampling (systematic) error, i.e. bias.

Sampling error

The aim of sampling is to draw a representative sample. A representative sample is one that has the same characteristics as the population from which it is drawn. How well a sample represents the target population depends to a large extent on the quality of the sampling frame, the method of selecting the sample from the sampling frame and the sample size (further information on sampling in Chapter 17). Sampling error is the variability that arises simply through the process of collecting data from a sample rather than every single individual in the population of interest, i.e. a census, which would give a sampling error of zero. By chance alone, it is likely that the sample selected will differ slightly in some way from the population. This difference, or sampling error, is one that can be quantified in the variables being measured by the survey. Thus, a survey sample will generate a sampling error greater than zero (as there will always be some error).

One way of reducing sampling error in a survey is by determining an appropriate sample size, as there is an association between size and error and one general rule holds true: the larger the sample size the smaller the sampling error (please see Table 17.5 for an example). However, calculating the sample size for a survey can be tricky. First, surveys will usually aim to provide estimates of a number of different characteristics. For instance, in a survey evaluating outpatients departments, you may want to assess patient satisfaction with the cleanliness of the clinic area, the attitude of the staff, the acceptability of the time spent waiting to be seen, the information they received, etc. The required precision for these different estimates is likely to vary, which in turn will affect the sample size required. Second, researchers will typically want to drill down into estimates for different subgroups within the sample, for example, what are the estimates of patient satisfaction for different outpatient clinical specialties such as cardiology or rheumatology? In such studies, the minimally adequate sample size needs to be determined not by the estimates for the total population, but rather for the smaller subgroups.

Systematic error

Non-sampling errors are those unrelated to the sampling process. They are subdivided into two main types.

Administrative errors

Administrative errors include errors made in the implementation of a sampling plan, or during data collection and analysis, such as incorrect recording of data or data entry mistakes, or even deliberate mistakes introduced by the researcher designed to fix, fake or misrepresent data. These errors are commonly due to researcher carelessness, confusion, neglect or omission. The majority of administrative errors can be minimised by having detailed procedural steps laid out for each task in the administration of the survey which are followed, checked off and double-checked as progress is made through each step of the survey.

Respondent error

This type of error is a major potential source of survey error of which there are two types: non-response bias and response bias. Non-response bias arises from the survey's non-respondents, i.e. those people in the sample who do not take part. This may be due to a number of reasons, from those who simply refuse to provide data, to those who did not receive the survey as they were in hospital for instance. There may also be participants who were unable to supply the required data due to other reasons such as illness, or low literacy skills that preclude their completion of the questionnaire.

Methods are available to minimise non-response bias. These vary by the mode of survey administration. For instance, telephone survey response rates benefit from having interviewers that are available to make appointments at times that are convenient to respondents, or by sending respondents an advance information sheet clearly informing them of the purposes of the project, and ensuring the confidentiality of their responses. For mail surveys, it is generally true that a professionally produced and attractive looking questionnaire with a prepaid reply envelope and clear instructions on how to complete the task will benefit response rates (McColl et al., 2001).

As important is the extent to which you follow up on non-responders. There is a balance to be struck, however, between a researcher's persistence with the aim of achieving a good response rate and a person's right not to feel coerced into participating or feel excessive intrusion into their lives from repeated attempts by the researcher to secure their participation. General common sense and researcher professionalism should prevail in this area, and the checks and balances made by an ethics committee provide a moderating function. There are also time and financial implications to following up non-responders, as can be seen in the case study.

Case study

A mail survey is to be carried out to ascertain people's satisfaction with their family doctor. To ensure that there is a representative sample of the population and to ensure that the analysis is fully powered, a sample size of 500 is needed. Following the initial distribution of the questionnaire, two reminders will be sent to non-respondents, the first of which will include another copy of the questionnaire. Reply-paid envelopes will be included with the initial mailing and the first reminder. It is anticipated that 40% of those contacted, i.e. 200 patients, will respond to the initial distribution. Of the remaining 60%, i.e. 300 patients, 90 participants (30%) will respond to the first reminder, while 40%, i.e. 84 participants, of the residual 30%, i.e. 210 participants, will respond to the second reminder.

Using this information the following resource requirements can be calculated:

- Number of questionnaires = 500 + 300 for initial mailing + first reminder
- Number of cover letters = 500 + 300 + 210 for all three mailings
- Number of large envelopes (to hold the questionnaire):
  a. for posting out = 500 + 300 for initial mailing + first reminder
  b. for returning completed questionnaires = 500 + 300 to be enclosed with initial mailing + first reminder
- Number of small envelopes = 210 for second reminder.

On top of this you must allocate substantial administration time, e.g. photocopying, putting in envelopes, etc. For more detailed guidance regarding the personnel, knowledge and resources required for implementing a survey please see McColl et al. (2001).

One metric for evaluating non-response is the response rate. The appropriate method for calculating a survey's response rate is to divide the number of people who complete and return the survey by the total number of people who were sampled and express this as a percentage. This is helpful to know, and studies should always report the response rate. There is no universally agreed standard for

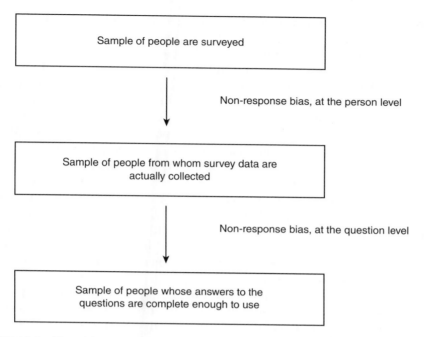

Sample of people are surveyed

Non-response bias, at the person level

Sample of people from whom survey data are
actually collected

Non-response bias, at the question level

Sample of people whose answers to the
questions are complete enough to use

FIGURE 12.1   Bias – the steps between the target population and the sample of data analysed

a minimum acceptable response rate, but it is clear that data from very low response rates for example, 5, 10 or even 20%, are likely to be systematically different from the target population of interest.

Response rate alone is not the complete picture, as studies have shown that it is not a good predictor of non-response error. To explore the impact of a non-response rate, some understanding of the bias from the non-responders needs to be assessed, i.e. how the non-responders may systematically differ from the responders. To do this, one might look at the basic demographics of the non-responders and compare them to the responders (for example, have more females than males responded?), and then assess the extent to which such a non-response is likely to impact on the survey estimates. Figure 12.1 shows where systematic bias can be introduced during the data-collecting period.

The second type of respondent error is response bias. Response bias occurs when respondents answer questions in a way that consciously or unconsciously misrepresents the truth. There are a number of different types or mechanisms of response bias to be aware of.

Acquiescence bias occurs when respondents tend to concur with a particular view or agree with all questions, specifically those positively phrased, regardless of their content. It is sometimes the tendency of a respondent to agree with a statement when they are in doubt or lack knowledge on a particular subject. Designers of questionnaires attempt to minimise the effect of this bias by employing a balance of positively and negatively phrased questions or switching the order of responses periodically in a measurement scale, for example, from 'Strongly agree – Strongly disagree' to 'Strongly disagree – Strongly agree'. Face-to-face interviews are more likely to provoke acquiescence bias than anonymous postal surveys.

Social desirability bias results from the desire of respondents to present themselves in the best possible light, in order to gain prestige, or appear in a different social role. It is manifest in the over-reporting of desirable behaviours, and under-reporting of undesirable behaviours, and is apparent in health-related surveys, for example, smoking habits, alcohol consumption, participation in exercise. Methods exist to help reduce this problem, including assurances of confidentiality and anonymity, checking responses against known 'facts' or objective measures, such as carbon monoxide readings for smoking, and indirect questioning. Social desirability bias may occur when behaviour questions are asked after knowledge questions on a related topic, presenting questions on personal dietary behaviour after items on knowledge of good eating practice for example. Social desirability bias is more likely to be a factor in surveys where there is social interaction with the researcher, such as face-to-face or telephone interviews, rather than surveys without direct interaction such as postal surveys.

If you are conducting your survey using interviews, bias can also be introduced by the interviewers who can not only affect response rates but also the extent to which respondents give inaccurate answers and other data inconsistencies. These anomalies are due to a number of potential reasons including interviewer training and experience, interviewer bias, i.e. opinion or prejudice of the interviewer which may influence the results, precision in recall and coding of responses. Training and supervision of interviewers, including peer observation, feedback and encouraging reflective practice, together with good survey design, can all help reduce these factors, as can choosing interviewers who represent the participant, such as similar ethnicity, age bracket or sex, or you may wish to recruit patients to collect this data (please see Chapter 16: 'Patient and Public Involvement').

Tools for collecting data

A search of the literature will show that there are literally thousands of surveys and questionnaires already in existence, each designed to measure particular beliefs, attitudes or opinions in a wide variety of health-related areas. Bowling's books *Measuring Disease* (2001) and *Measuring Health* (2004) are excellent starting points, as they provide an extensive list of questionnaire material in health-related areas. Both books summarise the essential background material on the construction, reliability and validity of each data collection tool.

It is far easier and preferable to use an existing questionnaire for a number of reasons. First, it takes time, resources and expertise to create a valid and reliable questionnaire (see Powell et al., 2009), so being able to side-step the development work is an obvious benefit. Second, it enables the selection of a reliable and valid questionnaire with tested and published psychometric properties (see Oppenheim, 2000, for details). This provides assurance to grant reviewers that any proposed new study is, in this respect, methodologically sound. Third, it will facilitate comparison of newly generated data with those previously published. There are potential disadvantages in utilising previously published questionnaires and these include: cost (the questionnaire may only be available to use under licence for a fee); copyright issues (permission may need to be sought from the author or holder of the copyright to use the questionnaire); and suitability (the questionnaire may be too general and may not be specific enough to answer your hypotheses or research questions). To be able to search for relevant survey tools, and to critically appraise them in order to determine their applicability to your research project, it is important that you become aware of the key terminology for the psychometric properties of questionnaires:

- *Test–retest reliability* – used to assess the consistency of a measure from one time to another. This is done by conducting the survey at two different time points with the same participants. The closer the results the greater the test–retest reliability.

- *Internal consistency reliability* – the extent to which items on a scale contribute to a single construct. Similar questions on a survey may well be used to gauge internal consistency reliability. For example, within a survey on depression, responses to the statement 'I always feel like crying' would be expected to correlate with responses to the statement 'I always feel sad', in order for the scale to demonstrate good levels of internal consistency reliability.

- *Face validity* – occurs where a survey appears to be valid to respondents.

- *Predictive validity* – the ability of a questionnaire to predict the results of an outcome or event in the future. For example, the ability to predict future health care utilisation using a health frailty scale.

- *Content validity* – the extent to which a questionnaire covers all of the constructs in the domain of the subject in question. This is established by referring the questionnaire to an expert panel. For example, in an obesity scale you would not only expect to see questions regarding diet, but exercise habits too.

- *Concurrent validity* – the extent to which a questionnaire correlates with another more established test that measures the same subject area. For example, if a new scale measured levels of depression, you may expect its results to correlate with those from the Hamilton Rating Scale for Depression (Hamilton, 1960).

- *Construct validity* – the degree to which a questionnaire measures the trait or theoretical construct that it is intended to measure. For example, you would expect a depression scale to identify clinically depressed patients.

- *Sensitivity (responsiveness)* – is the ability to detect relevant changes over time, such as detecting progressive memory impairment with a cognitive function questionnaire, in people with prodromal Alzheimer's disease.

Although it is recommended that you search the literature and use previously published questionnaires or survey tools rather than create your own, if you do need to develop new measurement scales you can refer to Streiner and Norman (2008), or if you are looking for further detail on questionnaire design for surveys involving health care staff and patients you can refer to McColl et al. (2001).

Modes of survey data collection

The choice of data collection mode, mail, telephone, face-to-face interview or internet, is an important step in the survey design process. Findings from the literature suggest that no single mode of administration is superior in all respects or in all settings. McColl et al. (2001) suggest, therefore, that the choice of mode of administration should be made on a survey-by-survey basis, taking into account the following.

Study population

Research looking at the health needs of the homeless would not be suited to postal, telephone or internet modes but more suited to face-to-face interviews at a homeless shelter, for example.

Survey topic

The more anonymous the mode, the more honest the answers, therefore surveys involving sensitive issues, such as illicit drug taking, are perhaps best approached with anonymous postal or internet survey modes and not conducted face-to-face in order to minimise bias.

Volume of data to be collected

A survey with many qualitative questions, or a lot of scales, is best conducted face-to-face or by telephone. This will help with the response rate.

Complexity of data to be collected

If a survey requires responses to scenarios or lengthy questions, then face-to-face or telephone interviews are preferable, where the participant can ask questions if they do not understand. If a participant does not understand a question on a self-completion questionnaire they will either not complete the survey, or omit questions.

Resources available

Your budget, length of time for your research and access to support staff will influence your choice of mode. For example, face-to-face surveys not only take the time of the interview itself, but also time and expense for the travel to the participant's home, whereas although postal surveys can be quicker, you need to budget for the photocopying and postage.

Table 12.1 sets out the advantages and disadvantages of each mode of collection.

TABLE 12.1 Main advantages and disadvantages of each mode of collection

	Face-to-face interviews	Telephone interviews	Self-completion/ postal questionnaires	Internet*
Advantages	• Ability to handle long questionnaires, complex questions and open-ended questions • Control over the interview is high • Use of visual aids • Low possibility of respondent misunderstanding • Missing data or item non-response is low • Achieve high-response rate	• High response rates • High relevance to the interviewee • Anonymity is moderate • Costs are moderate • Control over the interview is high • Missing data or item non-response is low • Easy to call back or follow-up respondents • Adaptable to computer technology • Ability to reach a large number of geographically spread population	• Low cost • Ability to reach a large number of geographically spread population • Interviewer bias avoided • Less open to social desirability bias • Adaptable to computer technology e.g. scanning of completed questionnaires • Anonymity high	• Low cost • Ability to reach a large number of geographically spread population • Targets individuals by email • Less open to social desirability bias • Anonymity high • Use of visual aids • Data entry is automatic • Ensures consistent data coding • Built in checks and prompts to ensure all questions are completed • Automatic 'routing' or signposting to appropriate questions
Disadvantages	• Can gather unnecessary data • Anonymity is low • Costs are high (interviewers, training and travel) • Open to interviewer bias • Open to social desirability bias	• Access or sampling problems with some target groups • No use of visual aids • Some possibility of respondent misunderstanding • Unable to ask long questions	• Low response rates • Questions are mostly closed • Possibility that respondents misunderstand questions • Administration time high • Missing data or item non-response high • No control over who completes the questionnaire	• Sampling issues e.g. construction of a sampling frame and non-probabilistic sampling • Low response rates • No control over who completes the questionnaire

*Readers can find further information on internet survey methods in Chapter 13: 'The Internet as a Research Medium'.

Researchers will often combine more than one mode of administration in order to increase the response rate. If you do choose more than one mode of administration, you must record which mode was used to collect that participant's data to allow post-hoc analysis to determine whether there are systematic differences between modes; as the case study illustrates, care should be adopted with this approach.

Case study

Erhart et al. (2009) studied the possible differences from using telephone and mail survey modes to measure health-related quality of life and emotional and behavioural problems in children and adolescents.

   Small but relevant differences were found from the responses generated by the different survey modes. The effects appeared to be different among children and their parents for some domains in the measures. They conclude that these effects could bias results when comparing children and parents. Moreover, these could be of practical relevance when estimating important public health measures such as the prevalence of mental health problems.

Survey administration and implementation

To successfully manage and implement a survey, a range of personnel, knowledge and resources are required (for further detail on this please see McColl et al., 2001). Once all of this is in place and you have determined the most appropriate and valid survey tool with which to answer your research question, you will need to obtain ethical approval after which you will need to ascertain its applicability to your target population is appropriate. This is done by a process called piloting.

Piloting

Piloting the whole survey process is highly recommended. This should include all of the key processes from drawing a sample from a dummy sampling frame, administering the questionnaire to a small number of volunteers, and entering and analysing data. Piloting of questionnaires is particularly important when bespoke questions have been developed, or when established questions or scales are to be used in a novel setting or with a novel population. McColl et al. (2001) note some of the main functions of piloting:

- To test the survey procedures overall under 'main survey' conditions
- To check how respondents cope with the questionnaire and instructions
- To check whether respondents understand the questions as intended
- To provide better estimates on which to base sample size calculations
- To estimate the rate of, and speed of, response to the main survey
- To smooth coordination and establish systems and routines.

Ethics

Before piloting your survey you will need ethical approval in place (please see Chapter 15: 'Designing and Conducting an Ethical Research Study'). It is acknowledged that your survey or procedure may change slightly after the pilot, however this is usually regarded as a minor amendment for which approval is given quickly by the chairman, rather than you having to go through the whole procedure again. There are a number of ethical issues with surveys requiring consideration and planning.

- Initial contact with a potential respondent, e.g. a covering letter, invitation to participate, etc., should be from a person with whom the respondent would expect correspondence, such as a member of their health care team, and not a researcher unknown to them.
- Returning a postal questionnaire is regarded as giving consent to take part in a research survey.
- Repeated reminders – more than three is generally considered unacceptable.
- Anonymity – there are two levels of anonymity to consider with postal or online surveys:

  ○ Fully anonymous means that there is no identifier on a questionnaire, i.e. there is no way to link a returned questionnaire with a respondent. This means that selective distribution of reminders to non-responders is precluded. Instead, reminders have to be sent to the whole sample which may annoy those whom have previously completed and returned their questionnaires.

  ○ Linked anonymous means that there is an identifier on a questionnaire, such as a participant number, that can be linked to the participant's contact details (held securely and confidentially on a database) by the researcher. Hence selective distribution of reminders to non-responders is possible.

- Confidentiality – if you assure confidentiality to your participants, this means that:

  ○ Only members of the research team can access participant details (such as name and address) or completed questionnaires and only for uses associated with the purposes or implementation of the survey.

  ○ Participant details and questionnaires will be stored in secure password-protected computer systems or locked rooms and cupboards.

  ○ Identifiable information of participants are not revealed to any third party.

Analysing survey data

Analysing survey data is performed to relate the results back to the original purpose of the survey, for example, to measure ..., to assess ..., etc. It is important to note that analysis should be conducted in accordance with the plan that was generated while designing the survey and not left as an after-thought once the data have been collected. This is to help ensure that the data collected and the planned analysis are coherent and facilitates interpretation of data and the drawing of conclusions. There should be no temptation to 'data-dredge' or go on a 'fishing expedition', looking for various interesting relationships within the data collected but you should stick to the original research question/hypothesis. If your survey is qualitative, or incorporates qualitative components, you would analyse the data according to whichever approach you have chosen (please see Chapter 20: 'Qualitative Analysis').

To analyse quantitative data, two main steps are required; first, the survey results are transformed into data files suitable for analysis (this step requires coding, data entry and cleaning), and second the analysis itself. Coding is the process of turning questionnaire responses into standard categories represented by numbers, for example, a five-point Likert scale coded as 'Strongly agree' = 1, 'Agree' = 2, 'Neither agree nor disagree' = 3, 'Disagree' = 4 and 'Strongly disagree' = 5. The coding scheme needs to be applied consistently and include standard codes for other eventualities such as missing data (often 9, 99, or 999), or 'not applicable' (often 8, 88, or 888). Do not choose a code that could be a genuine reply though, such as for 'age' you would not choose 99 to represent missing data if this age is a possible answer, instead you would chose 999. For each questionnaire, the coded response for each question is entered into a database or statistical software package. Such software can provide initial quality control measures, for example, permitting the entry of only legal codes in any particular field. However, even when using software, errors can occur in data entry.

Errors can be identified and rectified through data cleaning either manually by checking each entry, or automatically, for example by using software functions to check minimum and maximum values in fields. Other measures to check data reliability are also considered best practice such as review by multiple researchers or double data entry (Baerlocher et al., 2010), whereby the data is entered into two separate databases and when complete, merging the databases together to identify errors (if no errors are made they should merge perfectly). Checks for the consistency of variables can also be carried out. For instance the location of a general practice visited should not appear if the participant had already answered that they did not visit a general practice. Consistency checking is especially important for dates, for example to check that for a given hospital inpatient episode, the date of discharge from hospital comes no earlier than the date of admission, and the dates of all in-hospital tests and procedures do not fall outside these two dates. Another common error is ticking two option boxes, such as both 'Blue' and 'Green' for eye colour, when only one value may be specified. An invalid value should be changed to another value only if there is confidence as to the reason for the error, otherwise either the original value should remain or it should be recorded as 'missing data'. It is important that a log is recorded of all potential data errors, and how they were dealt with so that they are all traceable at a later stage if required.

Analysis of survey data draws on a number of different statistical methods (some specialised), for instance, calculating a response rate and adjusting for non-response; adjusting for items that were not answered; estimating sampling errors and calculating other statistics about the probable relationship between sample estimates and the characteristics of the population (Fowler, 2009); also assessing change over time using repeated cross-sectional surveys. These techniques are beyond the scope of this chapter and advice from a statistician is recommended.

Readers can also find further information on general approaches to quantitative data analysis in Chapter 19.

Summary

- The survey method is widely used in health services research; it offers an efficient and versatile approach.
- Surveys can be quantitative, qualitative or a mixture of both.
- There are various modes for survey data collection. Which one is appropriate for your project depends upon the research question, population and resources available.
- It is advisable to use an existing validated survey wherever possible, as survey design takes a lot of thought and effort.
- Successful implementation of this method requires knowledge of the main sources of potential error and how to minimise them.
- The advice of a statistician during the planning and analysis phases of a project which uses a questionnaire is strongly recommended.

Questions for Discussion

1. Achieving a useful response rate is often the most challenging element when undertaking a survey. What steps might you take during the planning and implementation stages of your survey to increase your response rate?

2. You are planning a postal survey using a questionnaire designed to gather data on patients' views on the quality of service they received in a hospital Emergency Department. What are the main potential sources of error and how could they be minimised?

Further Reading

Blair, J., Blair, E.A. and Czaja, R.F. (2012) *Designing Surveys: A Guide to Decisions and Procedures* (3rd edn). Thousand Oaks, CA: SAGE.

Fowler, F.J., Jr. (2009) *Survey Research Methods* (4th edn). Thousand Oaks, CA: SAGE.

References

Andrews, G., Henderson, S. and Hall, W. (2001) 'Prevalence, comorbidity, disability and service utilisation: overview of the Australian National Mental Health Survey', *British Journal of Psychiatry*, 178: 145–53.

Appleby, J. and Deeming, C. (2001) 'Inverse care law', *Health Service Journal*, 1110 (5670): 37.

Baerlocher, M.O., O'Brien, J., Newton, M., Gautam, T. and Noble, J. (2010) 'Data integrity, reliability and fraud in medical research', *European Journal of Internal Medicine,* 21 (1): 40–5.

Boyd, J. (2010) *Diabetes Patient Experience Project: Guidance Manual for Diabetes Patient Survey.* Oxford: Picker Institute Europe.

Bowling, A. (2001) *Measuring Disease: A Review of Disease Specific Quality of Life Measurement Scales* (2nd edn). Buckingham: Open University Press.

Bowling, A. (2004) *Measuring Health: A Review of Quality of Life Measurement Scales* (3rd edn). Buckingham: Open University Press.

DeCourcy, A., West, E. and Barron, D. (2012) 'The National Adult Inpatient Survey conducted in the English National Health Service from 2002 to 2009: how have the data been used and what do we know as a result?', *BMC Health Services Research*, 12: 71.

Dworkin, R.H., Turk, D.C., Revicki, D.A., Harding, G., Coyne, K.S., Peirce-Sandner, S., Bhagwat, D., Everton, D., Burke, L.B., Cowan, P., Farrar, J.T., Hertz, S., Maxi, M.B., Rappaport, B.A. and Melzack, R. (2009) 'Development and initial validation of an expanded and revised version of the Short-form McGill Pain Questionnaire (SF-MPQ-2)®', *Pain*, 144: 35–42.

Erhart, M., Wetzel, R.M., Krügel, A. and Ravens-Sieberer, U. (2009) 'Effects of phone versus mail survey methods on the measurement of health-related quality of life and emotional and behavioural problems in adolescents', *BMC Public Health,* 9: 491.

Fowler, F.J., Jr. (2009) *Survey Research Methods* (4th edn). Thousand Oaks, CA: SAGE.

Gartner, C., Scollo, M., Marquart, L., Mathews, R. and Hall, W. (2012) 'Analysis of national data shows mixed evidence of hardening among Australian smokers', *Australian and New Zealand Journal of Public Health*, 36 (5): 408–14.

Greco, M., Powell, R. and Sweeney, K. (2003) 'The Improving Practice Questionnaire (IPQ): a practical tool for general practices seeking patient views', *Education for Primary Care*, 14, 440–8.

Hamilton, M. (1960) 'A rating scale for depression', *Journal of Neurology, Neurosurgery and Psychiatry*, 23: 56–62.

Hart, J.T. (1971) 'The inverse care law', *The Lancet,* i: 405–12.

McColl, E., Jacoby, A., Thomas, L., Soutter, J., Bamford, C., Steen, N., Thomas, R., Harvey, E., Garratt, A. and Bond, J. (2001) 'Design and use of questionnaires: a review of best practice applicable to surveys of health service staff and patients', *Health Technology Assessment,* 5: 31.

O'Cathain, A., Murphy, E. and Nicholl, J. (2010) 'Three techniques for integrating data in mixed methods studies', *British Medical Journal*, 341: 1147–50.

Oppenheim, A.N. (2000) *Questionnaire Design*. London: Continuum.

Powell, R.J., Powell, H.J., Baker, L.H. and Greco, M.J. (2009) 'Patient Partnership in Care (PPiC): a new instrument for measuring patient-professional partnership in the treatment of long term conditions', *Journal of Management & Marketing in Healthcare*, 2 (4): 325–42.

Reeves, R. and Seccombe, I. (2008) 'Do patient surveys work? The influence of a national survey programme on local quality-improvement initiatives', *Qual Saf Health Care*, 17: 437–41.

Streiner, D.L. and Norman, G.R. (2008) *Health Measurement Scales: A Practical Guide to their Development and Use* (4th edn). Oxford: Oxford University Press.

13

THE INTERNET AS A RESEARCH MEDIUM

Penny Benford and Dawn-Marie Walker

Learning Objectives

- To explore aspects of the research process which may benefit from being conducted online
- To identify the pragmatic and methodological issues and challenges which should be considered in relation to online research methods
- To gain an understanding of specific internet-based research methods including online surveys, interviews, focus groups and gathering data from social media

Introduction

There are many potential benefits which can be conferred on traditional research procedures when implemented via the internet. Additionally, its unique qualities offer researchers new possibilities beyond those which would otherwise be achievable. The internet enables rapid digital data transfer, remote access to other computers and information stores anywhere in the world, and a range of possibilities for interpersonal communication including real-time text chat, audio/video conferencing, voice telephony, as well as email. Social network sites enable us to keep in touch with people, make new contacts and share with others our own thoughts, news, photos and videos. For the purposes of this chapter, we will mostly focus on internet-based research methods which are mainly textual in nature (rather than those which are predominantly audio-visual), since these formats perhaps offer the greatest degree of novelty, and potential to researchers, and are more widely used currently. However, internet technologies continue to evolve rapidly as we write. No doubt there is more for us to expect from the newer social media, as well as mobile technologies and other emerging phenomena.

What can the internet offer the researcher?

Economy and convenience

Clearly there are implications for time, cost and convenience at various points in the research process: participant recruitment, data collection, and data handling. Internet-based communication can reduce the necessity for travel, saving time and money; make it easier for participants to take part; and ensure the safety of both the researcher and the participant. Convenience of timing and location can also offer more privacy than, say, a face-to-face interview conducted in a participant's home, thereby allowing freer self-expression. Online methods can also speed up the rate at which data are returned, with particular benefits when data collection is repetitive or longitudinal in nature, and conferring economies in terms of postage, printing, data transcription and input. Such considerations may be particularly important for researchers with limited resources, projects requiring large data sets and preliminary studies in support of a funding application, such as pilot work. Additionally, the elimination of the process of transcription should reduce the potential for error and bias.

Participant access

Due to its size and geographical reach, the internet can put us in touch with a wide pool of potential research participants. Social network sites and online forums can help locate specific populations through pre-existing groups, or through the formation of new ones, and may be particularly useful for purposive or snowball sampling of hard-to-reach populations (Brickman-Bhutta, 2009). For some socially marginalised or hard-to-reach groups, the internet may provide a safe, accessible and, if desired, anonymous means by which they can participate in research from which they may otherwise have been inhibited from taking part. Researchers should remember, however, that internet access is not universally available and online methods may fail to reach all potential participants.

Research tool flexibility

The internet can provide flexibility in the way in which data collection tools are designed in order to offer alternative formats (audio, video or text) for participants according to personal need or preference. You can also include media, text, graphics, video, audio, etc., to enhance the content of a questionnaire or to enable experimental studies to take place online. Online questionnaires can be designed to minimise the burden on respondents, for example, questions can be automatically filtered, or 'branched', as a result of the answers selected to previous questions.

Interaction characterised by reduced presence

Internet-based communication can enable greater anonymity whilst at the same time allowing interactivity, which may be a more comfortable and acceptable way for participants to engage in research concerning sensitive subjects. Furthermore, the absence of non-verbal feedback, and the reduction of cues to social identity such as age, sex, social and ethnic background, may lessen the perception of a power differential between interviewer and interviewee. Theories of computer-mediated communication suggest that, due to its lack of social cues and relative anonymity, participants may be less inhibited and more open in their conversations when online (Walther, 1996).

A source of rich data

Online groups, blogs and social network sites offer a rich source of qualitative data produced by vast numbers of individuals, with personal experiences and insights on a vast array of topics, of which health issues are particularly prominent. Additionally, due to the reduction in time pressure and distractions characteristic of computer-mediated communication, particularly email, as well as the potential to reread the dialogue if typed, online interviews may produce data which combine the interpersonal nature of face-to-face interaction with the reflection of writing, making them excellent tools for qualitative research. It may even mediate between the qualitative–quantitative dichotomy (Seymour, 2001), with the potential to yield rich, reflective data whilst reducing researcher bias and the complicating aspects of non-verbal interaction.

Issues to consider

Technical requirements

The wide use of email and the availability of a range of specialised software have opened this approach to research to practically anyone with general computer literacy and equipment. Researcher-friendly tools are available to support online questionnaire design and construction, video or voice group conferencing, data processing and storage, and website design. Other tools that may be especially suitable for participants as they may already be using them are email, discussion boards, instant messaging, mailing lists and online chat rooms. As well as the technical requirements for designing the study, you should consider issues to maximise data security, including anti-virus and encryption software. A note of caution regarding survey software and administration sites is pertinent here: you should establish the security and ownership implications of the data collected, and whether they comply with your institution's guidelines. You will also need to consider the equipment and support requirements of your participants. A study may be compromised if the necessary hardware, software and skills are not already available or easily attainable to participants without causing undue inconvenience or disruption. Participants may have older computers with restricted bandwidth and speed of internet connection. Therefore try to use standard, widely available tools for data collection and bear in mind that current versions of software may not be available or easy to install on older machines with slower internet connection.

Sampling

Although there is a rapid growth in the size and activity of the internet population, there are discrepancies in its penetration between particular groups, the most digitally disadvantaged groups being people of lower income or educational level, people with disabilities, rural populations and the elderly (Dutton and Helsper, 2007). There is a risk therefore, of selection bias when using online research tools, and that their increased use will fail to include those people who are already subject to social exclusion offline. Nevertheless, the growing prevalence of the 'silver surfer' as the population ages, and the advent of smartphones and internet-ready televisions, should serve to reduce the 'digital divide', and internet users should become more representative of the general population over time. However, these more recent innovations require further development and standardisation to improve their potential to support online research methods. If you are going to collect data or recruit from a specific website, you should be aware of their user demographics. Users of social networking sites, for example, are typically younger (Lenhart, 2009), whilst mailing list users are more likely to be white, employed, married and parents (Best and Krueger, 2004).

Contacting potential research participants directly is more problematic via the internet than in more traditional types of research. Unless a sampling frame of internet users appropriate to your research question is available via another source, recruitment will most likely be achieved by posting information on websites, resulting in non-probability samples of participants (please see Chapter 17: 'Sampling'). This raises challenges regarding generalisability and bias, so that post-survey adjustments (weighting procedures) may be required. Furthermore, a lack of sampling frame can make it difficult to determine non-participant bias and rates of recruitment and attrition (please see Chapter 12: 'Surveys'). If approaching people via a social network site or an online group, you might get a general impression of sample frame characteristics from the number and demographic profiles of its users if available. However such data originate from self-identifying information supplied for the purposes of registration, and should therefore be treated with caution.

Approaching an organisation relevant to your target population to advertise and circulate the link to your research webpage may enable a more accurate estimate of the sampling frame size based on the size of their mailing list or number of members. Organisations may have certain requirements and/or charge for this service. The use of a counter to record visits to your research page may also help you estimate the proportion of people who opt to take part, after reading the study information although this may be skewed by multiple visits from single users. Attrition rates can also be difficult to ascertain when compared to a face-to-face situation since an incomplete survey could either be due to a technical disruption or the participant's wish to withdraw. Incorporating a 'withdraw' button into your interface may help to make this distinction. Similarly, a lack of response to a particular question could be due to not wanting to answer it, not understanding it or simply an omission. A 'decline' option could help you to differentiate between these, or having the survey designed so that participants cannot proceed if a question is unanswered.

Case study

A psychologist wants to conduct an exploratory study of the experiences of adults who go through the diagnostic investigations for Asperger syndrome (AS). AS is a high functioning form of autism, and individuals with AS are of average intelligence or above. Areas of difficulty typically include non-verbal aspects of social communication, and processing and retaining verbal information. However, due to their intellectual strengths and an ability to hide their impairment in straightforward situations, many individuals remain undiagnosed until late into adulthood. Arguably, the experience of an adult going through the diagnosis procedure is different to that experienced by a child.

As the participants are 'hard to reach' due to their difficulty with social communication, the internet may be a useful tool to locate participants, in addition to those who might be referred to the study by support services, as the internet has seen the emergence of a large number of online forums which put people with AS in touch with each other. The psychologist is aware that some people using these forums may not have a formal diagnosis, and are self-identifying themselves as having AS, or are considering undergoing diagnostic assessment. However, for this study, the perspectives of these individuals may enrich the data as well as providing the opportunity to follow some participants as they go through the process. To ensure that he obtains a sample reflecting a diversity of demographic factors, e.g. age, education, ethnicity, etc., he will also include traditional advertising via appropriate publications and organisations, such as support groups, further and higher educational establishments, specialised educational and employment providers, and residential and day support services. Organisations and charities which provide services for adults with autism will be also approached to advertise the study via their websites.

Online groups and netiquette

When approaching online groups for the purposes of recruiting participants and/or collecting data, researchers should be aware of the standards of online behaviour, i.e. netiquette, as this shows courtesy and respect, and should circumvent the possibility of alienation and non-responsiveness. Best practice is to ask the group moderator for permission to post to the group. Hewson (2003) provides some useful guidelines:

- Post participation requests to newsgroups or individual mailboxes – do not post study materials directly, as this can cause offence.
- State clearly the affiliation of the study to give it credibility and avoid hostile responses.
- Read postings to a newsgroup after posting a participation request in order to monitor whether the study is being discussed by members of the group (which could pose a threat to validity)!
- Send one or two follow-up postings (repeat requests) to newsgroups, as this has been found to generate further responses, but take care not to 'spam' a newsgroup or individual with repeated postings.

Referring to Hall et al. (2004), the Exploring Online Research Methods web resource (www.geog.le.ac.uk/orm, accessed March 2013) advises consideration of the following issues:

- The importance of the subject header used in any posting to a newsgroup, to assure no misunderstandings between the researcher and newsgroup members occur.
- Self-identification and self-presentation of the researcher are critical, as readers will form their evaluations about the credibility of the research and the researcher based on this. A formal verifiable, disclosed identity of the researcher, for example through a link to an institutional website, can increase this credibility (Madge and O'Connor, 2002), and shows respect and courtesy to members of the newsgroup.
- The ability to 'speak' the newsgroup's 'language', e.g. their use of jargon, acronyms, emoticons, etc., shows respect to the rules and conventions of the group.
- An awareness of the culture of the newsgroup should be attained through online acclimatisation or reading FAQs and archives prior to 'jumping in' in order to understand the nuances of group interactions. It will also prevent asking questions that could have been answered by an archive search.
- The researcher has an obligation to be 'up front' about the purpose, nature, procedures and risks of the research.

Validity, reliability and trustworthiness

Reduced researcher involvement and control

The main factor to consider in relation to the validity of data resulting from internet-mediated research is the level and nature of your involvement, and control over various aspects of the research process. However, these are also issues for other non-face-to-face methods of data collection, such as postal surveys. When compared to a face-to-face method, you will be less able to verify participant identity, or their level of engagement. If these factors are important for your study, consider other methods of data collection, which could still be internet-based, perhaps using video for example. There is also potentially less reliability in the way in which research interfaces are presented to participants due to variations in hardware and software. Differences in computers, monitors, browsers and internet connections may result in variations in the appearance and speed of the presentation of materials, with particular implications for studies which are more experimental in nature. Where variations of this type would be detrimental to your data, more traditional research designs may be more appropriate.

Hewson (2003) makes some useful recommendations to maximise the validity of data obtained by an online method. You should make it clear to participants when recruiting what is required in terms of software and hardware in order to take part. As with all research, clear, explicit instructions should be given to participants, and data collection tools should be piloted across a range of platforms. According to Hewson the most direct way of validating procedures is to conduct a comparative study using both internet and traditional modes of administration and then compare the data obtained. Additionally, the results from internet-mediated studies should be compared to expected trends as gained from the literature.

Online deception

Validity may also be compromised by *online disinhibition* whereby some people, due to a perception of online anonymity, act in ways uncharacteristic of their offline behaviour (Suler, 2004), which opens up the possibility of lying and deception by the participant. However, in his review of internet behaviour and virtual methods, Joinson (2005) argues that, when compared to offline formats, higher self-disclosure and lower social desirability (i.e. the tendency to present oneself in a positive light) characterises respondent behaviour in computerised research, particularly when sensitive topics are involved.

Ethical considerations

Online disclosure

Since participants cannot see the interviewer they may be more apt to disclose information they would not otherwise have done in other forms of communication

(Hiltz and Turoff, 1978; McCoyd and Kerson, 2006). This can be a concern for online interviews, in particular those which are less structured in nature and are conducted by email where the interaction between researcher and participant may continue over a long timescale, such that the participant may 'forget' that they are involved in research. Benford and Standen (2011) in their study involving email interviews employed various strategies to maintain participants' awareness of the online communication being research, including the use of an impersonal username in the interviewer's email address, for example, research.project@university.ac.uk rather than joe.bloggs@university.ac.uk; the inclusion of a link to the project website at the end of each email sent; and the use of wording pertinent to the interview process, for example, 'To continue with our interview ...'

Online privacy

Privacy is a widely debated issue amongst internet researchers, since the distinction between public and private domains online is not clearly defined, particularly if you want to use unsolicited data, for example, those contained in online discussions, blogs and social network sites. Even in those contexts which are seemingly public in nature (in that there are no access restrictions or explicit conditions restricting the reuse of materials by third parties), participants may have posted their comments and contributions with a different perception of privacy and most likely without the expectation that it could be used for research purposes. They may have the *illusion* of privacy since they may have had to become a member and obtain a password for participation, even though these may be easily attainable. Furthermore, they cannot see the people who read their messages. The key issue is whether the individual or group *considers* their postings to be public or private. It requires careful consideration and consultation to determine the complex issue of privacy in data such as these (please see Ess et al., 2002).

Although the internet can be a rich source of qualitative data, it is paramount that their use by researchers does not cause distress or disruption to the individuals or groups from which they originate. It is therefore recommended that the individual supplying the data, and where appropriate the site moderator, are contacted personally about the use of their data for research purposes.

Informed consent

Obtaining informed consent online can be convenient, economical and reduces the potential for coercion when compared to traditional interactions. However, the process is compromised due to difficulties verifying the identity and capacity of volunteers to give consent, and ensuring that they have accessed and understood the necessary information prior to giving consent. These issues are not unique to internet-based research however, and there are ways in which these issues may be addressed, such as presenting segmented information on different pages each requiring a click to accept before moving on. Participants may ask questions via email, phone or project website, although the extra effort needed for this may deter some participants. You should also consider whether it is sufficient for consent to be indicated electronically, by clicking an accept button on an online consent form, or whether legally verifiable signatures are required, in which case the option is for participants to download and print off the form to sign and return via email (scanned copy), fax or post, although the burden of doing this may reduce uptake.

Data security and confidentiality

Risks to data security online include: software viruses; human error resulting in data being sent to the wrong address; and access by hackers. It is therefore important that strategies to maximise data security are built in to the study design including:

- use of anti-virus software and password-protected databases;
- separating research data from personal identifying details, cross-referenced by unique identifying code numbers for the storage and transmission of data;
- monitoring access logs;
- prudent use of email, particularly those with attachments; instead use password-protected web resources to access study materials and research tools;
- use of encryption software for emails containing sensitive data;
- prompt transfer of data from the internet to your institutional secure server;
- regular back up of data files.

To protect the identity of participants, all personally identifiable details should be removed from the research data before reporting. This includes all names (personal, user, domain), email addresses, online pseudonyms, as well as references to specific places, people and events. It is possible that the location and identity of the author of web postings can be discovered with the use of search engines, therefore you may want to restrict the use of direct quotes in reports and publications resulting from your study.

Participant distress, withdrawal and debriefing

The voluntary nature of participation and the ability to withdraw from research at any time is core to the ethics of human research. It may be argued that participants in online studies are freer to do this due to the lack of presence of the researcher (Johns et al., 2004). The design of online studies should incorporate mechanisms for withdrawal, for example, building in a withdraw button in online questionnaires or synchronous interview interfaces. For email interviews, it is a good idea to set a time limit for responses after which an email will be resent, with an added statement enquiring whether the informant wishes to cease participation in the project.

When collecting data online there is a risk that the participant's emotional status is missed, or misinterpreted. Therefore when researching topics of a sensitive nature you may need to consider other study designs, or offer a choice of formats. It is also necessary to devise a way of debriefing your participants. This may involve ensuring they supply email or postal addresses so that they can receive debriefing materials, or the use of a debriefing screen which appears if they press 'withdraw', or upon conclusion of participation. You may also consider posting the research findings on your project website to which participants can be referred.

Using online methods

Supporting traditional methodologies

Internet methods may be used to support more traditional research designs, such as advertising and recruiting participants to a trial via websites. Respondents may be provided with a link to access an inclusion criteria survey, followed by the information sheet, consent form and then any self-completion instruments if appropriate. Randomisation, if required, may automatically occur once participants have submitted their online baseline data. Depending on the nature of the project, the internet may also facilitate ongoing data collection. For example, participants could submit results of self-administered biometric measures such as weight, or complete psychometric measures online. Diary data could be collected in the form of secure, password-protected blogs, which has the benefit that you can monitor progress on an ongoing basis. If post-intervention interviews are incorporated into your study, you may consider offering the option of an email or online chat format in which to conduct them.

Online surveys

Although online surveys take time initially to set up, they have the potential to collect large volumes of data cheaply and quickly. They can be conducted via email, either as an attachment or within the body of the communication, or via a webpage. Email questionnaires are more straightforward to implement, require less in terms of technical skill and can be sent directly to specific respondents rather than requiring participants to be guided to a webpage. However, web-based questionnaires offer more potential than email or traditional methods for attractive, flexible and user-friendly interfaces due to greater interactive, graphical and multimedia possibilities. They have more potential to maintain respondent anonymity if desired, and can enable the automatic export of data into databases and statistical packages.

When designing an online questionnaire, you should have an introductory page, containing: a welcome message; brief background information to the project; login/procedural instructions; and a link to a FAQs/study information page which participants may be required to indicate they have read before proceeding (see earlier discussion on informed consent). Specific instructions regarding how to answer questions should be provided at the point of need within the questionnaire. Various response formats are possible: text for open questions; dropdown menus, radio buttons or check boxes for closed questions; and slider bars for rating scales. To maximise the ease of navigation for the respondent, questions should be presented in cohesive groups on separate pages, and automatic filtering should be used as appropriate. The use of a 'progress bar' can keep respondents informed of their advancement through the questionnaire and may reduce attrition.

Specialised software can facilitate the design and construction of online question-naires, and some websites, for example, Survey Monkey (www.surveymonkey.com, accessed March 2013) offer 'start to finish' services for online survey administra-tion. For a more detailed technical discussion of software that supports survey construction please see:

Exploring Online Research Methods: www.geog.le.ac.uk/orm (accessed March 2013)

WebSM Portal: http://websm.org/ (accessed March 2013)

Online questionnaires should be piloted thoroughly across a variety of platforms and by a range of users to assess problems with access, page design, navigation and content.

Case study

The psychologist needs to collect some demographic information, i.e. sex, ethnicity, age, age at diagnosis (if applicable), professionals involved, educational and employment history and relationship status. He would also like to incorporate a measure of autistic traits, i.e. the Autism-Spectrum Quotient (Baron-Cohen et al., 2001). He knows that, due to the social communication difficulties of the respondents, putting these up online may prove more acceptable to them, in addition to being quicker and more convenient to process than postal surveys. The psychologist wants to circulate a link to the survey, so has chosen to use an online survey software. He will also offer postal questionnaires as an alternative if the participant wishes, which may enhance response rate and broaden the diversity of the sample. He will ensure that the content, wording and format of these two versions are as closely matched as possible to minimise the impact of any mode effect. The psychologist will also note in the data which method was used to enable post-hoc analysis.

Online interviewing

The internet can enable research interviews to be conducted using videoconferenc-ing technology, and this has potential benefits in terms of reduced cost, greater safety, as well as flexibility and convenience regarding location of the interaction. This may enable the inclusion of some individuals who would otherwise be unable or reluctant to participate. Alternatively you may decide to conduct an online inter-view via text, with the additional advantage that the need for transcription is eliminated. Compared to videoconferencing, these interviews are further from the traditional face-to-face interview format, with the loss of non-verbal data. However they offer more anonymity, may yield data of greater depth and reflexivity, and can be more conducive to the discussion of sensitive topics as well as more inclusive of hard-to-reach populations. Online interviews may be synchronous or asynchronous. Synchronous interviews take place in real time using tools such as instant messaging, and more closely resemble traditional interview formats, compared to asynchronous interviews which are typically conducted via email, interviewer and interviewee responding to each other in their own time. Asynchronous interviews take place over longer periods of time with questions being sent in stages rather than provided as a complete set at the outset.

Asynchronous email interviews are generally more straightforward to organise, requiring little or no technical training or support for participants. They offer more choice and flexibility over where, when and how participants make their responses, which may confer a greater sense of control and empowerment in the research process to the participant, compared to the synchronous situation, and may also reduce the impact of tedium, fatigue or interfering distractions. However, email interviews may suffer from a lack of momentum and continuity, which may result in paucity of data. The timescale involved in an email interview is not easily predicted but, depending on the rate of exchange of messages, is potentially long, which can increase attrition. You should consider that close and simultaneous involvement in several individuals' lives for extended periods of time could be comparable to a participant observation study, with a similar requirement on your energy to maintain an appropriate level of engagement.

Conversely the longitudinal nature of asynchronous interviews may be more conducive to the development of rapport and rich dialogue. They have the potential to yield data comparable to the personal narratives of diary accounts, and afford flexibility in the way the interview proceeds. As McCoyd and Kerson point out, 'Email interviews allow follow up questions in ways that face-to-face interviews do not' (2006: 401). There is also the possibility of incorporating new topics into the interview guide in response to the emerging data, consistent with a grounded theory approach (please see Chapter 20: 'Qualitative Analysis'). Additionally, the ongoing nature of the email interview may help you to become closer to the data during collection, thereby strengthening the iterative process characteristic of qualitative data analysis.

You should consider the issue of spontaneity of typed online interviews, where it is not known how much editing has occurred before posting, especially in email interviews. Chen and Hinton (1999) found that participants can be more measured in their responses than in face-to-face interviews, changing the nature of the data produced. Therefore online asynchronous interviews should be seen as providing mediated accounts (Gibson, 2010). Typed synchronous interviews incorporate more spontaneity, although the time pressure of typing may deter some from taking part and impede the quality of responses from participants less proficient in their keyboard/literacy skills. They also lack the flexibility for participants to choose when they respond. However, they are much shorter in timescale, reducing the likelihood of attrition, whilst still offering the potential for some reflection due to reduced researcher presence and their textual nature.

Loss of non-verbal data

Typed online interviews lack non-verbal cues, such as facial expression, tone of voice or gestures which can enrich data and help to establish rapport. Research has shown that relationships can and do develop online (Walther, 1992). However, rapport is not guaranteed in the online interview, and will be determined by the interactive skills of the interviewer, the focus of the research project and the way in which it is presented. For email interviews, Mann and Stewart (2001) see the provision of a schedule ahead of the interview as beneficial to the establishment of trust and rapport. Some online interviewers share personal information and photographs to help open up dialogue with their participants (Kivits, 2005; O'Connor and Madge, 2001). You will need to decide whether this is appropriate in the context of your research project, or whether it is preferable to maintain a certain distance and reduce the effect of cues to social identity on the interaction.

The email interview places greater demands on the interactive skills of the online interviewer due to the greater degree of discontinuity. As Kivits remarks, the email interview involves 'constant negotiation ... where motivations waver between establishing and keeping up an interpersonal and enjoyable talk with respondents and simultaneously installing a delineated research interview situation' (2005: 35). Responses will need to be adapted according to individual styles and needs. Online interviewers therefore need to develop the skill of listening and reassuring through words (Mann and Stewart, 2000). The experience of Benford (Benford and Standen, 2011) was that she developed a sense of how many follow-up questions to send and how quickly to respond to participants' emails in order to maintain momentum, whilst striving to avoid becoming a nuisance and overwhelming them with her enthusiasm (see also Bampton and Cowton, 2002).

The loss of non-verbal information may affect the process of analysis, which will be based solely on textual data. However, the significance of non-verbal information in qualitative interviews is debatable since the extent to which it is included in the transcripts of face-to-face interviews is highly variable and 'involves making assessments of participants' mood or intentions which may well be incorrect' (Mann and Stewart, 2000: 193).

Case study

As the psychologist is exploring the experiences of adults who go through the diagnostic investigations for AS, interviewing would be a good way of collecting these data. He believes that the internet will offer participants a potentially less stressful communication situation than an offline context, and one in which participants may find it easier to open up with their thoughts and feelings. The psychologist chooses an email interview method which is more flexible in terms of pace compared to real-time

(Continued)

(Continued)

text chat to help to alleviate any anxiety his participants may have. Prior to data collection, he puts the interview guide up on the project website and forwards the link to this to prospective participants. He has decided not to put personal information or photos on the website to maintain a certain distance. Due to the long-term nature of email interviews, as well as the potentially more intimate nature of online interaction (Walther, 1996), he fears that there may be a risk of dependency amongst his participants who may be socially isolated. He realises that sensitivity is needed on his part and careful handling in order to prepare participants for the end of the interview. The psychologist plans to organise the data by keeping two ongoing Word documents for each participant: one in which each email is pasted and as such the interview grows; the other, a record of ongoing thoughts and reminders, including future lines of enquiry and potential concepts for analysis. He will examine these documents and the interview guide on receiving a reply from a participant, which will allow for reflection before replying and continuing the dialogue. He will also offer an alternative interview format if the participant prefers.

Online focus groups

Similar to online interviews, online focus groups can be asynchronous or synchronous and share similar benefits and issues for consideration. The internet offers opportunities for the construction of focus groups which may be otherwise unfeasible due to the divergent needs and circumstances of the participants. Asynchronous focus groups can even mix individuals across time zones. Online focus groups, particularly in an asynchronous format, may be difficult to manage due to reduced researcher presence, resulting in off-topic discussion. Conversely, reduced researcher effect may allow for greater group independence, yielding rich, participant-driven data. This might be further enriched by a reduced tendency to conform compared to a traditional focus group (please see Chapter 7: 'Qualitative Data Collection').

Asynchronous focus groups can be mediated by group email lists, or web-based bulletin boards on which participants post responses and comments and read those from other group members. Bulletin boards may be designed and managed through a simple interface on the host website with password access if required. The URL for the board is then distributed to participants.

Synchronous online focus groups can be mediated by instant messaging software in a private password-protected virtual space, and more closely mimic the interactions of traditional focus groups. They do not require long-term time commitments from participants, and may be easier to manage, but risk being dominated by participants with superior typing speeds. Since interaction is essential for focus groups, the online format requires measures to establish group trust and rapport, for example through the inclusion of an introductory exercise by which participants familiarise themselves with each other, or by sharing photos of themselves prior to the group convening.

> ## ⌐ Case study ⌐
>
> Online focus groups may be less acceptable to people with AS due to the complexity of group interaction and concerns about the behaviour of strangers online. Although the psychologist considers approaching a pre-existing group from which to form a focus group, he decides not to as he thinks that the pre-established relationships may make it difficult for the participants to focus on the research topic, and is concerned that he might change the group dynamics by his presence.

Social media

The internet is host to a seemingly infinite number of online group discussions, blogs and social network sites containing personal reflections and experiences on a diverse range of topics, health issues being particularly well-represented. These qualitative data may be considered naturalistic in character in that they are not produced for the purposes of research and are not contaminated by any kind of researcher effect. However, due to the conscious or unconscious intention of the author to be perceived in a certain way, data should be regarded as 'semi-ethnographic'. There is also the possibility for a more quantitative approach to the data, including analysis of patterns of online interactions and communication as well as the content of messages, postings and tags associated with photos and videos.

Online groups

These may occur in real time within a chat room or they may be asynchronous, mediated by electronic mailing lists or bulletin boards. Membership may originate from established offline groups or be formed through online networking based on a common purpose or interest. Some groups may have rules for acceptable online behaviour, and a moderator who intercepts all messages before posting, filtering out those considered to be inappropriate, irrelevant or offensive. You may wish to participate in the group in order to collect data rather than analysing archived postings, but be aware of the 'observer effect' if you identify yourself to the group (please see Chapter 7: 'Qualitative Data Collection') or the ethical challenges associated with covert participation (please see Chapter 15: 'Designing and Conducting an Ethical Research Study').

Blogs

Blogs are ongoing online journals which are becoming increasingly popular amongst internet users. They can yield longitudinal reflective personal data. As sources of data, however, blogs may be limited due to the select population who keep them, i.e. people who are comfortable with, and motivated by this type of discourse. Blog search engines such as Google Blog Search (www.google.com/blogsearch, accessed Feb. 2013) may help you find suitable blogs for analysis. Snee (2010) recommends that blogs should be read online before being imported into a data analysis package, so that they have been seen in their original context. Alternatively a specific sample of participants could be recruited to maintain secure password-protected blogs in which to record data, for example, an exercise or mood blog.

Social network sites

Social network sites, such as Facebook, Linkedin, typically allow individuals to create a public or semi-public personal webpage or profile on which they upload content of their choice, for example, photos, music, etc. They may also have a list of users (or 'friends') with whom they share a connection, and communicate with them via posted comments or private messaging. Some sites include built-in blogging technology, for example, Twitter; video-sharing facilities, for example, YouTube; and the ability to form groups around a shared focus, for example, Facebook. They are potentially a source of personal narratives and demographic data and a platform for survey-based studies, as well as giving you the opportunity to observe networks of people who have something in common, such as being friends, working at the same place or being fans of this book (become our friend on the book's Facebook page). However, of concern are issues of validity, reliability and representative sampling, as well as ethical questions regarding informed consent and privacy, particularly concerning people who appear in a participant's list of friends (Redmond, 2010).

Case study

The psychologist conducts a lot of background work using social media sites. It helps him to design his interview schedule from the discussions members of an AS forum are having. He does not take part in any of the discussions as he thinks the forum's members might find this distressing and intrusive. Because the psychologist is hoping to gather data from some participants currently going through the process of being diagnosed with AS he has designed some individual, online, password-protected, blog spaces for them. He will ask these participants to complete a blog each with reflections of their experiences as they go through the diagnosis process.

Summary

- There are many potential benefits which can be conferred on traditional research procedures when implemented via the internet.
- Due to its unique qualities, the internet offers the researcher new possibilities beyond those which would otherwise be achievable.
- The web offers the qualitative researcher a seemingly infinite amount of unsolicited narratives and discussions from a wide range of personal perspectives and experiences.
- The researcher must consider whether online methods can sufficiently meet their requirements in terms of sampling, data validity and ethical practice.

Questions for Discussion

1. If you were to assess the appropriateness of an internet method of data collection for a study, what issues would you need to consider regarding the following?

   a. Your sample

   b. Ethical issues

   c. Technical requirements

   d. The platform/interface you wish to use

2. For the following groups of participants, what might you consider in assessing whether an internet method is appropriate for collecting data from them?

   a. People with no fixed abode

   b. Consultant surgeons working in secondary care

   c. Teenagers, 13–19 years of age

   d. Retired people aged over 60

3. Taking into account the issues identified for the participants in question 2, would you either choose a traditional method of data collection, or are there certain steps you could take prior to data collection to ensure your internet method's validity?

Further Reading

Bruckman, A. (2002) *Ethical Guidelines for Online Research*: www.cc.gatech.edu/~asb/ethics/ (accessed November 2013).

Couper, M.P. (2008) *Designing Effective Web Surveys*. New York: Cambridge University Press.

Dochartaigh, N.O. (2012) *Internet Research Skills*. London: SAGE.

Economic and Social Research Council (2012) *ReStore: Sustaining and Promoting Online Resources*: www.restore.ac.uk (accessed November 2013).

Economic and Social Research Council. *Exploring Online Research Methods*: www.geog.le.ac.uk/orm (accessed November 2013).

Fielding, N., Lee, R.M. and Blank, G. (eds) (2008) *Online Research Methods*. London: SAGE.

Hewson, C., Yule, P., Laurent, D. and Vogel, C. (2003) *Internet Research Methods: A Practical Guide for the Social and Behavioural Sciences*. London: SAGE.

Hine, C. (ed.) (2005) *Virtual Methods: Issues in Social Research on the Internet*. Oxford: Berg.

Johns, M.D., Chen, S-L. and Hall, G.J. (eds) (2004) *Online Social Research: Methods, Issues and Ethics*. New York: Peter Lang.

Kraut, R., Olson, J., Banaji, M., Bruckman, A., Cohen, J. and Couper, M.P. (2004) 'Psychological research online: report of the board of scientific affairs advisory group on the conduct of research on the internet', *American Psychologist*, 59: 105–17.

Mann, C. and Stewart, F. (2000) *Internet Communication and Qualitative Research*. London: SAGE.

Walker, D.-M. (2011) The emergence of online research methods. *British Medical Journal*: http://blogs.bmj.com/bmj/2011/10/28/dawn-marie-walker-the-emergence-of-online-research-methods/ (accessed November 2013).

Walker, D.-M. (2013) 'The internet as a medium for health service research Part 1', *The Nurse Researcher*, 20 (4): 18–21.

Walker, D.-M. (2013) 'The internet as a medium for health service research Part 2', *The Nurse Researcher*, 20(5): 33–7.

References

Bampton, R. and Cowton, C.J. (2002) 'The e-interview', *Forum: Qualitative Social Research*: www.qualitative-research.net/fqs-texte/2-02/2-02bamptoncowton-e.htm (accessed November 2013).

Baron-Cohen, S., Wheelwright, S., Skinner, R., Martin, J. and Clubley, E. (2001) 'The Autism-Spectrum Quotient (AQ): evidence from Asperger Syndrome/high-functioning autism, males and females, scientists and mathematicians', *Journal of Autism and Developmental Disorders,* 31: 5–17.

Benford, P. and Standen, P.J. (2011) 'The use of email-facilitated interviewing with higher functioning autistic people participating in a grounded theory study', *International Journal of Social Research Methodology,* 14: 353–68.

Best, S.J. and Krueger, B.S. (2004) *Internet Data Collection*. Thousand Oaks, CA: SAGE.

Brickman-Bhutta, C. (2009) *Not by the Book: Facebook as a Sampling Frame*: www.thearda.com/workingpapers/download/Not%20by%20the%20Book%20-%20Bhutta.pdf (accessed November 2013).

Chen, P. and Hinton, S.M. (1999) 'Realtime interviewing using the World Wide Web', *Sociological Research Online,* 4(3): www.socresonline.org.uk/4/3/chen.html (accessed November 2013).

Dutton, W.H. and Helsper, E.J. (2007) *Oxford Internet Survey 2007 Report: The Internet in Britain*. Oxford: Oxford Internet Institute.

Ess, C. and the Assocation of Researchers (2002) *Ethical Decision-Making and Internet Research: Recommendations from the AoIR Ethics Working Committee*: www.aoir.org/reports/ethics.pdf (accessed November 2013).

Gibson, L. (2010) *Using Email Interviews: Realities Toolkit 09*. ESRC National Centre for Research Methods: www.socialsciences.manchester.ac.uk/morgancentre/realities/toolkits/email-interviews/index.html (accessed November 2013).

Hall, G.J., Frederic, D. and Johns, M.D. (2004) 'NEED HELP ASAP!!!': A feminist communitarian approach to online research ethics', in M.D. Johns, S-L. Chen and G.J. Hall (eds), *Online Social Research: Methods, Issues and Ethics*. New York: Peter Lang.

Hewson, C. (2003) 'Conducting research on the internet', *Psychologist,* 16: 290–3.

Hiltz, S.R. and Turoff, M. (1978) *The Network Nation: Human Communication via Computer*. Cambridge, MA: MIT Press.

Johns, M.D., Hall, G.J. and Crowell, T.L. (2004) 'Surviving the IRB Review: institutional guidelines and research strategies', in M.D. Johns, S.-L. Chen and G.J. Hall (eds), *Online Social Research: Methods, Issues and Ethics*. New York: Peter Lang.

Joinson, A. (2005) 'Internet behaviour and the design of virtual methods', in C. Hine (ed.), *Virtual Methods: Issues in Social Research and the Methods*. Oxford: Berg.

Kivits, J. (2005) 'Online interviewing and the research relationship', in C. Hine (ed.), *Virtual Methods: Issues in Social Research and the Methods*. Oxford: Berg.

Lenhart, A. (2009) *Adults and Social Network Sites.* Washington, DC: Pew Internet and American Life Project.

McCoyd, J.L.M. and Kerson, T.S. (2006) 'Conducting intensive interviews using email: a serendipitous comparative opportunity', *Qualitative Social Work,* 5: 389–406.

Madge, C. and O'Connor, H. (2002) 'Online with the e-mums' *Area,* 34: 92–102.

Mann, C. and Stewart, F. (2000) *Internet Communication and Qualitative Research.* London: SAGE.

Mann, C. and Stewart, F. (2001) 'Internet interviewing', in J.F. Gubrium and J.A. Holstein (eds), *Handbook of Interview Research.* Thousand Oaks, CA: SAGE.

O'Connor, H. and Madge, C. (2001) 'Cyber-mothers: online synchronous interviewing using conference software', *Sociological Research Online,* 5: www.socresonline.org.uk/5/4/o'connor.html (accessed November 2013).

Redmond, F. (2010) 'Social network sites: evaluating and investigating their use in academic research', ICERI (International Conference of Education, Research and Innovation), Madrid, 15–17 Nov.

Seymour, W.S. (2001) 'In the flesh or online? Exploring qualitative research methodologies', *Qualitative Research,* 1: 147–68.

Snee, H. (2010) 'Using blog analysis', *Realities Toolkit.* ESRC National Centre for Research Methods: www.socialsciences.manchester.ac.uk/morgancentre/realities/toolkits/blog-analysis/10-toolkit-blog-analysis.pdf (accessed April 2012).

Suler, J. (2004) 'The online disinhibition effect', *Cyberpsychology and Behavior,* 7: 321–6.

Walther, J.B. (1992) 'Interpersonal effects in computer-mediated interaction', *Communication Research,* 19: 52–90.

Walther, J.B. (1996) 'Computer-mediated communication: impersonal, interpersonal, and hyperpersonal interaction', *Communication Research,* 23: 3–43.

14

SYSTEMATIC REVIEWS

Jo Leonardi-Bee and Olwyn M.R. Westwood

- To know the rationale for a systematic review and discuss the advantages and disadvantages of this method
- To be able to distinguish and critique the differences between a systematic review and a narrative review
- To have a good knowledge of the five main stages to a systematic review
- To appreciate when synthesising findings from studies may be appropriate
- To be able to build a team with the relevant expertise required to conduct a systematic review

Introduction

More than 2 million articles are published each year in biomedical literature. Therefore in our roles as researchers, health providers and policy-makers, we are inundated with unmanageable quantities of information from studies. How can we possibly make sense of all of this information so that we are able to inform practice? It would be impossible for us to keep up to date with all of the latest relevant research unless we could access a synthesised form of evidence, which has combined the critically appraised documents in an appropriate way so we have an objective outcome we can base our clinical judgement on. Traditional literature reviews is one such approach that synthesises studies. However, the methods used to conduct these are variable, with most published reviews containing very little information about the methods they used to identify the studies. Due to this lack of reporting, it is usually very difficult to tell whether the findings are based on an unbiased perspective of what all of the research is saying about a particular research question or hypothesis, or represent the author's prior beliefs. With a traditional literature review there is also no appraisal system, therefore the included papers may be of dubious quality.

Case study

A Nobel Prize-winning American Scientist, Dr Linus Pauling, was a firm believer that vitamin C was effective in preventing the common cold. He therefore took vitamin C every day and never got a cold, thus providing him with anecdotal evidence of efficacy. This led Pauling to review the evidence which assessed the relationship between vitamin C and the common cold, from which he produced a book to popularise his beliefs: *Vitamin C and the Common Cold* (1970). This book concluded that the majority of the included trials found vitamin C to be effective. Additionally, further research showed that there was a plausible biological mechanism by which vitamin C could prevent a person from getting a cold. The book was a massive hit with the public, and the sales of vitamin C soared. If the association was true, then this would be very important for public health and the economy if one considers all of the days taken off work due to the common cold. However, before implementation into clinical practice, his work needs to be assessed for bias and quality.

To do this we need to think about the studies he used to base his conclusions on. First, we need to ask ourselves; were the trials representative of all of the trials investigating vitamin C and the common cold that had been conducted, or could they have been selected because they found vitamin C to be effective? If he only included studies which found vitamin C was effective, then the conclusions of the review would also find vitamin C was effective. Second we need to ask ourselves; were the included studies conducted to the highest quality, or could the studies have been very poor, leaving the study's findings not valid or reliable?

At first glance it appears that the four included trials are good quality, being double blind RCTs. However, Pauling based his quantitative estimations on only one of them, a trial which found a 45% decrease in the number of colds in the vitamin C group

(Ritzel, 1961). Upon closer inspection, Ritzel's sample was not representative as they had low dietary vitamin C, and were a group of children in the Swiss Alps. Another of the four included trials also had a sample of schoolchildren with low dietary vitamin C.

Since the book, many clinical studies regarding vitamin C for preventing the common cold have been conducted, resulting ultimately in a systematic review (Hemilä et al., 2010). Hemilä and team analysed the results of 29 trials, involving approximately 11,000 participants. Only five of the trials showed a preventative effect of taking vitamin C, where incidence was halved. However the samples in these trials were atypical, consisting of marathon runners, skiers or soldiers on subarctic exercises! However although vitamin C is not effective for prevention, the duration of colds (calculated from a total of 9649 episodes) was reduced by an average of 8% in adults and 13% in children. The severity of the cold was also significantly reduced overall.

As you read this case study, your opinion might have changed from pledging to take vitamin C daily to getting some in for the next time you get a cold. This highlights the value of a systematic review. Previously you would have had to base your judgement on either Pauling's biased work, or have read and appraised all of the individual publications. Therefore the aim of systematic reviews is to give a complete and balanced overview of the available evidence concerning a specific research question. The question may relate to assessing the effectiveness of an intervention or treatment, such as the vitamin C example, but could also assess whether there is an association between an exposure and outcome, for example whether exposure to other people's smoking is associated with lung cancer in non-smokers. Systematic reviews are not only useful in evidence-based medicine, but also to inform future research, such as being able to identify and refine hypotheses; and ascertain, and ultimately avoid, the pitfalls encountered in previous research. However like any piece of evidence, the systematic review must be critically appraised as methodological quality can be highly variable, although reviews that are conducted by specialist groups such as Cochrane are generally more rigorous and better reported (please see Chapter 3: 'Critical Appraisal').

A systematic review is 'the application of scientific strategies that limit bias to the systematic assembly, critical appraisal, and synthesis of all relevant studies on a specific topic' (Cook et al., 1995: 167) which is done through 'an overview of primary studies which contains an explicit statement of objectives, materials, and methods and has been conducted according to explicit and reproducible methodology' (Greenhalgh, 1997). Therefore the essence of a systematic review is finding and collecting data from rich sources (published and unpublished), evaluating their quality and then summarising the results, which means that the process for a traditional literature review and a systematic review are extremely different. Whereas a traditional literature review may suffice in providing background knowledge for a publication or grant application, a systematic review is a piece of research in its own right (please see Table 14.1).

TABLE 14.1   Traditional literature reviews versus systematic reviews

Traditional Literature Review	Systematic Review
Prone to bias owing to subjective nature	Less prone to bias owing to objective nature
Literature search often inadequate	Comprehensive literature search
Usually lacks description of methods	Contains clear and reproducible methods
The review usually cannot be replicated or verified	Can be replicated and verified if wished
Difficult to judge the quality of the review	Contains strict inclusion and exclusion criteria and detailed assessment of the methodological quality of the studies is performed
Difficult to know what methodology the cited papers use	Often only include papers using one type of methodology, e.g. RCTs; or the methodology is cited
Conclusion is usually based upon a counting of studies	Conclusion is based upon synthesis of results, qualitatively or quantitatively
Grey literature usually ignored therefore conclusions can represent publication bias	A grey literature search strategy is usually incorporated

Conducting a systematic review

A systematic review may be a specific piece of work by a research team, or could be a work package within a larger project such as a multicentre randomised controlled trial (RCT). There are both advantages and disadvantages associated with this method (please see Table 14.2).

TABLE 14.2   Advantages and disadvantages of conducting systematic reviews

Advantages	Disadvantages
Systematic reviews are cheap pieces of research, e.g. no participant expenses, etc.	The process of designing and conducting a review is laborious and time consuming
Less bureaucratic. No ethical or research governance approvals to gain	The data gathered from various studies may not be easy to compare
The conclusions drawn are generally more reliable and accurate than discrete studies	
Generalisable conclusions for a broad population may be inferred from the data that is not achievable from the discrete investigations	

Key people required to conduct a systematic review

If you ever come across a piece of research which says it is a systematic review but only has one team member/author, be wary. Systematic reviews are a team effort, and must be to prevent bias. They are only successful if the correct people work together during the development of the protocol, through the stages of conducting the systematic review and during the writing up of the results. You do not have to be an expert in systematic reviews to do one, however, as long as at least one member of the team has experience in performing one, anyone can learn how to do one successfully and to the highest quality. The key players in conducting and producing a systematic review to the highest level are:

- clinical expert;
- information specialist expert;
- methodological expert;
- statistical expert (if quantitative papers are being included);
- usually one or two researchers to search screen and select the studies for inclusion.

Many systematic review teams now include a patient/public representative with an interest in the topic as an active team member. This is because the findings of systematic reviews often influence health care, so it is important that the results are relevant to patients/the public. Also there is usually a wide dissemination of systematic review results, therefore it is important that the published text of the review can be understood by an intelligent lay person, so they can make informed choices about their own treatment options (please see Chapter 16: 'Patient and Public Involvement').

Stages of a systematic review

Having ascertained that no current, empirical, systematic review for your specific research question exists, and that a systematic review is warranted, either due to an overwhelming or contradictory evidence base, the next phase is to design and conduct the systematic review, for which there are five main stages to complete:

Formulate a pragmatic research question

When deciding upon the question, it needs to be broad enough for an inclusive literature capture, for example, for the analysis of variation across the population of interest, yet sufficiently focused that a discrete and realistic number of papers can be located for analysis. For example 'How effective is cancer screening in the UK?' is too broad. A better question would be 'How effective are routine mammograms in detecting cancer in women aged 60 or older?' Questions can be also too narrow, which would not only limit the number of articles returned, but also the impact your results have on practice. If your focus is too narrow, your results would only be informative for a very small group of people, such as 'What is the evidence of increased survival rates in women aged between 50–65 years who are screened regularly for cervical cancer?' Perhaps here you could open it up to any woman aged 16 or older.

The question for a systematic review needs to be clearly defined, answerable and important enough to justify all of the hard work. In order to formulate the question, the research team need to deliberate:

- the nature of the information and data that will be obtained;
- the nature of the settings where the primary data were collected;
- the characteristics and demographics of the patients/samples;
- the categories of studies that will be included, such as randomised controlled trials or qualitative studies.

The types of questions answered by a systematic review are diverse and may necessitate qualitative, quantitative or a mixed-method approach to the data analysis, depending on the anticipated outcomes. Thus your question should also guide you towards the various methods for the analysis. Here are some examples of the types of questions that could be employed:

- A health economic question with significance to managers/policy-makers, e.g. the impact of introducing keyhole surgery for hernia repairs in secondary health care with regards to patient stay, costs and patient outcomes.
- An epidemiological study of disease, e.g. examining aetiological factors that affect a named disease and its progression (a classic study was the link between tobacco smoking and lung cancer).
- Finding a prognostic indicator of disease progression, e.g. examining the weighting of the co-morbidity factors in cardiovascular disease.
- The efficacy of a diagnostic intervention on a disease, e.g. assessing the impact of mammography for detection of breast cancer in a specific age range.
- Comparing the precision and accuracy of two methods, testing the same physiological measurement or analyte, e.g. the use of telemedicine in blood pressure monitoring versus hospital outpatient appointments.
- Comparing the effectiveness of different medications/treatments for a named disease, e.g. comparing the efficacy of the various medications available to treat gout.
- If the best medication/treatment for a certain disease is known, the question might be to ascertain the optimal regimen, e.g. 'What should the delivery pattern of cognitive behavioural therapy be for treating mild depression?'

Identifying the relevant literature through an extensive search

Unlike the traditional literature review where we just run a basic search and look at a selection of papers, for a systematic review we have to look at all of the available evidence that has answered the question of interest. This requires a comprehensive search strategy which is usually very time consuming to develop and implement. However, the literature search is a significant phase of activity and those who are conducting the searches need to be systematic and inclusive in order to capture the important and relevant studies. This can be achieved from searching a wide range of sources, including several electronic databases that represent the type of literature needed, such as for health you may use Medline and EMBASE (please see Chapter 2: 'Finding the Evidence to Support your Research Question'). The research question should offer an essential steer for the decision regarding which of the databases should be examined.

You may also want to 'hand search' specific relevant journals, by reading the indexes to ensure you have not missed any relevant papers. For example, if your review was regarding an intervention for type I diabetes, you may consider hand searching a journal such as the *British Journal of Diabetes and Vascular Care*. You may also want to hand search relevant journals which are not indexed in your chosen electronic database.

With this phase of searching comes the potential for bias, for example, *language bias*. Electronic databases are often restricted to including only published research which is written in English. This may result in biasing the findings of the review. Translation costs may deter you from appraising publications in other languages; however it is important, as Egger et al. (1997) found that positive findings were more likely to be published in English-speaking journals (as higher prestige), whereas negative findings would be published in local journals. Therefore a thorough search of non-English language databases needs to be performed, such as using the LILACS database to identify papers in journals from Latin America and Caribbean region, which includes Portuguese and Spanish languages.

When you and your research team are drafting the search strategy, you should also consider how you will identify 'grey literature'. This is unpublished data, such as what you might find in a trial registry, from pharmaceutical companies or charities, or by contacting eminent authors in the field. Websites of research councils may also have their list of successful applicants and abstracts of projects funded. Other forms of grey literature include evidence presented at symposia or conferences, theses or as restricted reports – as such they are not so readily accessible (please see Chapter 2: 'Finding the Evidence to Support your Research Question' for some ideas of how you might source this data). It is advisable for you to contact the author of the grey literature with a description of your review and why you are contacting them, together with a request for the information you need. However, be warned that some authors may not be willing to share their unpublished data.

Implementing a grey literature strategy will also help prevent *publication bias* becoming an issue in your review. This is the tendency for papers with positive results to be published, whereas negative or null hypothesis results are almost never published. A review by Dwan et al. (2008) found that there was strong evidence for publication bias on two levels: (i) a study-level problem, where the paper is either not submitted, or submitted but rejected, as Dwan and team found that studies that report positive or significant results were more likely to be published; and (ii) an outcome-level problem where there is selective non-reporting of outcomes within published studies. Here they found that outcomes that are statistically significant have higher odds of being fully reported in the publication. It would therefore follow that the content found by electronic databases is likely to be skewed towards a 'positive bias'. You can attempt to balance this out via your grey literature search strategy, for example, detecting trials from the registry, which often are updated with their outcomes, even though they may not result in publication.

The next step in drafting your literature search is to write down your list of search terms (once again, Chapter 2 has more detail about this). Your list needs to be exhaustive so as not to miss any relevant papers, therefore you need to be aware of all of the nuances in vocabulary and spelling (synonyms):

- Different words which have the same or similar meanings, such as death, mortality, survival statistics, and so on, rather than restricting the focus to the precise terminology of the agreed research question.
- The difference between spellings of keywords, e.g. randomised controlled trial or randomized controlled trial or even the use of the acronym RCT.

Your initial search may well identify different terminology that you were not aware of, and can direct you to further information sources, for example, searching the Citation Index on relevant papers you have retrieved may springboard you into different journals or undiscovered articles, as arguably, since they have cited your retrieved paper, they may be relevant to your review. Equally, a general inspection of the bibliography or reference list on your retrieved papers should also uncover further data, and can be good at helping to identify grey literature, as they may have discussed a book chapter or theses.

Assessing the methodological quality of the appropriate studies

This is an important aspect of any systematic review. Some studies are poorly conducted and/or reported; leaving it questionable as to whether these studies should inform practice. Therefore it is a vitally important step for the retrieved literature to be assessed for methodological quality. The method of assessment you use to judge the quality of an individual study depends on the type of study you are assessing. What you are trying to assess is whether the study was conducted sensibly and whether the results are credible or valid. You can do this by identifying the strengths and weaknesses of the study, and determining whether the study is at a high risk of bias. This should be a standardised approach and can be done by using a critical appraisal tool to ensure this process is fair and unbiased (please see Chapter 3: 'Critical Appraisal' for further description).

Extracting the data, summarising the evidence; interpreting the findings and delivering a meaningful conclusion

Once we have identified and obtained all of the relevant literature regarding our research question, and ensured the quality of all evidence which fits the inclusion criteria, we then need to extract the data and summarise all of the information in a coherent synopsis. This can be done either qualitatively using a descriptive format, for example, 'When looking at the included studies, it does not appear that exposure to cigarette smoke consistently increases the risk of lung cancer in non-smokers' (surprising but true; please see Blot and McLaughlin (1998) for an interesting debate on this); or quantitatively, using a statistical method called meta-analysis. A meta-analysis can be used to calculate a pooled measure of an effect by statistically combining the numerical results from several studies. A measure of effect, such as odds ratios, and an estimate of precision, such as the standard error, are extracted from each study and entered into the meta-analysis.

The primary role of a meta-analysis is to improve the precision of these measures of effect by statistically combining the data from the studies together and estimating a new pooled measure of effect. Therefore a meta-analysis can pick up small, but real effects otherwise lost in single trials. Each study is weighted in the meta-analysis based on the precision of its measure of effect, such as the standard error, so that the more precise studies have more weight in the meta-analysis than the smaller sized studies which usually have imprecise findings, resulting in a larger standard error. A meta-analysis can also inform future research such as using the estimates obtained as a measure of effect when calculating a sample size; and can identify important factors which need further research to assess definitively whether they impact on the effectiveness of a treatment (effect modifiers), or the course of the disease.

It may also be that your review will combine different study designs. Therefore the research team also has the essential task of planning how to collate and present the data so that logical and authentic outcomes might be demonstrated. Based on the synthesised results, meaningful conclusions should be then determined and agreed by all research team members.

Drafting a protocol

A well-defined protocol means that the research team have had to reason, discuss and agree the above steps. Once this has been done, you will need to draft your protocol. The underlying principle of a systematic review is that a protocol, which contains strict inclusion and exclusion criteria for the literature, is drafted prior to the search commencing. The inclusion criteria usually consist of a description of the following: types of studies to be included (such as RCTs, cohort studies and so on), types of participants or populations (e.g. women, children), types of interventions or exposure (e.g. screening for cervical cancer, antidepressants), and types of outcomes measures (e.g. mortality, efficacy). It is usually recommended that the exclusion criteria are minimal so that the findings from the review are generalisable to a wider population. The protocol will also contain explicit details regarding how the literature will be searched and any search terms that will be used, the methods for screening literature for eligibility, data extraction and quality assessments, and the methods that will be used for analysis. In preparing the protocol, a number of functions will be accomplished:

i. The formulation of a well-defined timeline detailing the different levels of activity, and which team members have agreed to be involved at which stages. A systematic review typically takes around 12 months to complete and your team should be committed to the duration of the project.

ii. You will have deliberated and decided upon on the most reliable methods to use such as ascertaining what critical appraisal tool you are going to use, etc.

iii. You will also have discussed the impact your conclusions might have on the defined area of health care.

As a systematic review is a massive undertaking, it is imperative that the protocol is detailed and well thought out. Therefore it is worthwhile looking at previous successful protocols in order to gain a sense of what is needed, such as on the Cochrane website.

Conducting a systematic review

A well drafted protocol will prove invaluable when you are conducting a review, as you can refer back to it with any queries, and all of the research team can carry out the tasks according to protocol and therefore the process is standardised. As mentioned previously, conducting a systematic review is a team effort not only due to the varying expertise needed and the inordinate amount of work required, but also to eliminate the possibility of subjective bias which may be introduced when you are working on your own. It is therefore usual for two researchers to independently screen the papers identified from the searches, using either a two-stage or three-stage process. In a two-stage process, each paper from the search is checked for eligibility against the inclusion and exclusion criteria, using first the titles and abstracts, and then the full text of the papers that are deemed potentially eligible based on their titles and abstracts. In a three-stage process, first the titles are screened, then the abstracts, and finally the full texts. Any disagreements in eligibility at the different stages are usually resolved through discussion and consensus; this therefore validates the conclusions offered from your review. At the beginning of your searches, it is pragmatic to be more inclusive – an over-enthusiastic initial 'cull' of chosen papers should be avoided in favour of a more liberal approach so as not to discard ones that could turn out to be appropriate. Once you begin your searches, there may be some 'fine-tuning' of the inclusion and exclusion criteria previously agreed, either because your searches are not returning many items, or it is returning too many irrelevant ones. If you do change your criteria, the searches need to be repeated and the studies you have included/excluded prior to the change need to be revisited to see if they remain in that same category.

Given the extensive nature of the medical and health care literature, this stage is demanding as there are likely to be a huge amount of studies returned that are identified by the searches. However, following screening against the inclusion and exclusion criteria to check eligibility, very few studies may be a precise 'fit' for your research question, therefore you will be appraising a small sample of the total number initially identified. At each stage of the process you need to keep a log of the numbers of studies identified (after removing duplicates, as the same paper might be returned from different electronic databases), excluded and included. You may find keeping a Preferred Reporting Items for Systematic Reviews and Meta-Analysis (PRISMA) (Moher et al., 2009) flow chart a useful organisation tool for your numbers (please see Figure 14.1).

As part of the quality evaluation, and to ensure you are using a standardised procedure, thus keeping the process as free from bias a possible, a previously

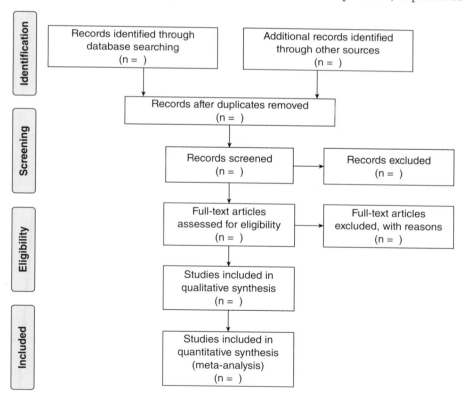

FIGURE 14.1   Preferred reporting items for systematic reviews and meta-analysis: the PRISMA statement (Moher et al 2009)

defined scoring system is normally used for the assessment of the literature. Many scoring systems, or critical appraisal checklists, have been developed over the years, and the majority of these ask questions to assess whether bias that could be prevalent within the study design have been minimised. Therefore, there are different systems and checklists depending on the study design being appraised (please see Chapter 3: 'Critical Appraisal' for more detail on this topic).

In general, however, if your review is including randomised controlled trials, their scientific rigour is usually assessed based on the following components: (i) whether the method used to generate the randomisation sequence was adequate; (ii) whether the randomisation sequence was blinded from the researcher before the patients were randomised (allocation concealment); (iii) whether the physician/researcher, patient and outcome assessors were blinded to the trial arm the patient was in (blinding); (iv) whether the drop-out rate in each arm was low and whether the rate differed between the trial arms (attrition bias); and (v) whether the intention to treat principle was used during statistical analysis (where patients are analysed based on the intervention they were randomised to, rather than the intervention they subsequently received). (Please see Chapter 11: 'Clinical Trials' for a more complete description.)

The quality of comparative epidemiological studies is usually assessed based upon the following criteria: (i) whether the sample was representative (selection bias); (ii) whether the ascertainment of the disease and the exposure were adequate (information bias); (iii) whether the cases and controls, exposed and unexposed were comparable (confounding); and (iv) whether the non-response rates (non-response bias) or follow-up rates (attrition bias) were sufficiently low. (Please see Chapter 10: 'Epidemiology' for a more complete description.)

Please remember when assessing methodological rigour that few research papers are without flaws and teams should assume a professional and respectful attitude to assessing the quality of work of others.

Data extraction

Once the papers to be included are agreed, based upon your inclusion criteria and consensus when necessary, two or more researchers should then independently extract the data from these studies and compare their extractions and, once again, reach a consensus. The team might opt for a manual approach and use a data extraction form for this. With a vast literature search, diverse styles for presentation of data are inevitable, so these forms serve as a mechanism for standardising the data reporting for your review. In turn, this should help identify any 'patterns' or relationships in the data. It is recommended that the data extraction form is piloted on a small number of studies to ensure suitability before being used for the remaining studies.

Analysis

The findings from the studies can either be summarised qualitatively, for example, 'When looking at the studies, it does not appear that vitamin C supplementation can prevent a cold; however, a massive dose of vitamin C could slightly decrease the duration of the common cold.' Qualitative descriptions such as these are used when the quantitative data cannot be pooled and analysed using a meta-analysis. If the included publications are quantitative and similar in type, such as all being RCTs, you may be able to analyse the pooled data using meta-analysis, which gives a new estimate of the effectiveness of an intervention or of an association between an exposure and disease. For example, 'Vitamin C supplementation can significantly reduce the risk of developing one or more cold episodes during treatment (pooled Odds Ratio 0.98, 95% confidence intervals 0.95 to 1.00).' (Please see Chapters 10: 'Epidemiology' and 19: 'Quantitative Analysis' for further description.)

Results from a meta-analysis are presented using a forest plot which contains the numerical data from the individual studies together with their confidence intervals. The studies are usually presented in the plot in order of first author's name or chronologically based on date of publication. Figure 14.2 is an example of a forest plot which summarises six trials assessing the effectiveness of Mefloquine for the prevention of diarrhoea as compared to a control. The number of people experiencing diarrhoea in each treatment group are presented, i.e. 'events', along with the number of participants in each treatment group, i.e. 'total'. The odds ratio and 95% confidence interval for each study are presented both numerically and graphically. The squares represent the odds ratio for each study, and the horizontal lines represent the 95% confidence intervals. You will notice that some of the squares are bigger than others, this is because each of the studies included in the meta-analysis is weighted so that the more precise studies, i.e. the ones with the smaller confidence intervals, are given more weight (also given numerically in the 'weight' column as a percentage of the total that study adds to the overall result). The vertical line shows where the odds ratio is 1, i.e. no association between treatment and outcome. The studies to the left of this show that Mefloquine reduces the odds of

Study or Subgroup	Mefloquine Events	Total	Alternative-Control Events	Total	Weight	Odds Ratio IV, Fixed, 95% CI	Odds Ratio IV, Fixed, 95% CI
Arthur 1990	64	134	58	119	25.1%	0.96 [0.59, 1.58]	
Boudreau 1993	16	203	19	156	12.5%	0.62 [0.31, 1.24]	
Croft 1997a	58	183	103	176	32.8%	0.33 [0.21, 0.51]	
Čroft 1997b	25	247	25	224	17.8%	0.90 [0.50, 1.61]	
Koliaritsch 1997	22	60	9	60	7.9%	3.28 [1.36, 7.92]	
Ohrt 1997	7	68	4	67	3.8%	1.81 [0.50, 6.49]	
Total (95% CI)		895		802	100.0%	0.71 [0.56, 0.91]	
Total events	192		218				

Heterogeneity: Chi² = 28.01, df = 5 (P < 0.0001); I² = 82%
Test for overall effect: Z = 2.68 (P = 0.007)

0.2   0.5   1   2   5
Favours Mefloquine   Favours Control

FIGURE 14.2   Mefloquine versus a control for the prevention of Diarrhoea

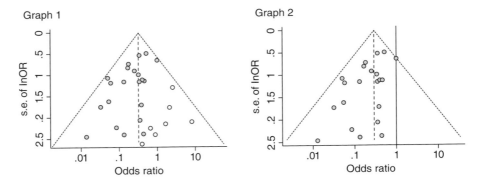

FIGURE 14.3   Funnel plots (Egger 1997)

diarrhoea occurring. The studies which are to the right of the vertical line show that the control (over Mefloquine) reduces the odds of diarrhoea occurring.

At the bottom of the forest plot there is a diamond. The centre of the diamond represents the pooled odds ratio, and the horizontal corners of the diamond are the 95% confidence intervals for the pooled odds ratio. As the diamond is to the left of the vertical line, this shows that Mefloquine reduces the odds of diarrhoea. Addition-ally, as the edges of the diamond are all to the left of the vertical line, the association is statistically significant. The pooled odds ratio is 0.71, which indicates Mefloquine significantly reduces the odds of diarrhoea by 29%. Additionally, the 95% confidence intervals are (0.56 to 0.91), indicating we are 95% confident that the true odds ratio relates to between a 9% (0.91) and 44% (0.56) reduction in the odds of diarrhoea.

You can also assess publication (or selection) bias through meta-analysis via a fun-nel plot. In Figure 14.3, the dark dots represent published data, whilst the open dots or circles represent unpublished data. Due to the inverse standard error scale on the y axis, i.e. the vertical axis, you expect to see larger more powerful studies towards the top with smaller studies scattered along the bottom. The outer dashed lines of the funnel represent the area in which 95% of the studies are expected to lie if there is no bias. The solid line represents no effect size, i.e. an odds ratio of 1, whereas the dashed vertical line represents the effect size found in the meta-analysis. In graph 1 you can see a symmetrical scattering of dots, however graph 2 shows a funnel plot with gap in the bottom right-hand corner containing no dots. This represents bias, and the meta-analysis may therefore overestimate the intervention effect.

Software packages are available for analysis, for example, RevMan from the Cochrane Collaboration for quantitative data, which will produce forest and funnel plots as above, or SUMARI from the Joanna Briggs Institute for use with qualitative data. The utility of these software packages is that a range of screens can be employed with several functions for data input and scrutiny.

Qualitative metasynthesis

If the papers you are including are mainly (or solely) qualitative, there are methods suitable for combing the data. One such method is framework synthesis, which is based upon the framework approach (please see Chapter 20: 'Qualitative Analysis' for a description). This involves finding a pre-existing framework which best fits your question, then extracting the data from all of the included papers and entering them into the framework. You may also generate new themes in this manner. Or you may decide that rather than use a framework that you will develop a set of brand new themes which emerge from the amalgamated qualitative data. If you would like to use this type of analysis, there are a couple of suggestions for further reading at the end of this chapter.

Case study

The systematic review of trials assessing the effectiveness of vitamin C for the common cold (Hemilä et al., 2010) as outlined previously, has been performed adhering to the Cochrane Collaboration guidelines. This study will be used to exemplify the stages of a systematic review as described above.

Framing the question

The authors of the review state a clear question in their aim: to assess whether an oral dose of at least 0.2g/day vitamin C supplementation reduced the incidence, duration or severity of the common cold when used every day to prevent onset, or as therapy after the onset of symptoms. The authors set out clear inclusion and exclusion criteria.

Identifying the relevant literature

This version of the review is an update, and searched for literature from 2006 up to 2010 that could be added to the literature already identified in previous versions of the review, of which there were three (Douglas et al., 1998, 2004, 2007). All together, the review comprises evidence from the past 60 years in total. The authors searched a wide range of electronic databases, and imposed no language or publication type restrictions.

Assessing the methodological quality of the included studies

The authors assessed each of the included studies for methodological quality based on allocation concealment, double-blinding, randomisation, placebo, incomplete outcome data and selective reporting of outcomes. The authors did not perform any analyses that assessed the effect of methodological quality on the findings of the summarised results though.

Summarising the evidence; interpreting the findings

The authors summarised the findings from the studies qualitatively and quantitatively, using meta-analysis (utilising RevMan), and interpretation of the findings of the analyses.

Dissemination

For your systematic review to have an impact in the medical and health care community, the results, outcomes and conclusions need to be presented in a logical and cogent format (see Table 14.3). The use of tables, graphs and diagrams generally are the clearest and most concise arrangement for exhibiting substantial quantitative data sets, and clear and succinct writing should be used for discussing any compelling evidence.

TABLE 14.3   Presentation of data in a systematic review

Methods used for the search:

- Search engines investigated and the headings used in the search
- Methods for identification of studies in the 'grey literature'

The number of papers:

- That were found
- Screened at the different stages
- Studies that were finally included
- Duplicated data – earlier cited studies but based upon the same data set which are excluded to avoid bias
- Excluded studies – reasons for exclusion, including full text not being retrievable and where papers could not be translated

Characteristics of the studies assessed for inclusion/exclusion:

- The participants – their demographics
- Sample size
- Disease/disorder
- Methodologies used
- Number and type of interventions
- Nature of any intervention[s], e.g.

  o classification of drug, therapeutic regime, dose of treatment
  o non-pharmaceutical interventions, exposure levels, ascertainment of exposure

- Description of the outcomes, including definitions used for ascertainment, timing of the outcomes

Quality of the data – where each paper is given a score on the quality of the output via the critical appraisal process:

- Median and ranges of your quality score
- Median scores for particular components of your quality assessment
- Discussion on any possible heterogeneity in the papers retrieved and a hypothesised explanation for this
- A discussion around publication bias

Impact of the intervention[s]:

- Results of the review/meta-analysis, including levels of heterogeneity/effect of intervention[s] found in the groups
- Subgroup analyses based on *a priori* defined groups
- Sensitivity analyses based on restricting the results based on *a priori* defined groups

For instance, you may have conducted an epidemiological review which suggests that the progression of your named disease occurs in a wide variety of environmental contexts. Your conclusion for dissemination would be that the disease was either (a) independent of, or (b) transferable between, the different environmental settings. Conversely, you might find that your named disease is affected by specific environmental factors. In both of these cases your review would recommend further primary research to ascertain the true epidemiological profile of this disease.

Summary

- Systematic reviews provide a comprehensive and unbiased synthesis of the available evidence regarding a focused research question.
- The key players involved in a systematic review are: clinical or topic expert, information specialist, methodological and statistical expert.
- There are five stages to a systematic review: (i) formulating a question, (ii) identifying literature, (iii) assessing the quality of the evidence, (iv) summarising the findings and (v) interpreting the findings into a meaningful conclusion.

Questions for Discussion

Access the following systematic review from the Cochrane Database of Systematic Reviews website (http://www.thecochranelibrary.com): Wiysonge CS, Shey MS, Kongnyuy EJ, Sterne JAC, Brocklehurst P. (2011) Vitamin A supplementation for reducing the risk of mother-to-child transmission of HIV infection. *Cochrane Database of Systematic Reviews*, 19(1): CD003648.

Use the review to answer the following questions:

1. Have the authors identified a need for the review?
2. Is sufficient background information presented?
3. What are the inclusion criteria for the studies?
4. Is the literature search comprehensive?
5. How is the methodological quality of the retrieved studies assessed?
6. What process do the authors use to extract data?
7. What data synthesis is performed, if any?

Further Reading

Barnett-Page, E. and Thomas, J. (2009) 'Methods for the synthesis of qualitative research: a critical review', National Centre for Research Methods: http://eprints.ncrm.ac.uk/690 (accessed Sept. 2012)

Dixon-Woods, M., Agarwhal, S., Jones, D., Young, B. and Sutton, A. (2005) 'Synthesising qualitative and quantitative evidence: a review of possible methods', *Journal of Health Service Research Policy*, 10 (1): 45–53.

Dixon-Woods, M., Agarwhal, S., Young, B., Jones, D. and Sutton, A. (2004) *Integrative Approaches to Qualitative and Quantitative Evidence*. London: Health Development Agency: http://www.nice.org.uk/niceMedia/pdf/Integrative_approaches_evidence.pdf (accessed Sept. 2012).

Gough, D., Oliver, S. and Thomas, J. (2012) *An Introduction to Systematic Reviews*. London: SAGE.

Greenhalgh, T. (1997) 'How to read a paper: papers that summarise other papers (systematic reviews and meta-analyses)', *British Medical Journal*, 315: 672.

Higgins, J.P.T. and Green, S. (2011) *Cochrane Handbook for Systematic Reviews of Interventions*. Version 5.1.0. The Cochrane Collaboration: www.cochrane-handbook.org (accessed Aug. 2012).

Paterson. B.L., Thorne, S.E., Canam, C. and Jillings, C. (2001) *Meta-Study of Qualitative Health Research*. Thousand Oaks, CA: SAGE.

Pogue, J. and Yusuf, S. (1998) 'Meta-analysis', *The Lancet*, 351: 47–52.

Below are the URL links to three reusable learning objects that use multimedia technology: www.nottingham.ac.uk/nmp/sonet/rlos/ebp/systematic_reviews/index.html (accessed Aug. 2012): steps in conducting systematic reviews.

www.nottingham.ac.uk/nmp/sonet/rlos/ebp/meta-analysis (accessed Aug. 2012): introduction to meta-analysis.

www.nottingham.ac.uk/nmp/sonet/rlos/ebp/meta-analysis2 (accessed Aug. 2012): presenting and interpreting meta-analyses.

Websites

Campbell Collaboration, www.campbellcollaboration.org (accessed Aug. 2012).

Centre for Reviews and Dissemination, www.york.ac.uk/inst/crd (accessed Aug. 2012).

Cochrane Collaboration, www.thecochranelibrary.com (accessed Aug. 2012).

Critical Appraisal Skills Programme www.casp-uk.net (accessed Aug. 2012).

International Clinical Trials Registry, http://apps.who.int/trialsearch (accessed Aug. 2012).

Joanna Briggs Institute, www.joannabriggs.edu.au (accessed Aug. 2012).

NHS Health Technology Assessment Programme, www.ncchta.org (accessed Aug. 2012).

References

Blot, W.J. and McLaughling, J.K. (1998) 'Passive smoking and lung cancer risk: what is the story now?', *Journal of the National Cancer Institute*, 90 (19): 1416–17.

Cook, D.J., Sackett, D.L. and Spitzer, W.O. (1995) 'Methodologic guidelines for systematic reviews of randomized control trials in health care from the Potsdam consultation on meta-analysis', *Journal of Clinical Epidemiology*, 48: 167–71.

Douglas, R.M., Chalker, E.B. and Treacy, B. (1998) 'Vitamin C for preventing and treating the common cold', *Cochrane Database of Systematic Reviews*, issue 1.

Douglas, R.M., Hemilä, H., D'Souza, R., Chalker, E.B. and Treacy, B. (2004) 'Vitamin C for preventing and treating the common cold', *Cochrane Database of Systematic Reviews*, issue 4.

Douglas, R.M., Hemilä, H., Chalker, E. and Treacy, B. (2007) 'Vitamin C for preventing and treating the common cold', *Cochrane Database of Systematic Reviews*, issue 3.

Dwan, K., Altman, D.G., Arnaiz, J.A., Bloom, J., Chan, A.-W., et al. (2008) 'Systematic Review of the Empirical Evidence of Study Publication Bias and Outcome Reporting Bias', *PLoS ONE,* 3 (8): e3081.

Egger, M. (1997) 'Bias in meta-analysis detected by a simple graphical test', *British Medical Journal,* 315: 629.

Egger, M., Zellweger, Z., Schneider, M., Junker, C., Lengeler, C. and Antes, G. (1997) 'Language bias in randomised controlled trials published in English and German', *The Lancet,* 350: 326–9.

Greenhalgh, T. (1997) 'How to read a paper: papers that summarise other papers (systematic reviews and meta-analyses)', *British Medical Journal,* 315: 672.

Hemilä, H., Chalker, E. and Douglas, B. (2010) 'Vitamin C for preventing and treating the common cold', *Cochrane Database of Systematic Reviews,* issue 3.

Moher, D., Liberati, A., Tetzlaff, J., Altman, D.G. and the PRISMA Group (2009) 'Preferred reporting items for systematic reviews and meta-analysis: the PRISMA Statement', *PLoS Med* 6(6): e1000097.

Pauling, L. (1970) *Vitamin C and the Common Cold.* Basingstoke: Freeman.

Ritzel, G. (1961) 'Kritische Beurteilung des Vitamins C als Prophylacticum und Therapeuticum der Erkältungskrankheiten' [Critical analysis of the role of vitamin C in the treatment of the common cold], *Helv Med Acta,* 28: 63–8.

Part IV

CONDUCTING VALID AND ETHICAL RESEARCH

15

DESIGNING AND CONDUCTING AN ETHICAL RESEARCH STUDY

Mary Patricia Tully and Gordon Taylor

- To understand the basics in the application of consequentialism, duty-based deontology and rights-based deontology to conducting ethical health services research
- To list some of the common codes of research ethics used in health services research
- To understand how to answer seven key questions, covering common ethical issues, which researchers should ask themselves about their research
- To understand how to apply the key ethical issues that also need to be considered when the study is ongoing

Introduction

Often, when researchers think of research ethics, their hearts sink. Images of interminable forms, aggressive committees and unexplainable revisions requiring months of rewriting flash before their eyes. However, it need not be like that! Being aware of the common ethical issues which are present in research with participants, and the kinds of factors that ethics committee members will be assessing in research studies, can help ease the process by enabling you to address many of the common pitfalls that researchers encounter in demonstrating how they will conduct their research ethically.

Research with human participants has contributed enormously to the welfare of our societies. Although most research does considerable good with little or no potential for harm, it can also pose significant risks and the possibility for things to go wrong. It is really only in the past 60 years that codes and guidelines have been drawn up as to how ethical research should be conducted. The first full statement of the human rights of participants in research was drawn up in 1947 as part of the judicial decision against prominent German doctors and scientists who were on trial for experimenting on humans who were held in the concentration camps (Katz, 1996). The Nuremberg Code outlined 10 requirements for ethical research on humans (Table 15.1).

This code was drawn up in response to the types of research conducted by the Nazi doctors; therefore, it focuses on governing non-therapeutic research on humans. Subsequent ethical guidance extends this to other types of medical research. In 1964, the Declaration of Helsinki drew a distinction between non-therapeutic and therapeutic research. Recent revisions, we are now on the sixth (2008), have broadened the scope to include research on identifiable human tissue and data (World Medical Association, 2008). This Declaration forms the basis of the ethical guidelines for medical research. However, not all academic disciplines relevant to health services research use the same guidelines. The British Psychological Society have their own Code of Human Research Ethics, for example, which

TABLE 15.1   A summary of the key principles in the Nuremberg code, 1947 (Katz, 1996)

1	The voluntary consent of the participant is essential.
2	The research should be expected to yield fruitful results.
3	The research should be justified by previous research.
4	The research should avoid all unnecessary physical and mental suffering and injury.
5	There should be no expectation that death or disabling injury will occur.
6	The degree of risk should never exceed the humanitarian importance.
7	Prior arrangements should be provided to protect participants from injury, disability or death.
8	Research should be conducted only by scientifically qualified people.
9	During the research, the participant should be able to withdraw.
10	During the research, the researcher can terminate the study, if the risk of injury, disability or death is too high.

includes sections on social responsibility in the use of research findings and the ethical conduct of research involving deception (British Psychological Society, 2010). The latter occurs where the participant is wilfully misled initially about the research question, because knowing the real purpose would enable participants to modify their reactions and thus invalidate the findings. The Social Research Association *Ethical Guidelines* recognise that there are similarities and differences between ethical guidelines and requires multidisciplinary researchers to reach an agreed ethical framework for their joint research study, incorporating the principles from each of the disciplines as necessary (Social Research Association, 2003).

There are three distinct perspectives that are commonly taken, regardless of academic discipline, based on well-known ethical theories. First, the end must justify the means, i.e. the ethical theory of consequentialism. This approach does not consider what is going to happen during the research, but only what the expected outcome is. Taken to its extreme, it could thus be argued that a research study with considerable morbidity for a small number of participants, but with a large-scale reduction in morbidity for many thousands of patients in the future, is morally justified. Second is the perspective that no harm should come to the research participants, regardless of how good an outcome might be expected, i.e. duty-based deontology, which considers what will actually happen during the research study. Third is the perspective that the participants should have the right to autonomy, i.e. rights-based deontology. This means that people have the right to consent to take part in research if they wish, which may have some personal risk,, provided they have been given adequate information about what will happen to them if they consent, and they have the freedom to choose whether to take part or withdraw.

Ethical review of a research study seeks to ensure that all three of these perspectives are considered together. Designing research that only considers the consequences of a successful outcome, with no thought given to possible harm or informed consent, would be regarded as unethical, and approval would not be granted. On the contrary, never considering the value of the research and only considering the prevention of harm to the participants would mean that nothing other than the most risk-free research would ever be done, which in the long term, would have a detrimental effect on overall evidence-based medicine. For each individual study, a balance needs to be drawn between all three perspectives. It is in achieving this balance that the potential for disagreement between the researcher and the ethical approval board can occur. The NHS ethics service, for example, are told to prioritise duty-based and rights-based deontology: 'the interests of researchers and research are always secondary to the dignity, rights, safety and well-being of people taking part in research' (Department of Health, 2011: 14), whereas researchers submitting applications for review may prioritise consequentialism.

Designing an ethical research study

Most researchers who are doing health services or clinical research will have to submit an application to an ethics committee at some point in their career. Regardless of whether you use your health or university ethics service, there are fundamental decisions that you need to make about the design of your research study which can impact on the ethics. Below is a series of questions that you should ask yourself about your study. This will not only make the completion of the ethical approval form easier, but also your grant proposal, as funders usually ask, as part of their award application, if there are any ethical considerations associated with your proposal, and often will not release the grant until ethical approval is in place.

Is the research of potential value?

The expectation that research should yield fruitful results is the foundation of ethical research. There are two aspects that you should consider when answering this question: (i) the potential outcome of your research, and (ii) the 'return on investment' of the resources required for its conduct. When the research outcome is considered from a consequentialist perspective, you should be convinced that conducting the research is more likely to maximise the benefits to mankind than not conducting the research. Not every piece of research is necessarily going to maximise societal benefit in the same way. The benefit from conducting the research could simply be new knowledge that has value because it underpins the next piece of research. The impact of the research on direct patient care may only occur following a sequence of preliminary studies leading to a definitive study, each with varying kinds of values. It is up to you to explain the value of conducting the work in a way that is comprehensible to the ethics committee members.

In particular, a very clear justification needs to be given for research that might be otherwise argued as having a relatively minor impact. The outcome of conducting a study might not be related to the research findings themselves, for example. A small-scale study investigating patients' information requirements, replicating a previous small-scale study that had been conducted elsewhere, could be argued as having little potential value. However, because it is conducted by an undergraduate student, the value of the research is in its training capacity, which could be considered more useful than the study findings.

The 'return on investment' of the research is underpinned by similar ethical arguments. Due to the scarcity of research funding and the strict budgets imposed, the best use must be made of available resources. It would be hard to argue that a trivial study was a good use of such resources. The investment is not just money, however. Research participants, who are willing to risk inconvenience or harm, often do so because they believe that the research results will benefit a larger group of people. If a study cannot deliver on this implied promise, it removes the rights of participants to be fully informed about what will happen, not just to themselves, but to the results of the study.

Will the research be conducted in a methodologically robust manner?

This question addresses whether the research design chosen is capable of fulfilling the project's aims and objectives. Without this, the research cannot deliver any benefits and, from a consequentialist perspective, it is thus unethical. More worryingly, the wrong method can result in findings that can be misinterpreted. A fatally flawed research study could erroneously state that, for example, drug A is appropriate for the treatment of a particular disease state, leading to its introduction into practice. Many patients would thus be exposed to an ineffective treatment that may have unpleasant side effects, and be costly to the health provider. From a duty-based deontology perspective, this is clearly unethical. Although an ethics committee is not a peer-review body itself, many of its members are experienced researchers. If members notice that a study is methodologically flawed, this will be highlighted and the committee will propose that it would be unethical for the study to be allowed to progress without appropriate amendment (Angell et al., 2008). In addition, NHS and university committees expect evidence that peer review of the study design has been conducted, commensurate with the scale of the research.

There are certain aspects in the choice of study design that raise specific ethical problems (Brabin et al. 2009; Roberts et al., 2009; Tully et al., 2009; Vail et al., 2009). One of these is whether it is ethical to use randomisation in clinical trials of therapeutic agents such as medicinal products or surgical techniques (please see Chapter 11: 'Clinical Trials'). Consequentialism would argue that a randomised clinical trial is the best possible method to answer the question as to which of two or more therapeutic options is more effective. Any other research method would therefore be unethical. Duty-based deontology, on the other hand, would argue that doctors are required to offer their patients the best care that they can. But how can they offer the best care when the patient is being randomised to one of several arms of a study and not being explicitly offered 'best care'? However, the trial should be conducted because there is limited evidence as to whether any the options is better than the other, i.e. community equipoise. This is when the opinion of the scientific community at large is considered, rather than the belief of the individual doctor as to which intervention is best. If that uncertainty did not exist, it would be an unethical study. Thus, it is argued, if the body of evidence allows no certainty as to which option is best, the doctor can discharge their duty of care by giving the patient any of the options to which they could be randomised, as without the evidence, all are possibly the 'best care'. There is some debate, however, as to how such equipoise is applied in clinical trials (Gifford, 2000), as individual doctors still have to consider their own personal values when recruiting their patients to specific clinical trials.

With placebo-controlled studies, achieving equipoise can be even more challenging as the doctor has to be uncertain whether the intervention being tested is no better than doing nothing. In the Declaration of Helsinki, the use of placebo-controlled studies is limited to occasions where there is either no proven or no available treatment (World Medical Association, 2008). In the USA, the Food and Drug Administration requires that the comparator for any new drug seeking market authorisation is a placebo, except in life-threatening situations. The Medicine and Health Products Regulation Authority in the UK does not require this, however. This can lead to a major ethical dilemma for international studies conducted in the UK, when there is the belief that proven treatments are already in existence and that it would be unethical to use placebos as the comparator. Therefore, in such situations, the researcher needs to explicitly justify the choice of a placebo-controlled study to the ethics committee.

Does the research have an acceptable risk-benefit ratio?

The risk-benefit ratio of the research study must be both justifiable and acceptable. Consequentialism highlights the importance of the study having value overall, although not necessarily to the individual participant. For example, a new drug treatment must be properly validated with randomised, placebo-controlled clinical trials in which some participants who are randomised to the intervention arm may get benefits, or side effects, from the new treatment being tested. Others will be randomised to the control arm where they receive a placebo, which will give them only the placebo effect. Without conducting such a trial, however, it would not be possible to get a potential valuable new treatment onto the market. A before and after study, for example, would expose all participants to the same benefits and risks, but robust and valid results regarding efficacy and harm would not be obtained. Duty-based deontology, on the other hand, considers whether the risk to participants is justifiable and acceptable.

Deciding whether the risks and benefits of an individual study are justifiable and acceptable considers both of these ethical perspectives. If the potential risk of study participation is that the patient may lose their hair, for example, this would need to be put in the context of the hypothesised overall benefit of the study. If the study was to investigate a new shampoo to treat head lice more quickly, this harm may not be considered either justifiable or acceptable, even if head lice eradication was quicker. However, if the study was to investigate a new treatment to reduce mortality in liver cancer, the harm is comparable to other chemotherapeutic agents and the benefit, if it did indeed reduce mortality, would be considerable. Thus the risk could be considered both justifiable and acceptable.

Perceptions of risk need to be considered by both the researchers and the participants, who are likely to value risks and benefits differently to each other. Public and patient involvement in the research design stage can be invaluable for identifying patient values (please see Chapter 16: 'Patient and Public Involvement').

Are the research participants recruited in a way that protects their right to privacy?

In order to recruit participants to a research study, they first have to be identified and then approached. In any study, researchers are looking for participants who fulfil certain inclusion criteria; therefore, prior to being approached, the researchers need to know which patients are likely to fulfil the inclusion criteria. This raises some issues regarding confidentiality as it is an expectation of patients that their health records are kept confidential by their doctors. There are a number of potential ways around this problem which allow people the right to confidentiality, whilst researchers identify potential participants. The most common method is for people who would normally have access to health care records as part of their job, for example, practice nurses, family doctors, etc., to identify potential participants and contact them on behalf of the researchers. Please bear in mind, however, that some practices will charge for this type of service. Alternatively, people can give their consent for their records to be accessed by the researchers themselves. They could give this consent as part of a screening questionnaire, for example, sent indiscriminately to all people attending a particular service on behalf of the researchers. Active teams of researchers may initially ask patients if they are willing to participate in research in general, rather than for a specific study. Data can then be collected as to what disorders they have, and their contact details and consent for access to their records added to a research register owned by the team. Potential participants can then be contacted at a later time about specific research studies. The creation and maintenance of such registers does not require an ethical opinion in the UK.

Do the participants have autonomy to provide freely given, informed consent?

Rights-based deontology argues that the consent process is fundamental to the conduct of ethical research. The consent process is more than just asking a participant to sign a sheet, however. Consent must be freely given, i.e. the participant is not coerced into agreeing to participate and they have the option to say no if they wish. Although researchers forcing participants into joining their study is generally unheard of, a perception of coercion can exist in the mind of the potential participant, which can be just as powerful as actual coercion. Such a perceived lack of free will could occur in a number of situations. Subordinates, such as junior researchers, may feel pressurised into participating in studies recruiting healthy volunteers. They may be asked by the person who will write their performance review, or by the colleague who participated in their own study six months ago. Elderly patients may not feel powerful enough in the relationship to say no to their doctors if asked to participate in a clinical trial they are running. Concerted effort, therefore, needs to be made so that such pressure is identified and avoided. For example, rather than asking the junior researchers to participate in person, you could use adverts for your project where they have the freedom whether to respond or not. Or rather than patients being asked by their own doctors to participate in studies (although they could introduce your study), consent could be obtained by an independent person to whom they felt able to say no, without worrying that it will impact negatively on their future care.

For consent to be valid, it must also be informed. For the majority of studies, this will mean the provision of a participant information leaflet (PIL) and, where possible, going through this with potential participants to ensure that they understand it. A PIL should tell potential participants what the study is aiming to do, why they have been approached and, if they do participate, what they will have to do and/or what will happen to them. It must be written using language that potential participants can understand (once again, patient involvement can be a useful tool to help you with this). In studies with children, it is commonplace to have an age-appropriate PIL for the child, in addition to the one for the parent or guardian who will be giving formal consent. Such PILs can make extensive use of illustrations or cartoons so that the child can understand what would happen to them if they took part. Information can also be provided via alternative media, such as by audio or video recordings. These may be appropriate for people who are unable to read or are visually impaired. Regardless of the medium chosen for your PIL, a copy of it should be given to the participant so that it can be referred to when desired. Detailed advice on the content and layout of PILs can be found on the National Research Ethics Service website (NRES, 2012). Potential participants need to be given adequate time to read and understand the PIL and, if they wish, discuss the research with others before making a decision. Twenty-four hours for this is common. Shorter times would need to be clearly justified but can be acceptable, such as needing to obtain consent from women for an obstetric trial when they are admitted onto a maternity ward in labour.

Although seeking and obtaining consent is clearly the ideal, there are many types of research that could not be done at all if this was an absolute imperative, such as studies into new treatments for people unconscious after head trauma or with advanced dementia. For people who have no capacity to consent, it is important that the research that is being conducted is related in some way to their condition. It could be argued that it is a violation of these people's autonomy if the research could just as easily be conducted with people who do have capacity to consent. People who have a temporary loss of capacity, such as those who are unconscious, can be consulted about the study when they have regained capacity. At that time, if they do not wish to participate in the study, their data can be removed, although it may not be possible to reverse research interventions they have had whilst lacking capacity. In England and Wales, the Mental Capacity Act (2005) gave a legal framework as to what to do when seeking to involve adults in research who cannot consent for themselves. The NRES website provides detailed information about how to adhere to this legislation, which may give helpful guidance for studies recruiting participants who cannot give informed consent for whatever reasons.

As well as ensuring that people who do not want to participate are given the opportunity to refuse, it is just as important to ensure that the people who do want to participate in research are given that opportunity. It has been argued that participating in scientific research is a moral duty (Harris, 2005; Shapshay and Pimple, 2007). Therefore, care should be taken to include, wherever possible, people with a broad range of ages, disabilities, sex, sexual orientations, race, cultures and religions when recruiting participants, reflecting the cultural diversity within society (Department of Health, 2005). For example, this could involve translating PILs into different languages or providing the information in alternative formats (there is more discussion about inclusive recruitment in Chapter 18: 'Recruitment and Retention'). However, there can be perfectly legitimate scientific reasons for excluding certain groups of people, such as when there would be an unacceptable level of risk to them. Pregnant women being ineligible for studies investigating new medicinal products is one example. There may be other methodological reasons, such as when using validated questionnaires which are only available in English as your outcome measure the study may have to exclude people who cannot communicate fluently in that language. Any exclusion criteria you choose, however, must be rationalised and explained to the ethics committee, so that it is clear that you have given some thought to ensuring diversity in your recruitment.

There are types of research where gaining informed consent is not feasible at all and decisions have to be made as to whether the consequences of doing the research outweighs the rights of the people to consent to their participation. One example is observational research of groups of people (such as in a waiting room), where prior consent is not possible without changing behaviour and seriously compromising the quality of the data (please see Chapter 7: 'Qualitative Data Collection'). Another is when analysing large health care databases, where obtaining consent from each and every patient whose details are in the database would take longer than doing the actual study! Researchers need to explicitly weigh up the importance of the public interest in doing the research versus the rights of the patients to control the use of data about themselves (Brown et al., 2008; Parker, 2005).

Are there procedures to protect the well-being, privacy and dignity of the participants?

One of the key things that should be addressed is the protection of research participants from predictable harm. Well-being is not just physical, but also mental. In many research studies, some physical and/or mental health side effects are predictable. A randomised controlled trial to assess the efficacy of a new non-steroidal anti-inflammatory drug, for instance, may cause gastric bleeding, as this is a common side effect in similar drugs, so might be predictable for a new one. Similarly, a questionnaire containing sensitive questions might be expected to cause upset to the participant. In both of these examples, what would normally be expected is that processes are put in place to ensure that these predictable consequences are identified and addressed. Safeguards could include conducting laboratory, physical or psychological tests and having prearranged procedures in place as to what would happen if these tests show adverse events have occurred. Researchers normally describe in the protocol how they will recognise and address adverse events for participants in the intervention arm of a study, however they may be less explicit at describing the processes to safeguard those participants in the placebo arm of the study. These people will not be receiving treatment, and should therefore be monitored for the effects of, for example, worsening disease.

It is also possible that the battery of tests (whether physical, psychological, or both) a study participant receives means that some hitherto unknown health problem comes to light. For example, if people's hearing levels are being assessed to ensure that only people within a predefined hearing range are recruited to the study, what would you do if you found that someone has hearing loss, who hitherto believed that their hearing level was 'normal'? Again, such eventualities are predictable, so a plan of what you would do if this circumstance arose should be drafted prior to starting the study. This could simply be to give the potential participant a letter to take to their family doctor outlining what was found (or to contact the family doctor directly, with the patient's consent). With the exception of some legal obligations, the information you obtain from a participant is confidential and should only be shared with other identified members of the research team. Participants have the right to expect the data they give you to be protected; therefore, reasonable precautions should be taken to safeguard the data. Any identifiable data and raw data, for example, completed questionnaires, interview recordings, etc., need to be carefully stored as the data could be linked back to the actual research participants.

It is not unusual for researchers to consider reusing data from one research study for another study. Perhaps they want to compare data from different time points, or want to compare their data with data from another research group. If this is a possibility for your project, you need to be explicit with your participants about what might happen to their data after the study ends. If their data are going to be retained and used by a wider research group, then you cannot promise the participants that their interviews, for example, will only be accessed by the interviewer alone. Explain what type of research could be done with the data and who would have access to it. This is particularly the case for data that are going to be shared with researchers outside of the country of origin. Participants will want reassurance that the other researchers would take similar care of their data as the research team they had originally given it to.

Is there a dissemination strategy for the research findings?

The publication of research results is not just for the benefit of the researcher's CV. Consequentialism argues that the research must be 'for the greater good'; publishing the results ensures that this can be realised. Health professionals can then decide whether to implement your findings in their clinical practice. Failure to disseminate thus takes away the goal-based justification for having done the research in the first place. Research that has not been published or made available by other means is no different than research that has not been conducted. The resources expended, including the time and effort and goodwill of the research participants, will have been wasted. This need to publish research is clearly made in section 30 of the Declaration of Helsinki (World Medical Association, 2008), which states that authors have a duty to make the results of their research on human subjects publicly available and that they are accountable for the completeness and accuracy of their reports. This does not just apply to studies with positive results. Studies with negative or inconclusive results must also be published, although it is acknowledged that this is more difficult due to publication bias (please see Chapter 14: 'Systematic Reviews'). With the emergence of open access repositories, trial databases and funders publishing the results from their awards on their websites regardless of the findings, this issue is becoming less problematic however (please see Chapter 21: 'Dissemination').

Case study

A pharmaceutical company has identified a potential new asthma inhaler drug. The drug is similar to other drugs already in use for asthma and looks promising after being tested in healthy volunteers. The company is therefore now looking to conduct an effectiveness study in patients with asthma. This will be a double-blind, crossover randomised controlled trial, which will be conducted in primary care. After consent, there is a short washout period of one week where participants do not receive any treatment at all, then for the next three months they are randomised to receive either the new inhaler drug or the standard treatment. There is then another week of washout, before participants receive three months of the alternative treatment they had not received in the first stage.

Is the research of potential value?

The pharmaceutical company needs to argue that there is a need for a new inhaler drug and that there is an advantage to the new drug over the others already available. From a consequentialist point of view, it would not be ethical to produce a drug with no hypothesised advantages over those currently available. One might argue, however, that another drug would create greater competition and therefore market forces would keep the price down, providing a benefit to the health care system.

Will the research be conducted in a methodologically robust manner?

From a consequentialist perspective, a randomised clinical trial is the best possible method to answer an effectiveness question. However, doctors are required to offer their patients the best care that they can, i.e. duty-based deontology. Therefore, for the research to be ethical, there needs to be uncertainty regarding whether the new inhaler is better than the currently prescribed one, i.e. community equipoise. The proposed study will compare the new inhaler with the one currently regarded as best practice. No placebo will be used, as this could be detrimental to the participant's health over the three months trial duration. The participant is also their own control, as data will be collected from them after using both the new inhaler and the usual care inhaler. The study also has predefined stopping rules if the interim analysis shows that there are serious adverse effects.

Does the research have an acceptable risk-benefit ratio?

Patients will not receive any medication during the washout periods, which puts them at potential risk of asthma attacks, so some appropriate safeguards need to be put in place.

Are the research participants recruited in a way to protect their right to privacy?

The researchers are recruiting patients with asthma requiring inhaler treatment from primary care. The study will be introduced to the patients via their family doctors and

(Continued)

(Continued)

posters will be placed in the waiting rooms. The researchers also have money to pay for one mail-out to all patients on the family doctor's database who fits their inclusion criteria. If patients are interested in taking part, they will be asked to contact the researcher whose details will be on any information.

Do the participants have autonomy to provide freely given, informed consent?

The family doctor will not be asked to take consent, to avoid the patient feeling coerced. Instead, consent will be obtained by a study nurse.

Are there procedures to protect the well-being, privacy and dignity of the participants?

As mentioned above, stopping rules are drafted and included in the trial, and all data collected for analysis will be anonymised. Participants will be advised that they can withdraw at any time, and taking part (or not) in the trial, or withdrawal, will not affect their health care provision. As it is predicted that there may be a chance of risk during the washout periods, a helpline number will be given so that they can talk to a nurse if required.

Is there a dissemination strategy for the research findings?

This trial is run by a pharmaceutical company, so publishing in academic journals is not the main objective. However, the trial and its results will be available on an open access trial register. They will also disseminate their findings at appropriate conferences, and to commissioners and patients via charity websites such as Asthma UK.

As can be seen in this case study, research may have to be terminated early if the risks of an intervention are shown to outweigh the benefits following interim analysis. Although it would seem unethical to keep people in the study if an interim analysis shows a large benefit of one of the interventions, there is a risk of overestimating the impact of the intervention by not completing the study according to the original protocol (Montori et al., 2005).

Conducting an ethical research study

Conducting research ethically is something that should be part of the study throughout its lifetime and is a responsibility for anyone conducting research with people. Research ethics is often seen as a hurdle that one has to overcome before study starts, and is just one of the approvals that needs to be obtained so that the researcher is allowed to start the study, and is then forgotten about. An ongoing study obviously needs to adhere to what was agreed at the time it received an ethical opinion, such as the recruitment and consent procedure of the participants. However, there are specific ethical issues that crop up during the study and which need to be considered also, such as participants being able to not only freely enter into the study, but freely withdraw also. There should be no pressure applied to keep someone in the study, nor should participants worry that, if they tried to withdraw, such pressure would be applied or their health care would be affected in anyway. Researchers should be prepared for the unexpected; in particular, junior researchers should have a clear mechanism for contacting and involving senior researchers if something goes wrong. In the next case study, for example, what would the interviewer do if a junior doctor described some serious malpractice?

Case study

Researchers are conducting a qualitative research study about the causes of prescribing errors in hospital practice. A lot is known about the prevalence of such errors – they occur with about 9% of prescriptions and for over 50% of hospital admissions. However, much less is known about *why* they happen. The researchers will recruit 30 junior doctors to the study by email and short recruitment presentations. They will be interviewed about any recent prescribing errors they had made, concentrating on the detail of what had happened and what was going on prior to the error occurring.

Is the research of potential value?

Knowing how such errors were caused would help to design an effective intervention in order to prevent them. In other words, this research would inform the next piece of research in this area.

Will the research be conducted in a methodologically robust manner?

As this is a *why* question, with lots of possible reasons to discover, qualitative methodology is appropriate.

Does the research have an acceptable risk-benefit ratio?

There is little physical risk associated with this project. If the team think that some of the interview questions could be emotive however, they need to put in a safeguard, such as providing leaflets for their employer's counselling service. Also, participants may feel that there are professional risks where, if they admit to making prescribing errors, they may be disciplined.

(Continued)

(Continued)

Are the research participants recruited in a way to protect their right to privacy?

The researcher would not have a legitimate right to access the human resources records of all staff in the hospital in order to produce a list of only the junior doctors so that they can email them. A gatekeeper, such as the postgraduate tutor, may be willing to send out an email on behalf of the research team. Presentations at pre-existing teaching sessions or in the doctors' mess (especially if the team can afford to pay for some food), posters and word of mouth would work better.

Do the participants have autonomy to provide freely given, informed consent?

Yes. The junior doctors will be invited to contact the researcher if they are interested, so there would be no coercion issues.

Are there procedures to protect the well-being, privacy and dignity of the participants?

Interviews rather than focus groups are appropriate, as discussing prescription errors could be regarded as private and emotive, and the participant may fear criticism or reprisal for their errors. Assurances should be made regarding the confidentiality of the data.

Is there a dissemination strategy for the research findings?

This is the first project of a programme of work whose ultimate objective is to design an intervention tool. Therefore, the results will support any ensuing grant applications. However, it is also envisaged that a peer-reviewed publication will be produced.

Scientific research fraud happens. Not often, but not never! Such misconduct undermines the entire purpose of doing any research – the gathering and analysis of data in order to advance knowledge. The 'greater good' is not achieved and the rights of participants to engage in an activity towards that greater good are denied. A systematic review of the international literature found that 2.6% of scientists surveyed admitted to fabricating or falsifying research data and 9.5% admitted other questionable research practices, such as removing parts of the data set or misleading the reporting of results (Fanelli, 2009). In addition, 12.3% and 28.5% respectively had personal knowledge of fabrication or falsification, or questionable research practices made by others. Junior researchers may be in the difficult position of knowing that such misconduct is occurring and having to decide what to do. The UK Research Integrity Office (www.ukrio.org) provides a helpline for the confidential discussion of suspected research misconduct if individuals feel that they cannot report it to the relevant governance structures within their organisation.

Summary

- Research is expected to be designed so that it is of potential value, conducted in a methodologically robust manner and have an acceptable risk-benefit ratio.

- Research participants should be recruited so as to protect their right to privacy and they should have the autonomy to provide freely given, informed consent prior to participation and to withdraw from the study at any time.

- During the conduct of research studies, there should be procedures put in place to protect the well-being, privacy and dignity of the participants, particularly from predictable risks.

- It should be possible to terminate a study early if there is an unacceptable risk to the participants or a suspicion of research fraud.

- When a study is complete, there should be an appropriate dissemination strategy for the research findings.

- The emphasis given to different ethical considerations will depend on your perspective: consequentialist, duty-based deontologist or rights-based deontologist.

Questions for Discussion

1. It is a principle of data protection that data should only be used for the purpose that it was collected. However, family doctors regularly consult their patient databases, collected for the purposes of treatment, in order to identify potential participants for research studies. Discuss whether this is a justifiable use of the data.

2. There is a clear power imbalance between the family doctor and their patient and therefore, from the point of view of the patients' autonomy, family doctors are not a good choice for consenting patients into studies. However, due to confidentiality issues, external researchers would not have access to the patient in order to consent them into the study. What steps might be taken to mitigate this situation?

3. What steps would you take to ensure that consent in the above case studies was both freely given and informed?

Further Reading

Foster, Claire (2001) *The Ethics of Medical Research on Humans*. Cambridge: Cambridge University Press.

Long, Tony, and Johnson, Martin (2007) *Research Ethics in the Real World: Issues and Solutions for Health and Social Care*. Edinburgh: Churchill Livingstone.

Rachels, James (2003) *The Elements of Moral Philosophy* (4th edn). New York: McGraw Hill.

References

Angell, E.L., Bryman, A., Ashcroft, R.E. and Dixon-Woods, M. (2008) 'An analysis of decision letters by research ethics committees: the ethics/scientific quality boundary examined', *Quality and Safety of Health Care*, 17 (2): 131–6.

Brabin, L., Roberts, S., Tully, M., Vail, A. and McNamee, R. (2009) 'Methodological considerations in ethical review – 1. Scientific reviews: what should ethics committees be looking for?', *Research Ethics Review*, 5: 28–30.

British Psychological Society (2010) *Code of Human Research Ethics*. Leicester: British Psychological Society.

Brown, L., Parker, M. and Dixon-Woods, M. (2008) 'Whose interest? British newspaper reporting of use of medical records for research', *Journal of Health Services Research and Policy*, 13(3): 140–5.

Department of Health (2005) *Research Governance Framework for Health and Social Care* (2nd edn). London: Department of Health.

Department of Health (2011) *Governance Arrangements for Research Ethics Committees: A Harmonised Edition*. London: The Stationery Office.

Fanelli, D. (2009) 'How many scientists fabricate and falsify research? A systematic review and meta-analysis of survey data', *PLoS One*, 4 (5).

Gifford, F. (2000) 'Freedman's "clinical equipoise" and sliding-scale all-dimensions-considered equipoise', *Journal of Medical Philosophy*, 25 (4): 399–426.

Harris, J. (2005) 'Scientific research is a moral duty', *Journal of Medical Ethics*, 31: 242–8.

Katz, J. (1996) 'The Nuremberg Code and the Nuremberg Trial: a reappraisal', *Journal of the American Medical Association*, 276 (20): 1662–6.

Montori, V.M., Devereaux, P.J., Adhikari, N.K.J., Burns, K.E.A., Eggert, C.H., Briel, M., Lacchetti, C., Leung, T.W., Darling, E., Bryant, D.M., Bucher, H.C., Schunemann, H., Meade, M.O., Cook, D.J., Erwin, P.J., Sood, A., Sood, R., Lo, B., Thompson, C.A., Zhou, Q., Mills, E. and Guyatt, G.H. (2005) 'Randomized trials stopped early for benefit: a systematic review', *Journal of the American Medical Association*, 294 (17): 2203–9.

National Research Ethics Service (NRES) (2012) 'Consent guidance': http://www.nres.nhs.uk/applications/guidance/consent-guidance-and-forms (accessed June 2012).

Parker, M. (2005) 'When is research on patient records without consent ethical?', *Journal of Health Service Research Policy*, 10 (3): 183–6.

Roberts, S., Brabin, L., Vail, A., Tully, M.P. and McNamee, R. (2009) 'Methodological considerations in ethical review – 4. Research conduct', *Research Ethics Review*, 5 (4): 143–6.

Shapshay, S. and Pimple, K.D. (2007) 'Participation in biomedical research is an imperfect moral duty: a response to John Harris', *Journal of Medical Ethics*, 33 (7): 414–17.

Social Research Association (2003) *Ethical Guidelines*. London: Social Research Association.

Tully, M.P., Vail, A., Roberts, S., Brabin, L. and McNamee, R. (2009) 'Methodological considerations in ethical review – 3. Sampling and data analysis', *Research Ethics Review*, 5 (3): 121–4.

Vail, A., Tully, M., Brabin, L., Roberts, S. and McNamee, R. (2009) 'Methodological considerations in ethical review - 2. Are the study aims justified and is the design appropriate?', *Research Ethics Review*, 5: 85–8.

World Medical Association (2008) *Declaration of Helsinki: Ethical Principles for Medical Research Involving Human Subjects*: http://www.wma.net/en/30publications/10policies/b3/17c.pdf (accessed Nov. 2012).

16

PATIENT AND PUBLIC INVOLVEMENT IN YOUR RESEARCH

Raksha Pandya-Wood and Andrew Robinson

Learning Objectives

- To understand the theory behind patient and public involvement in research
- To be able to apply the public and patient involvement theory into your own research
- To understand what appropriate involvement is
- To gain some understanding about the impact of patient and public involvement in research

Introduction

Patient and public involvement in research is research being carried out 'with' or 'by' patients or members of the public rather than 'to', 'about' or 'for' them. This includes, for example, working with research funders to prioritise research, offering advice as members of a project steering group, commenting on and developing research materials and undertaking interviews with research participants (INVOLVE website, 2012).

The move towards the involvement in research of patients and the public began with participatory action research which over the years, has gained power based upon its growing evidence base and validity, and been described as 'a powerful strategy for advancing scientific knowledge and achieving practical objectives' (Whyte, 1989: 367). In the UK in the 1980s when there was a Conservative government in power, the idea of market economies was being introduced into health and social care and consumerism became a focus of health care. In 1991, the Citizens Charter was introduced promoting the patients' voice, and by the year 2000, patient involvement featured in the Department of Health's Research and Development policy. Over the last decade there have been some huge policy changes to encourage involvement in all aspects of health research, such as the National Institute for Health Research funding an advisory group, INVOLVE, whose role it is to advance involvement and to promote it as an integral part of research.

There are many reasons for involving people in research. First, an underpinning philosophy is that involvement of people in research gives the research greater clarity, focus and relevance, and is therefore potentially better quality (Brett et al., 2009). Second, a pragmatic point is that research funders take involvement seriously and a lack of patient and public involvement in a grant application may negatively influence the funding decision. The Director General of NHS Research and the Chief Medical Officer have recently stated that involvement should be the norm not the exception (Staniszewska et al., 2011). A third reason is that involving people in health research holds a moral and ethical stance. People living with a health condition have a right to contribute to the research. Most government-funded research is paid for with money collected through taxation, and the public are the taxpayers.

Impact of patient and public involvement in research

In 2009, Staley conducted a review of hundreds of papers exploring how the impact of patient and public involvement appeared in health and social care research literature. The work aimed to explore the different types of impact noted at different stages of the research journey: pre, during and post research. Staley concluded that it was:

> ... difficult to assess the impact of involvement or to predict where involvement would have the greatest impact [and that] more work is needed to clarify the added value of involvement in different research contexts. (2009: 9)

A different review, incorporating a meta-analysis, explored the issues around measuring the impact from involvement. The researchers found that there was an inconsistency in how impact was understood and measured, and concluded that:

There is a clear need to develop a much more consistent and robust base by enhancing the quality of reporting to enable impact to be fully identified and evaluated. (Brett et al., 2010: 114)

The Brett team's conclusion was supported by another review that explored the impact of user involvement on NHS delivery which surmised that there was a 'lack of valid and reliable tools to capture the impact' (Mockford et al., 2011: 37). Based upon these conclusions, Staniszewska et al. (2011) developed the Guidance for Reporting Involvement of Patients and the Public checklist to help researchers determine the issues that should be reported when writing about patient and public involvement and its impact on the research process for journals.

Who are the patients and the public?

There are many names for people who use health and social care services such as 'user', 'lay person', 'client' or 'consumer' (McLaughlin, 2009). Table 16.1 gives an overview of some of the different types of people, groups and communities that are

TABLE 16.1 Who are the patients and the public?

Group	Who they are and what they can offer
Patients	Including past, current and potential patients gives researchers direct access to the views and experiences of the people the research aims to benefit.
Carers	Informal, or unpaid carers, look after people with a variety of illnesses or conditions. They offer invaluable insights into the needs of the people they care for but, equally importantly, also their own needs and perspectives of what it's like to be a carer.
Public	This may include people who have a particular interest in a specific area of health, or who have an opinion on certain health-related issues, including public health. Involving members of the public can be useful in obtaining a more objective perspective.
Parents and guardians	It may not be possible to directly involve children in research, depending on the age of the child and the task required. However, it may be possible to involve parents and guardians who have invaluable insights into the needs and experiences of their children.
People from diverse and vulnerable communities	This term may be used to describe many different types of people, such as people from black and minority ethnic communities or people with learning disabilities. These people are not always given the opportunity to be involved, but can add a great deal to the research when they are. For example, people with learning disabilities may live with a variety of long-term conditions and experience many barriers in accessing mainstream health services. Their views can prove invaluable if researchers engage them in an appropriate way, with accessible formats of communication.
Community support groups, charities, voluntary sector organisations	These support a large number of people with specific illnesses and conditions, as well as their families and carers. Accessing people through them can give the researcher access to a wide range of perspectives and experience, and also validate your research project, and so can confer trust.

included under the term 'patient and public' and what they can add to the research process through being involved.

Case study

Due to side effects of treatment, survivors of head and neck cancer are often faced with a limited ability to swallow which impacts on the type of food they can eat, with some survivors having to rely on sip feeds or having feeding tubes into their stomachs. These factors impact on their overall quality of life, including their ability to travel and socialise. Therefore, a project was designed to explore the issues surrounding food and eating with the aim of producing a booklet including recipes, anecdotes, cooking techniques and advice, which would help survivors cope and therefore improve their quality of life.

In developing the project, including formulating the research questions and determining outcomes, the researchers wanted to understand more about the issues faced by survivors of head and neck cancer in relation to food, and how these issues impacted on their quality of life. Involving patients helped them understand issues such as taste alteration, problems with certain food textures, functional difficulties of eating and the related emotions surrounding these.

In an article in an INVOLVE newsletter, the researchers wrote,

The proposal is more meaningful and patient/survivor-focused in its questions, research processes, planned milestones, outcomes and methods of dissemination than it would have been without the [patient and public involvement] ... Everyone's expertise has been placed on an equal footing during this process, and as a result this project is 'ours' in the full sense. It belongs to everyone involved in its journey so far. (Burges Watson et al., 2011: 10)

Levels of involvement

Figure 16.1 shows the spectrum of involvement, from consultation through to user-driven, and it highlights the power relationship that people have with the principal researcher (Hickey and Kipping, 1998). Consultation is the minimum level of involvement as it does not promise the acceptance of the suggestions that the patients and the public make (Kirby, 2004). Although consultation can provide useful comments and feedback that can be used to inform research, it can also encourage tokenism (Fleming and Hudson, 2009). Moving along the spectrum is collaboration, which is about having an active partnership between the researchers and the patients and the public. True collaboration takes time, and training, for the research team (Vijayakrishnan et al., 2006), and financial commitment (INVOLVE, 2010) but can have real measurable impact on the research. User-driven research is the last point on the spectrum. Here the users are in charge of the research. This takes extremely good mentoring skills from the academic/clinical co-applicants and can take a longer time to complete. It is also very difficult to secure funding for a user-led project, and is therefore rare (Shea et al., 2005).

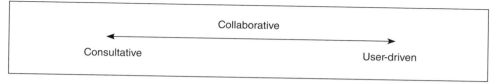

FIGURE 16.1   Spectrum of involvement (adapted from Hanley et al., 2004)

There is no optimum level of involvement, as it is whatever's appropriate and has impact for that particular project. Nor is it necessary to use the same level of involvement throughout the project. For example, it may be appropriate to work in collaboration with patients and members of the public during the design stage of a project, such as determining the outcomes in a focus group, and then consultation in the following stages, such as asking them to review recruitment information. It is also possible to combine two levels of involvement in the same stage – when designing your project, you might involve people through collaboration as mentioned above, whilst also consulting at the same time by presenting your protocol to a group of patients and asking for feedback.

Case study

The researchers in the head and neck cancer project worked in collaboration with survivors and their partners throughout the project. If the researchers had consulted instead, by developing the research question and subsequently asking for feedback, they would have been unlikely to have fully understood the issues faced by survivors, and the research outcomes may not have been as relevant, or as likely to improve their quality of life. Patient involvement stressed the importance of food in relation to overall well-being and quality of life, as opposed to purely in relation to health and nutrition.

To inform the development of the research question and outcomes, the researchers ran a series of 'food play' workshops. These were designed by survivors and their partners, through a pre-workshop questionnaire asking them about issues that affected their eating, and the foods that they missed. The results of the questionnaire fed into a discussion with a chef who applied different cooking techniques to the foods that were identified as difficult to eat, to enable them to be palatable again. Data from the discussions and food demonstrations were then used to formulate the research questions, which were refined in collaboration with survivors.

All of those who had attended the workshops remained involved throughout the project as members of an expert reference panel. This panel helped develop information for participants, and helped to collect and analyse the data, for example, facilitating focus groups, and determining themes in the qualitative analysis. The panel were also involved in the dissemination strategy, playing a pivotal role in the development of the key research outcome, the booklet.

One of the survivors was also a co-applicant and a member of the project steering group, acting as a link between the steering group and the patient reference panel. This person acted as the recruitment coordinator, leading the recruitment process by actively engaging his peers, making sure they had all the information they needed, and then recruiting them as participants.

Barriers and challenges to involvement

Patient and public involvement does not come without its challenges. In Table 16.2, we have attempted to group these into three categories. The challenges for clinicians and academics may be focused around the presumption that the research is too scientific for a patient to get involved in. Similarly, the patients and public may think that the researcher is not listening to their views. The third category of challenges may be that the whole research process is slowed down as a result of the involvement, due to the added bureaucracies and complexity.

Ethics and patient and public involvement

Currently, patient and public involvement for research design does not require ethical approval unless those who become involved have direct contact with

TABLE 16.2   Challenges to effective patient and public involvement in research

Clinicians and academics	Patients and public	General research process
• Giving control about the research to patients and the public	• Clinicians involving patients and the public is a token gesture	• Only a few studies have been funded to patient and public organisations when user-driven research has been planned
• Fear that patients and public too close and may get hurt	• Patients and public may feel intimidation	• Involving users adds costs
• Finding suitable patients and the public to involve	• There is a lack of guidelines on the area	• Adds complexity
• Lack of consensus with patients and public about research	• Expectations not fulfilled	• Adds time
• Colliding worlds	• There is a lack of clarity of roles	• Adds bureaucracy
• Patients and public are seen as inexperienced to involve in research	• Language (differences and jargon)	• Lack of funding for pre-protocol work
• Involving is costly	• May feel under trained	• Lack of relevant training/ mentoring provision
• Involvement is time consuming	• May feel under paid	• Lack of clarity of roles
• There are too many bureaucracies associated with research already, why add another layer?	• May receive negetive media coverage	• Finding new people to involve, not the 'usual suspects'
	• Personal circumstances (such as lone parent, long working hours)	• Involvement policy assumes that people want to be involved and this is not the case
		• Motivations can be diverse for getting involved

research participants, such as collecting interview data. A joint statement was released between INVOLVE and National Research Ethics Service (2009: 1):

> The active involvement of patients or members of the public does not generally raise any ethical concerns for the people who are actively involved, even when those people are recruited for this role via the NHS. This is because they are not acting in the same way as research participants. They are acting as specialist advisers, providing valuable knowledge and expertise based on their experience of a health condition or public health concern.
>
> Therefore ethical approval is not needed for the active involvement element of the research (even when people are recruited via the NHS), where people are involved in planning or advising on research, e.g. helping to develop a protocol, questionnaire or information sheet, member of advisory group, or co-applicant.

Developing a patient and public involvement plan

Developing an involvement strategy requires thought regarding what is appropriate for your project, and for which activities throughout the time span of the project. It may be appropriate to involve people in every stage of the research, or only in certain parts. There are various points where involvement can happen in the research cycle (Figure 16.2).

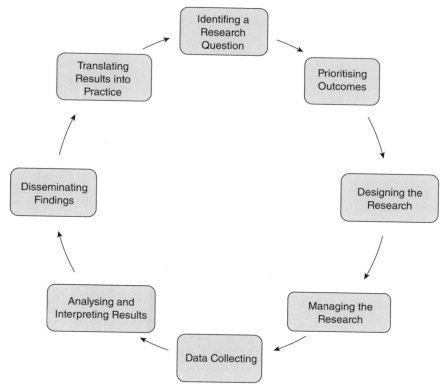

FIGURE 16.2   Cycle of Involvement (adapted from Hanley et al., 2004)

The involvement plan will be unique to that project. It may not be necessary to involve people in every stage of the research cycle as involvement is only necessary when the process will have an impact on the research. If the involvement has no impact, it may be regarded as tokenistic. It is also helpful to talk to people about which research tasks they would like to take part in and where they feel their skills and experience would be most useful. Some people may be interested in developing a project, for example, but not in collecting the data or disseminating the results. The most effective involvement comes from including relevant people in parts of the research in which they have an interest, and in which their participation will have an impact (Figure 16.3).

Involvement is easier and cheaper to incorporate in certain stages of the research, such as service users attending steering group meetings, or in the development of recruitment strategies, ensuring that recruitment is sensitive to the needs of the participants, such as making sure that the patient information contains everything that they need to know. Therefore involvement may enhance your recruitment rates. At other stages of the research process, involvement may be appropriate and have impact, such as for collecting data, but you may need to provide training for them which has time and cost implications. Therefore, when thinking through the different stages of the research cycle and developing your patient and public involvement plan, think about the time and resources that you have available in relation to that involvement.

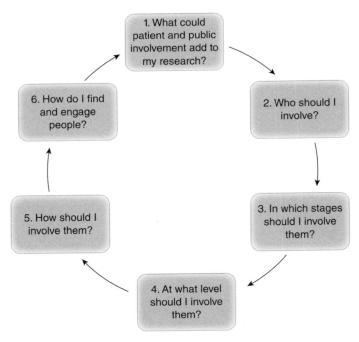

FIGURE 16.3   Cycle of patient and public involvement planning

> **Case study**
>
> To ensure that the research findings were relevant to survivors of head and neck cancer, and would improve their quality of life, the researchers involved survivors and their partners throughout the project. Involvement was especially important in the early stages of the research: in particular, the development of the research question and outcomes, the design of the recruitment strategy and determining the methods used. As the researchers had no personal experience of head and neck cancer themselves, many of the issues and priorities identified through the involvement would not otherwise have been considered.
>
> Survivors of head and neck cancer were also involved in the preparation of the NIHR Research for Patient Benefit funding application. The team included a hyperlink to a video in the 'Patient and Public Involvement' section on the form, which showed extracts from the "food play' workshops.

How do I find and engage people?

Who you should involve in your project is whoever the stakeholders of the research process and outcomes are. For example, if your study is to design an intervention that will be delivered by an occupational therapist to help people who have suffered a stroke, you would not only involve stroke patients, but also the therapists who have to deliver the intervention. Having determined who the stakeholders are that should be involved, a proactive and targeted approach to finding and engaging with them becomes achievable. As Figure 16.4 shows, there are various ways that you can find people to involve.

Ask patients, carers and members of the public with whom you already have contact	Search the internet for relevant community groups and charities	Advertise your positions on the People in Research web page
Contact your local Council for Voluntary Service which supports hundreds of local community organisations	Look in local directories of community groups and voluntary sector organisations	Contact patient and carer groups linked to topic specific research networks, e.g. Mental Health Research Network, etc.
Look on the INVOLVE web site for tips and further contacts	Link with primary care patients through GP practice patient forums	Put posters and flyers in out-patients clinics and public places such as libraries

FIGURE 16.4   How to find people to involve in research

Having identified potential people suitable for involvement in your project, consider how to engage them. This should be done in a proactive way. Rather than emailing your project information to the people/group, go to a meeting and talk to them about your research, ensuring that your information is sensitive and accessible to the people you are presenting to. If you want to engage people with learning disabilities you are unlikely to do this successfully if you send them written information, whereas talking to them using simple language and pictures is likely to prove productive.

When recruiting patients or public for involvement, you should explain exactly what it is you want them to do. Having a draft of a role description, which is negotiable, may be helpful as it will ensure that you are all aware of the required commitment and support offered. Both the researcher and the involved person could then sign a copy and keep one for future reference. Therefore, you need to think carefully about what you want the people to do during their involvement. You may know, for example, that you want to collaborate with patients in the design stage of your research because this will ensure that the research is both relevant to patients and accessible to potential participants. But what exactly are the patients you involve going to do, and who is going to work with them?

You must also keep the people you involved informed about the progression of your project. Service users are often left feeling frustrated as a project progresses, or even finishes, and they are not informed. This frustration can be avoided by involving them in the dissemination strategy (please see Chapter 21: 'Dissemination'). However, if your funding application is rejected, you must feed this outcome back to anyone who has been involved also.

Case study

One of the members of the research team is a speech and language therapist who has access to head and neck cancer patients. She was able to tell them about the project and asked them if they would be interested in getting involved and if so, what their role would be. Using a snowball method (please see Chapter 17: 'Sampling'), the patients were invited to contact other survivors of head and neck cancer they knew, to ask if they were interested in getting involved also. This method proved successful and in total 15 survivors expressed an interest. Due to the differing needs and experiences of each survivor, this meant there was a good cross-section of perspectives, and a diversity of experiences to inform the research. Had it been necessary to find further survivors of head and neck cancer to involve, this could have been done through community support groups and charities that support head and neck cancer patients.

The researchers knew that they wanted to involve past and current head and neck cancer patients to understand the needs and priorities of survivors which may change over time, and with different treatments. It became clear to the researchers, after discussions with the survivors, that it was also important to involve patients' partners in the research, as survivors talked about the direct effect their problems with food had on their partners, especially if the partners regularly did the food shopping and preparation of meals for survivors. Partners therefore had an invaluable insight into how food-related issues affected the survivors.

Involving diverse and vulnerable communities

It is not uncommon for researchers to find the process of recruiting people from diverse and vulnerable communities complex. Ensuring that your involvement is diverse indicates that you have included the expertise and opinions from a broad and varied, group of people. For example, if your project was regarding type 2 diabetes, more south Asians will be affected by this than white members of the community (Webb et al., 2011). Therefore if you were developing an intervention to prevent the onset of type 2 diabetes, it would be imperative that you involved members of the south Asian community. Depending on your project, efforts should be made to involve any vulnerable stakeholders too. This term includes small children and older people, the poor, people living with chronic illnesses, people from minority groups, and captive people such as refugees or prisoners (Spires, 2000). A study by Pandya (2007) looked at the drug and alcohol misuse in unaccompanied minors (young refugees who arrive into a country alone without guardians). The researcher was not a refugee herself and did not speak the languages that the young refugees did, so to hear their perceptions of why substance misuse was occurring in their group, it was important to build trust with them. She did this by working with refugee community organisations and youth services who were already working with this population, who then introduced her to the community of interest. She then gained the trust of a couple of members from that community who spoke some English. Through them she was able to access a larger group as these involved refugees were then able to introduce her to others, conduct some translation, whilst also offering her authorisation. Due to the nature of this project regarding illicit drug use, it was not deemed appropriate to give financial payment for their time, instead food and sweets were distributed.

Payments and expenses

When planning to involve patients and public in research it is important to think about payments and expenses. Those involved should not be out of pocket and therefore should have all of their travelling expenses reimbursed, for example, fuel and parking fees, train fares, etc. as a minimum. It is also good practice to pay people for their time, skills and expertise, in the same way that other members of the research team are paid for theirs. It may be necessary to make other payments to facilitate involvement also, such as paying for child care to enable guardians to take part in activities related to your research. However, payments and expense reimbursements may affect people's benefits and have tax and national insurance implications. Therefore you should let people who are interested in becoming involved in your research know about this and advise them to seek appropriate advice if they are likely to be affected. For more details about payments and expenses please refer to the INVOLVE Payment Guide (2010).

Training and support

It is important that those involved in your research have adequate training and support to help them carry out their role appropriately. Needs can be assessed by talking to them about the type of training and support that would be helpful to them before they become actively involved. This will then give you time to allocate support, or find training prior to involvement. In some cases, this may include emotional support. For example, people may find some of the issues you are researching distressing due to their own personal experiences, so you would need support mechanisms for this in place. It is also important to think about the format of the training and support, and to relate its format to the needs and abilities of those involved. For example, people whose first language is not English would need a translator, or for the training to be conducted in their language. Training does not necessarily need to be formal, however, such as regarding research methodology. Indeed, the prospect of such formal training may act as a barrier to some people becoming involved. The importance of patient and public involvement revolves around the skills, perspectives and experiences of people, as opposed to their knowledge of the research process itself.

Funding applications and patient and public involvement

Research funders want to see that the lay summary, the patient and public involvement strategy, the methodology, the management, the dissemination plans and the budget all marry together in a coherent manner. For example, if you say in the patient and public involvement section that you will involve patients in the dissemination of the research, you must come back to that point in the dissemination section. If you omit this, the reviewer may think that you only wrote it in the patient and public involvement section to make it look better. You also need to think about the support involved members may need and who out of your research team will be responsible for this. Similarly, if you say that you will offer your patients training, your budget will need to reflect the cost of that training. An appropriate budget for patient and public involvement should always be included in a research funding application. Involvement is now recognised as an integral part of the research process, and funding bodies are happy to fund it, as long as the projected costs of involvement are made explicit and are justified.

Summary

- There may be challenges associated with involvement; preinvolvement consideration of these may reduce them.
- Involving people in research design does not require ethical approval.
- For involvement to be meaningful, the researcher needs to identify:
    - What it will add, i.e. its impact and how you will measure this
    - The levels of involvement at which stages of the project
    - Who to involve and where to find them
    - How to involve them and what support or training will they require.

- Researchers must pay, mentor and train the patients and the public appropriately.
- Throughout the project the involved people must be kept informed regarding any developments.
- All research applications should have patient and public involvement woven through them, not just in the patient and public involvement sections.

Questions for Discussion

1. What benefits do you think the patient perspective adds to research that other research team members cannot?
2. What are the main challenges in involving patients and the public, and how might these be avoided?
3. Using the case study (or your own project) draw a timeline or Gantt chart, beginning from the start of the project to the end. Along this plot where, and when, you would involve patients, detailing their tasks and ensuring that it is meaningful, considering issues such as training, support and budget also.

Further Reading

Arnstein, S.R. (1969) 'A ladder of citizen participation', *Journal of the American Institute of Planners,* 35: 216–24.

Beresford, P. (2002) 'User involvement in research and evaluation: liberation or regulation', *Social Policy and Society,* 1 (2): 95–105.

Beresford, P. (2003) 'User involvement in research: exploring the challenges', *Nursing Times Research,* 8 (1): 36–46.

Carr, S. (2004) *Has Service User Participation Made a Difference to Social Care Services?* London: Policy Press.

Entwistle, V.A. (2007) 'Differing perspectives on patient involvement in patient safety', *Qual Saf Health Care,* 16 (2): 82–3.

Hogg, C.N. (2007) 'Patient and public involvement: what next for the NHS?', *Health Expectations,* 10 (2): 129–38.

INVOLVE (2012) http://www.invo.org.uk/ (accessed July 2012).

Martin, G.P. (2008) '"Ordinary people only": knowledge, representativeness, and the publics of public participation in healthcare', *Sociology of Health and Illness,* 30 (1): 35–54.

Tritter, J.Q. and McCallum, A. (2006) 'The snakes and ladders of user involvement: moving beyond Arnstein', *Health Policy,* 76 (2): 156–68.

References

Brett, J., Staniszewska, S., Mockford, C., Seers, K., Herron-Marx, S. and Bayliss, H. (2010) The PIRICOM Study: A systematic review of the conceptualisation, measurement, impact and outcomes of patient and public involvement in health and social care research. *UK Clinical Research Collaboration.* London: UKCRC.

Burges Watson, D.L., Lewis, S. and Buckley, J. (2011) 'John's cheese sandwich: taking on PPI, with relish', *INVOLVE newsletter* (autumn): 9–10.

Department of Health (2000) *Research and Development for a First Class Service: R&D Funding in the New NHS*. London: Department of Health.

Fleming, J. and Hudson, N. (2009) 'Young people and research participation', in J. Wood and J. Hine (eds), *Work with Young People: Theory and Policy for Practice*. London: SAGE, pp. 136–51.

Frazer, E. (1999) *The Problems of Communitarian Politics: Unity and Conflict*. Oxford: Oxford University Press.

Hanley, B., Bradburn, J., Barnes, M., Evans, C., Goodare, H., Kelson, M., Kent, A., Oliver, S., Thomas, S. and Wallcraft, J. (2004) *Involving the Public in NHS, Public Health and Social Care Research: Briefing Notes for Researchers*. Eastleigh: INVOLVE Support Unit.

Hickey, G. and Kipping, C. (1998) 'Exploring the concept of user involvement in mental health through a participation continuum', *Journal of Clinical Nursing*, 7: 83–8.

INVOLVE (2010) *Payment for Involvement: A Guide for Making Payments to Members of the Public Actively Involved in NHS, Public Health and Social Care Research*. Eastleigh: INVOLVE.

INVOLVE (2012) *Briefing Notes for Researchers: Involving the Public in NHS, Public Health and Social Care Research*. Eastleigh: INVOLVE.

INVOLVE/NRES (2009) *Patient and Public Involvement in Research and Research Ethics Committee Review*: http://www.invo.org.uk/posttypepublication/patient-and-public-involvement-in-research-and-research-ethics-committee-review (accessed July 2012).

Kirby, P. (2004) *A Guide to Actively Involving Young People in Research, for Researchers, Research Commissioners and Managers*. Eastleigh: INVOLVE.

McLaughlin, H. (2009) 'What's in a name: client, patient, customer, consumer, expert by experience, service user: what's next?', *British Journal of Social Work*, 19 (6): 1101–17.

Mockford, C., Staniszewska, S., Griffiths, F. and Herron-Marx, S. (2011) 'The impact of patient and public involvement (PPI) on UK NHS healthcare: a systematic review', *International Journal for Quality in Health Care*, 24 (1): 28–38.

Pandya, R. (2007) 'Work with black young people', in M. Sallah and C. Howson (eds), *Working with Young Refugees and Asylum Seekers through Participatory Action Research in Health Promotion*. Lyme Regis: Russell House Publishing.

Shea, B., Santesso, N., Qualman, A., Heiberg, T., Leong, A., Judd, M., Robinson, V., Wells, G., Tugewll, P. and the Cochrane Musculoskeletal Consumer Group (2005) 'Consumer-driven health care: Building partnerships in research', *Health Expectations*, 8 (4): 352–9.

Staley, K. (2009) *Exploring Impact: Public Involvement in NHS, Public Health and Social Care Research*. Eastleigh: INVOLVE.

Staniszewska, S., Brett, J., Mockford, C. and Barber, R. (2011) 'The GRIPP checklist: Strengthening the quality of patient and public involvement reporting in research', *International Journal of Technology Assessment in Health Care*, 27 (4): 391–9.

Spires, J. (2000) 'New perspectives on vulnerability using emic and etic approaches', *Journal of Advanced Nursing*, 31 (3): 715–21.

Vijayakrishnan, A., Rutherford, J., Miller, S. and Drummond, L.M. (2006) 'Service user involvement in training: the trainees' view', *Psychiatric Bulletin*, 30: 303–5.

Webb, D.R., Khunti, K., Srinivasan, B., Gray, L.J., Taub, N., Campbell, S., Barnett, J., Henson, J., Hiles, S., Farooqi, A., Griffin, S.J., Wareham, N.J. and Davies, M.J. (2011) 'Screening for diabetes using an oral glucose tolerance test within a western multi-ethnic population identifies modifiable cardiovascular risk: the ADDITION-Leicester study', *Diabetologia*, 3: Epub.

Whyte, W.F. (1989) 'Advancing scientific knowledge through participatory action research', *Sociological Forum*, 4 (3): 367–85.

17

SAMPLING

Nick Taub, Abdel Douiri and
Dawn-Marie Walker

- Be aware of the differences between nonprobability and probability sampling methods, and for what type of research each of these approaches is suitable
- Know the value of simple random sampling, from a sampling frame, being the basis of methods to obtain a representative sample
- Understand the use of strata to make a sample more representative, and the use of clusters and systematic sampling for ease of sampling
- Be aware of how sample size calculations are used to control the extent of random error

Introduction

In quantitative research we are generally interested in drawing a valid conclusion about a whole 'target population' of people. Often the target population includes people spread out over a wide geographical area, such as 'all the people with chronic arthritis, resident in the UK'. One might think that it would be ideal to carry out a census, that is, to gather the information required for the study from every single person in the target population, which has the advantage that all possibilities of error and bias will have been avoided. In practice, however, the task of collecting all information from such a large group would be extremely costly and time consuming, especially in the case of those people who did not initially respond to our request for information and thus need chasing up. Any non-response could cause selection bias in our census, a major problem in quantitative research, since certain types of individual, such as homeless people and non-English speakers, may be less likely to respond than others, thus rendering the study sample non-representative of the study's target population, and therefore the results of a quantitative study would be inaccurate. Another commonly seen example of selection bias is when, at least up the age of 60 years or so, older people are more likely than younger people to respond to a request for information.

In quantitative research, in an attempt to avoid bias, and in qualitative research, due to the need for only a small number of participants, we collect data just from a sample of the target population (Figure 17.1). Usually it is people who are being sampled, but sampling may also be used for individual treatment episodes, households or elements of the health care system such as general practices, clinics or hospitals. Choosing an appropriate sample is a crucial step for any piece of research, whichever methodology is being used.

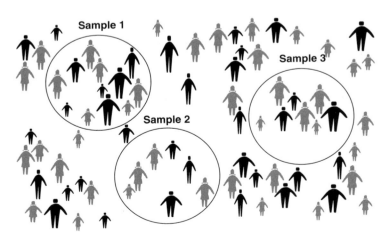

FIGURE 17.1   Three samples taken from a target population

Sampling approaches

The choice of sampling method for any study will depend on the research questions that are being asked and the overall study design that has been chosen. There are two general approaches to sampling. Nonprobability sampling, which is used in qualitative studies where there is no need to obtain a representative sample (see Chapter 7: 'Qualitative Data Collection'), or for those quantitative studies where speed and convenience are high priorities, and probability sampling which uses the 'random sampling' approach and aims to ensure that the sample is representative of your study's target population.

Nonprobability sampling

Nonprobability sampling is the method often used in qualitative studies where the rationale is to develop understanding around a complex issue through the collection of in-depth, rich data as might be collected via interviews or focus groups (please see Chapter 7: 'Qualitative Methodology'). Therefore, sample sizes tend to be small, with bias unavoidable. This is often not regarded as a problem in qualitative research, however, where participants are chosen who can provide insight into the topic, rather than represent any general population of people. For example, if you wanted to explore the use of complementary medicine for back pain, your target population would be those who have presented at their doctors, reporting back pain. If you randomly selected from this population, then it is quite possible that you would end up with a sample of people who have never used complementary medicine for back pain! Therefore, intensity sampling, a form of purposive sampling, may be used, where the selected participants are rich in information but are not extreme or deviant, i.e., you would recruit people who have used complementary medicine for their back pain. Alternatively, you may wish to select cases that represent the extremes on some dimension, i.e. extreme case sampling, where you actively recruit participants who are highly unusual in terms of the phenomenon of interest. For example, if you were conducting a study to ascertain attitudes to healthy eating in children, you might want to include some children whose parents are vegan. Otherwise, you may use negative case sampling, which is where you select cases that contradict your theory, which thus deepens your understanding of a topic. For a more detailed description of sampling for qualitative work please see Emmel (2013) in the further reading section of this chapter.

There are various different nonprobability sampling methods available:

- Snowball sampling works through the construction of a network of contacts. First, a small number of people from the target population are consented into the study, who are then asked to identify other people from the target population. In turn, these new participants are checked for membership of the target population and if appropriate, are asked to suggest their contacts and so on. This method can be useful when the target population is hard to reach or identify, such as studying prostitution (e.g. Cusick, 1998), and illicit drug use (e.g. Avico et al., 1988; Boys et al., 2001; Kaplan et al., 1987).

- Convenience sampling merely means that you collect data from those who are the easiest to reach, e.g. colleagues, friends, etc. This is the least rigorous or costly method and is therefore useful for when resources are limited.

- Quota sampling is convenience sampling carried out within each of a number of categories needed in the study.

- Purposive sampling is where participants are selected according to criteria relevant to your research objectives to try to ensure that you cover all the important perspectives. For example, you might expect there to be differences in attitudes towards healthy eating according to socioeconomic status (SES). Therefore you would need to ensure you collect data from all SES categories. Purposive, rather than quota sampling, is used when the number of participants is a target rather than a requirement, which makes it a common method in qualitative work, as one would cease data collection once saturation has been reached.

- Theoretical sampling is a method used solely for qualitative work as it is iterative. Samples are formed through theories emerging from the data as it is being collected, i.e. new samples are formed to develop or challenge emerging hypotheses (Glaser and Strauss, 1967).

If you are using a nonprobability method for recruitment, to ensure that all of the characteristics that you need are represented in your sample, a sampling grid can be developed containing all of the criteria you believe could influence the participant's beliefs or experiences (please see the case study). However if your qualitative project is using focus groups, it may be more appropriate to use homogeneous sampling, where the participants are more similar and compatible with each other, otherwise the discussion may either fail, or result in an argument!

Case study

A qualitative study was conducted to understand the health-related beliefs and experiences of gypsies and travellers (Van Cleemput et al., 2007). Their initial sampling grid comprised 269 gypsies and travellers who were already participating in a parallel health-status study whose inclusion criterion was any gypsy or traveller who had recently accessed health services. They used the maximum variation variant of the purposive method, meaning that cases were selected that would give a wide range of beliefs and experiences, and they then drafted a sampling grid with which to select 27 participants to interview (Table 17.1).

As you can see, the researchers identified a variety of criteria that they felt may influence the health-related beliefs and experiences of that population. This included not only sex, age and geographical location, but also whether the participant had attended school regularly as a child, perhaps because those who did attend school could be expected to be more socially assimilated and previously had had access to the school medical facilities. The researchers also thought that if a participant had a child under the age of 16 then this might affect their beliefs, arguably because their

TABLE 17.1   Sampling grid (Van Cleemput et al., 2007)

	Male
Sex	Female
Age group	16–25
	26–45
	46–65
	>65
Accommodation	Council site/private site
	Unauthorised roadside site
	Housed
	In temporary (homeless)
Location	Northampton
	Sheffield
	Bristol
	Norfolk
	London
	Leicester
Attended school regularly as a child	Yes/No
Have children <16 years	
Travelling patterns	All of the time
	Part of the time
	Rarely

child may be at school and/or accessing health services. The researchers also thought that travelling patterns may affect health-related beliefs due to social exclusion, and this might plausibly be more prevalent in people who spend a large part of their time travelling.

Nonprobability sampling can also be useful for quick and informal quantitative work when there is a lack of the funding needed for probability sampling, such as with small-scale project or pilot work. It may also be the only option open to you if you have a hard-to-reach population.

Probability or random sampling

In this approach every person in the target population will have a known chance, determined by the researcher, of being selected for the sample. This will help minimise selection bias and provide a sample representative of its population.

Sampling frame

Probability sampling requires the use of a sampling frame (except in the special case of systematic sampling, see below). A sampling frame is constructed by first making a list of the individuals in the target population (or as good an approximation to this as you can get), and then giving each individual a unique identifier to go into the sampling frame. The actual sampling will take place when random numbers are generated, using a computer package, which are then used to identify by number certain people listed in the sampling frame. These then are the people who have been selected for the study sample.

In practice it can be difficult to obtain a good sampling frame due, for example, to the continuously changing nature of most target populations, and many routinely available lists and directories, including the electoral role, being out of date. A typical example of the difficulties involved occurs if you are trying to sample from the population of all hospital outpatients. People attending sexual health clinics are not included in standard lists because the systems for these services are separate from the main hospital systems in order to meet the requirements of the Data Protection Act. Therefore either this group of patients would need to be excluded from the study's target population, or authorisation would need to be obtained to use these additional lists, which would then be merged into the main sampling frame.

For research, regarding people with specific medical conditions, it is often best to use an existing disease register as your sampling frame. Many of these registers are maintained for research and/or administrative reasons, although extra care should be taken before deciding to make use of an administrative register which may not be suitable for research purposes. Regardless of how you form your sampling frame, take note of how you did it, as when reporting the results of a study that used random sampling, it is important to describe how the sampling frame was constructed, and what its advantages and disadvantages were.

Simple random sampling

Simple random sampling is the most basic form of probability sampling and thus forms the basis of more complex probability sampling methods. Each individual in the sampling frame has the same probability of being randomly selected as others in the frame. For example, a researcher from occupational health wants to know the average level of job satisfaction of the managers of mental health units, as measured by a scale from 1 (strongly dissatisfied) to 100 (strongly satisfied). Each unit has one manager, and in total there are exactly 100 units across England (Figure 17.2), and the researcher decides to use simple random sampling. Each of the 100 mental health units is given a unique identifier (from 1 to 100) so that each manager has a 1% chance of being chosen.

Let us assume that the study design specifies that a sample of size 10 will be used (this is for illustration only as it is a very small sample size for quantitative work). The researcher obtains a random sample of 10 managers by first putting all of the numbers

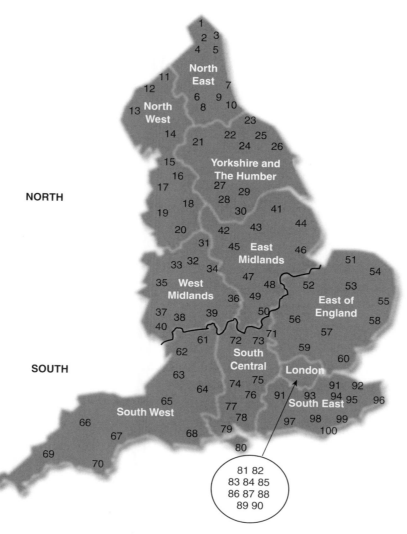

FIGURE 17.2 Geographical representation of the sampling frame

into a sampling frame (Table 17.2), and then uses computer-generated random numbers to select the managers. Suppose that the random digits produced by the computer, presented as pairs, are 20 94 95 76 80 48 65 16 24 96. These digits are then applied to the sampling frame: 20 = row 2, column 0, 94 = row 9, column 4, 95 = row 9, column 5, and so on. Note that when a random digit pair '20' appeared, then we select manager 30, not 20, since with the design of this sampling frame, row '2' represents 20 and column '0' represents 10, which sum to 30. Thus, our researcher ends up randomly selecting the managers 30, 94, 95, 76, 90, 48, 65, 16, 24 and 96. For the purposes of this example, the satisfaction level of each manager happens to be equal to their

TABLE 17.2   Sampling frame, for simple random sampling

Second digit

		1	2	3	4	5	6	7	8	9	0
First digit -	0	1	2	3	4	5	6	7	8	9	10
	1	11	12	13	14	15	16	17	18	19	20
	2	21	22	23	24	25	26	27	28	29	30
	3	31	32	33	34	35	36	37	38	39	40
	4	41	42	43	44	45	46	47	48	49	50
	5	51	52	53	54	55	56	57	58	59	60
	6	61	62	63	64	65	66	67	68	69	70
	7	71	72	73	74	75	76	77	78	79	80
	8	81	82	83	84	85	86	87	88	89	90
	9	91	92	93	94	95	96	97	98	99	100

identifier-number, therefore manager 1, who is in the 'North East' region, has a score of 1 indicating that they are strongly dissatisfied – and manager 100, at the bottom of the map in the south, has a score of 100 indicating that they are strongly satisfied. The true value of the target population's satisfaction level is 50.5 which is the mean, i.e. average of the numbers from 1 to 100. Whereas our sample's mean satisfaction score is: $(30 + 94 + 95 + 76 + 90 + 48 + 65 + 16 + 24 + 96) \div 10 = 634 \div 10 = \underline{63.4,}$ substantially different from the true mean figure which we know to be 50.5.

No matter how carefully a random sample has been selected, the result will (almost) never be exactly the same as the true population result. There are three important criteria to determine how useful the results from your sample are:

- If an infinitely large number of samples like this were taken, and the mean calculated for each one, then the average of these all together would be equal to the true value, therefore the sampling method would be 'unbiased'.

- The results must be presented together with their confidence interval, representing the precision, i.e. the margin for random error (please see Chapter 19: 'Quantitative Analysis').

- The degree of precision must be good enough for the purpose for which the result will be used.

Stratified random sampling

It is often the case that the target population for an investigation divides 'naturally' into subgroups of participants, or strata, meaning levels. The accuracy of the sample is improved by ensuring that people are sampled from each of the strata in the same proportions as they appear in the target population, i.e. proportionate stratified sampling. In the healthy eating project as mentioned earlier, for example, you could have strata based on the highest level of education achieved. You would expect to sample fewer people in the stratum denoting postgraduate qualifications than in the stratum for school-level qualifications, as more of the population will have school-level qualifications as their highest level of education. Stratification is particularly valuable when the sample is not large, or when there are one or more smaller strata with markedly different characteristics from the others, as it helps to remove some of the variability in the sample, and thus error. Therefore stratification according to education would make sense in the healthy eating project as health literacy, which is the ability to read, understand and make decisions based on certain special types of information, may correlate with levels of education, resulting in different attitudes towards diet.

To conduct stratified sampling, it is necessary that the sampling frame lists not only the identifier for each member of the target population, but also which stratum it is in. Simple random sampling is then carried out separately for each stratum. In the example of the medical unit managers, the population could be divided into two strata: the north and the south as the 50 managers in the northern half of the country have lower levels of satisfaction than the managers in the south. A stratified sampling frame (Table 17.3) is then produced similar to that for simple random sampling.

TABLE 17.3 Sampling frame, for stratified random sampling

North Stratum		Second digit - 1	2	3	4	5	6	7	8	9	0
First digit -	0	1	2	3	4	5	6	7	8	9	10
	1	11	12	13	14	15	16	17	18	19	20
	2	21	22	23	24	25	26	27	28	29	30
	3	31	32	33	34	35	36	37	38	39	40
	4	41	42	43	44	45	46	47	48	49	50

South Stratum		Second digit - 1	2	3	4	5	6	7	8	9	0
First digit -	5	51	52	53	54	55	56	57	58	59	60
	6	61	62	63	64	65	66	67	68	69	70
	7	71	72	73	74	75	76	77	78	79	80
	8	81	82	83	84	85	86	87	88	89	90
	9	91	92	93	94	95	96	97	98	99	100

As our occupational health researcher still requires an overall sample size of 10, the first task is to take a simple random sample of five managers from the north and then combine these with five sampled likewise from the south, taking five from each stratum because the population is equally divided between the north and the south. The random computer generated digits for the north are 45 17 40 14 89 25. Any digits representing manager identifiers greater than 50 are ignored as these denote identifiers belonging to the south stratum. These ignored numbers will be disregarded and not used in future sampling. Therefore the chosen north stratum managers with identifiers (ignoring 89) are 45, 17, 50, 14 and 25. For the south stratum, the random digits generated are 65 70 30 12 24 75 67 71. This time numbers lower than 50 are ignored as these will belong to the north stratum. Thus the south stratum managers chosen are: 65, 80, 75, 67 and 71. To calculate the mean satisfaction score of this sample, like before, we add all the numbers up and divide by 10. From this stratified sample, the total mean satisfaction score is calculated to be 50.9 points. This is closer to the known true value (50.5), and more accurate than the simple random sample, which will generally be the case when using stratification. This is because the standard deviation (or variability) of each stratum is 14.6 points, compared with 29.0 points for the entire population, and so there will be less error in a stratified sample.

Cluster sampling

Often a target population for a study naturally forms subgroups, i.e. clusters, that are geographically close together or otherwise relatively easy to contact together, such as the members of a household, students at a school, employees at a place of work, or patients attending a specialist outpatient clinic. In this type of situation, there can be great efficiency savings made by carrying out cluster sampling (also known as two-stage sampling). As well as reducing the travel time needed by researchers, cluster sampling can allow random samples to be taken in situations where a sampling frame of all the individuals in the target population would be inefficient or difficult to compile. For instance, if your target population consists of patients attending a specialist outpatient clinic, of which there are 200, the effort involved in compiling a sampling frame for all the patients attending each of the 200 clinics would be unreasonable. Therefore using the cluster sampling method, where each clinic is a cluster which you then choose at random, would be more practical.

To conduct cluster sampling, first, a sampling frame of the clusters needs to be created, from which a random sample of clusters is chosen. After this, a second sampling plan is created for selecting the individuals from within the randomly selected clusters. Depending on the aims of the study and the practical issues, this second stage might be a 'mini-census' inviting all of the individuals in the chosen cluster to take part in the study. Alternatively, it may involve a second stage of random sampling, for which individual sampling frames will need to be created for each selected cluster that contains identifiers for each potential participant who is a member of that cluster.

TABLE 17.4   Sampling frame, for cluster random sampling

Single

digit	Region										
0	North East	1	2	3	4	5	6	7	8	9	10
1	North West	11	12	13	14	15	16	17	18	19	20
2	Yorkshire	21	22	23	24	25	26	27	28	29	30
3	West Midlands	31	32	33	34	35	36	37	38	39	40
4	East Midlands	41	42	43	44	45	46	47	48	49	50
5	East of England	51	52	53	54	55	56	57	58	59	60
6	South West	61	62	63	64	65	66	67	68	69	70
7	South Central	71	72	73	74	75	76	77	78	79	80
8	London	81	82	83	84	85	86	87	88	89	90
9	South East	91	92	93	94	95	96	97	98	99	100

As in proportionate stratified sampling, the sample chosen from a cluster will often be similar in proportion to the size of the cluster in the target population. However, cluster sampling has implications for the precision and efficiency of a sample that contrast with those of stratified sampling. In stratified sampling, precision is improved because the individuals in each stratum are similar to each other but different from people in other stratum on a certain factor. In other words, the strata are homogeneous within, but heterogeneous between. Although clusters themselves should be similar to each other, within each cluster, individuals should be different from each other i.e. homogeneous between, and heterogeneous within. However, as with other probability sampling methods, the larger the sample the greater the precision.

In the example of the medical unit managers' study, it might be considered that the satisfaction scores could most conveniently be collected within each of the 10 national regions shown in Figure 17.2; therefore each region forms a cluster. A corresponding sampling frame is drafted from which clusters are chosen using single random digits in the same manner as in simple random sampling (Table 17.4). Once the researcher has randomly selected their clusters, they may wish to conduct a mini census or sample from the cluster.

If appropriate, you can combine stratification and clustering. You may wish to stratify the clusters to distinguish between the clusters of general hospitals, teaching hospitals and health care centres for example, or stratify individuals within the clusters, such as stratifying according to severity of the patient's condition, or subtypes of diagnoses. An example of combining stratification and cluster sampling methods can be seen in the case study.

⌐ **Case study** ⌐

Many patients suffering with psychosis fail to take their prescribed medication, for reasons including adverse effects from the medication, denial of their condition, and lack of organisation, and thus are liable to suffer a relapse and require emergency admission to hospital. Multidisciplinary 'assertive outreach' teams have been established nationally in order to monitor these patients and encourage them to take their medication as prescribed. These teams typically consist of psychiatrists, nurses, psychologists, social workers and support workers, and may also include staff with other expertise. A survey was carried out to estimate the level of 'failure', defined as the number of days participants spent as a hospital inpatient, during the two years following the start of their monitoring (Brugha et al., 2012). First, a census was established in order to list all such teams working in England, from which a cluster sampling design was used to ease the collection of patient information held centrally at each site where the assertive outreach team was based, i.e. each assertive outreach team was a cluster. It was thought that the outcome of admission to hospital might be more likely for patients in the care of an assertive outreach team which had been established more recently, and therefore had had less chance to become fully effective. The sampling frame of clusters was therefore divided into two strata: stratum 'A' consisting of teams that had been established for less than two years, and stratum 'B' for the older teams. The total number of teams was 186, and 102 of these (55%) had been established for less than two years. Therefore a stratified sample of 100 teams would need to contain 55 teams from Stratum A, and the remaining 45 from Stratum B, i.e. proportionate stratified sampling.

Systematic sampling

Systematic sampling is where members of the population to be sampled are given sequential identifier numbers, 1, 2, 3, 4, etc. Sampling is made by first randomly selecting a starting point in this list, between 1 and then whatever '_th' interval you decide, for example, 5th, 10th, 12th, 17th, etc. You then choose every person who appears on the list at that interval. The interval size is chosen according to the size of the sampling frame and the size of the sample that is required. In the example of the medical unit managers' study, a systematic sample of 20 could be obtained by first using the simple random sample frame (Table 17.2), then calculating what the interval should be in order to identify 20 managers: 100 ÷ 20 = 5. Then randomly selecting a starting number in the range 1–5, let us say 4, and then select every fifth manager (4th, 9th, 14th, and so on) up to the 99th. Systematic sampling is useful when lists are too long to easily or quickly enter into a computer, so long as there is no possibility of the individuals in the list varying according to your chosen interval, which would then introduce systematic error. An example of this would be if your chosen interval was every 7th patient, and it just happens to be that every 7th person is female.

Systematic sampling may also provide a method for situations where no sampling frame can be compiled, but where potential participants present sequentially in time, and where there is no danger of a time variation in any import characteristic of these people, which, once again, would introduce systematic error. For example, if you were recruiting people attending an Accident and Emergency Unit, then you would have to be careful what period of time you would recruit in as you would expect systematic error if you were sampling only around 11pm on a Saturday night, unless your project was regarding alcohol consumption and injury! You could also combine systematic sampling with another form of sampling. In this Accident and Emergency example, you might wish to cluster time periods over the week (e.g. Monday am, pm, evening; Tuesday am, pm, evening; etc.), randomly pick the required number of clusters and then use systematic sampling within the chosen cluster's time frame.

Sample size

If you are conducting a qualitative project, you will be looking to obtain an informative data set, and perhaps reach saturation with your sample, i.e. when no new themes are emerging (please see Chapter 20: 'Qualitative Analysis'). The sample size, therefore, cannot be obtained by a calculation but instead will be chosen depending on the type of qualitative analysis to be used, and the experiences gained from previous qualitative research on that topic. However, quantitative researchers are hoping to obtain statistical validity so they can generalise from their sample to the target population as a whole. They will also want to control the amount of random error in the results, which is done by choosing a suitably large number of people to include in the sample, i.e. sample size. It would be tempting to say that by having an appropriate sample size we could avoid any bias or random error, but that could be achieved only by carrying out a census with a 100% response rate, which is usually impossible.

If a study recruits a much larger number of patients than is necessary, then the waste of resources is clear. It is, in practice, much more common that a study recruits too small a number, and then it is likely that the research question, the object of the study, fails to be answered adequately. In this case, not only the financial and staff resources, but also any distress and inconvenience for the participants who have taken part may have been wasted. This is only partly offset by the possibility that a future systematic review (please see Chapter 14: 'Systematic Reviews') will combine the study's results with those of other studies, and produce a useful combined result.

Increasing the size of the sample increases the precision of the results. For instance, if you wanted to estimate the mean value of a score in a single group of people, then as you increase the sample size, (i) the standard error of the mean becomes smaller, causing (ii) the margin for random error to become smaller, so that the width of the 95% confidence for your result becomes narrower, meaning that (iii) your result becomes more precise (please see Chapter 19: 'Quantitative Analysis'). For example, if you wanted to measure the mental well-being in people who have been unemployed for six months or more, you would have a more accurate estimate of well-being having collected data from 200 people versus 50. However,

TABLE 17.5. Example of the approximate margin of random error that can be expected when estimating a proportion, such as 'good mental well-being', from a sample

| Sample size | Proportion of participants recording 'good' mental well-being | | |
| | 10% | 20% | 30% |
	Margin of random error (plus or minus)		
25	11.8%*	15.7%*	18.0%*
50	8.3%*	11.1%*	12.7%*
100	5.9%	7.8%	9.0%
200	4.2%	5.5%	6.4%
500	2.6%	3.5%	4.0%
800	2.1%	2.8%	3.2%
1000	1.9%	2.5%	2.8%
1500	1.5%	2.0%	2.3%
2000	1.3%	1.8%	2.0%

* only rough approximations, due to the small numbers involved

there are diminishing returns regarding improving the margin of error from increasing the sample size. As can be seen in Table 17.5, the decrease in the margin of error obtained by increasing the sample size is large when the samples are still small, but tails off the larger the sample gets. Therefore it may be uneconomical to collect data from a massive sample, for minimal benefit gained. As you can see using Table 17.5, if 20% of your sample of 100 participants reported that they had good well-being, the true proportion of the population with good well-being could vary by approximately ±7.8%, i.e. the true proportion of your population with good well-being could (from the 95% confidence interval) be as low as 12.2% (20 − 7.8) or as high as 27.8% (20 + 7.8). However if you increased your sample size to 1000 people, your margin of error falls to ±2.5%, so the 95% confidence interval is now from 17.5% to 22.5%. Thus the results would be much more precise.

If you are conducting a descriptive study, a common approach to calculating sample size is for a researcher to decide on a margin of error that is required and then use an appropriate formula or table (Table 17.5 is shown as an illustration of what you may find) to determine the sample size needed to achieve the desired level of precision.

Sample size is often calculated when comparing a proportion of some yes/no characteristic, or a mean value of some measurement, between two groups of people.

You will need to bear in mind prior to calculation:

i. the value for the P-value result of a statistical test, below which the result is considered to be statistically significant. This is usually set at 5%, so that test results with $P<0.05$ are considered to be significant.

and;

ii. the chance that you detect a difference between the groups, usually the smallest difference that you believe would be clinically important, given that such a different actually exists in the population. This is known as the 'statistical power' and is commonly set to either 80% or 90%.

The values needed for calculating sample sizes are usually obtained from either pilot data or published studies that have used the same outcome or who had a similar population. Great care must be taken in estimating these values and in providing justification for them. Other important considerations for determining your sample size will include the resources available (financial or staff), the length of time you have before the results are required and the availability of patients.

Many tables, formulas and online calculators exist for carrying out sample size calculations, however, it is strongly recommended to seek the advice of a medical statistician, or an experienced quantitative researcher with similar expertise. This is primarily because a sample size calculation is a crucial aspect of study design, in that a sample that is too small can cause a study to fail to detect a treatment effect or risk factor that would be of clinical or scientific benefit. It is likely that such an oversight would be picked up at the stage of applying for research funding or ethical approval, and thus merely cause a delay in the research programme until it was corrected. Otherwise, if such a study was actually carried out, then it could easily cause many thousands of pounds of medical research funding, and large amounts of staff and participant time to have been wasted.

Population parameters and sample statistics

To help describe how representative of the target population your sample is, sample statistics can be conducted and population parameters obtained. Sample statistics are estimates of means, and proportions, calculated on an outcome of interest such as the height or weight of participants. This can then enable us to make calculated inferences about the population parameter, i.e. a characteristic of the population. For example, in the well-being project, from your sample of 100 participants, you estimate that the mean well-being score is 7; this is a statistic calculated using your sample. From this you estimate that the target population, i.e. people who have been unemployed for six months or over, will have a mean well-being score of 7 also; this is a population parameter which you have determined through statistical inference. In practice however, no matter how carefully you select a random sample, the sample mean or parameters are unlikely to be exactly the same as the true target population's parameters.

Summary

- There are two approaches to sampling: nonprobability sampling which is based on selection criteria and is used for where generalisability of results is not sought, and probability/random sampling where the probability of every person in the target population being selected can be calculated in advance.

- The main methods for nonprobability sampling are: snowball; quota; convenience; purposive; and theoretical.
- The main methods for probability/random sampling are: simple random; stratified random; cluster random; and systematic.
- For simple random sampling, a sampling frame needs to be constructed which contains an identifier for each member of the target population. The sample is then picked randomly from the sampling frame.
- The size of a probability sample allows you to control the extent of random error in the results.

Questions for Discussion

1. You would like to explore the various pathways to access health care that people who are homeless use.

    a. What type of nonprobability sampling method would you use?

    b. What criteria might you want to include in your sampling grid?

2. What random sampling frame(s) might you use for the below projects, and give the rationale for your choice. Would a nonprobability approach be more appropriate for any of these project? If so, which ones and why?

    a. To study the health of elderly people living in residential care homes.

    b. To consider possible methods of transmission for a newly discovered disease, thought to be infectious, about which very little is known.

    c. To examine the regional variation in survival for patients diagnosed with oesophageal cancer.

3. What are the main advantages and disadvantages of:

    a. simple random sampling

    b. stratified sampling

    c. cluster sampling

    d. systematic sampling?

Out of the methods in question 3, which sampling design would be most appropriate to study the mental health of people serving terms in prison?

4 What are the main advantages, and disadvantages, of choosing a large sample size?

Further Reading

Daniel, J. (2012) *Sampling Essentials: Practical Guidelines for Making Sampling Choices.* London: SAGE.

Emmel, N. (2013) *Sampling and Choosing Cases in Qualitative Research*. London: SAGE.

Groves, R.M., Fowler Jr, F.J., Couper, M.P., Lepkowski, J.M., Singer, E. and Tourangeau, R. (2004) *Survey Methodology*. Hoboken, NJ: Wiley.

References

Avico, U., Kaplan, C., Korczak, D. and Van Meter, K. (1988) *Cocaine Epidemiology in Three European Community Cities: A Pilot Study Using a Snowball Sampling Methodology.* Brussels: European Communities Health Directorate.

Boys, A., Marsden, J. and Strang, J. (2001) 'Understanding reasons for drug use amongst young people: a functional perspective', *Health Education Research,* 16 (4): 457–69.

Brugha, T.S., Taub, N., Smith, J., Morgan, Z., Hill, T., Meltzer, H., Wright, C., Burns, T., Priebe, S., Evans, J. and Fryers, T. (2012) 'Predicting outcome of assertive outreach across England', *Social and Psychiatric Epidemiology,* 47 (2): 313–22.

Cusick, L. (1998) 'Female prostitution in Glasgow: drug use and occupational sector', *Addiction Research and Theory,* 6 (2): 115–30.

Dworkin, R.H, Turk, D.C., Wyrwick, K.W., Beaton, D., Cleeland, C.S., Farrar, J.T., Haythornthwaite, J.A., Jensen, M.P., Kerns, R.D., Ader, D.N., Brandenburg, N., Burke, L.B., Cella, D., Chandler, J., Cowan, P., Dimitrova, R., Dionne, R., Hertz, S., Jadad, A.R., Katz, N.P., Kehlet, H., Kramer, L.D., Manning, D.C., McCormick, C., McDermott, M.P., McQuay, H.J., Patel, S., Porter, L., Quessy, S., Rappaport, B.A., Rauschkolb, C., Revicki, D.A., Rothman, M., Schmader, K.E., Stacey, B.R., Stauffer, J.W., von Stein, T., White, R.E., Witter, J. and Zavisic, S. (2008) 'Interpreting the clinical importance of treatment outcomes in chronic pain clinical trials: IMMPACT recommendations', *Journal of Pain,* 9 (2):105–21.

Glaser, B.G. and Strauss, A.L. (1967) *The Discovery of Grounded Theory: Strategies for Qualitative Research.* New York: Aldine Publishing.

Kaplan, C.D., Korf, D. and Sterk, C. (1987) 'Temporal and social contexts of heroin-using populations: an illustration of the snowball sampling technique', *Journal of Mental and Nervous Disorders,* 175 (9): 566–74.

Thompson, S.K. (2012) *Sampling* (3rd edn). London: Wiley.

Van Cleemput, P.V., Parry, G., Thomas, K., Peters, J. and Cooper, C. (2007) 'Health-related beliefs and experiences of gypsies and travellers: a qualitative study', *Journal of Epidemiology and Community Health,* 61: 205–10.

18

RECRUITMENT AND RETENTION

Victoria Hall Moran and Diane Whitham

Learning Objectives

- Identify the importance of recruitment and retention in research
- Understand the rationale behind, and need for, a cohesive, well-thought-out strategy to maximise recruitment and retention
- Consider the factors involved with choosing the most appropriate sites for recruiting participants
- Understand the challenges to successful recruitment and retention

Introduction

Recruitment and retention of participants is an essential task in any empirical research study and is one of the most significant challenges faced by investigators. It is important because recruiting and retaining a specific sample of participants in a study determines how well the target population is represented. Recruitment procedures that fail to adequately sample the population of interest can potentially skew study results or threaten external validity by reducing their generalisability to the target population from which the sample was drawn. Poor recruitment can result in an underpowered study, which may erroneously fail to find statistically significant clinically relevant effects, i.e. type II error (please see Chapter 17: 'Sampling'). A non-significant finding increases the risk that an effective intervention will be abandoned before its true value is established, or that there will be a delay in demonstrating its value while more trials or meta-analyses are done. Also, exposing participants to an intervention with uncertain benefits due to the trial being underpowered, raises ethical issues if the researchers are unable to conclude whether the intervention does more good than harm on completion of the trial (Treweek et al., 2010). Studies may have to be extended due to poor initial recruitment, which increases costs and could have an adverse impact on the commitment of those who have already been recruited to the study (Gul and Ali, 2010) and could result in the premature termination of the study (Hunninghake et al., 1987).

Enhancing the conditions to ensure optimal participation is a key aim in research studies and the recruitment and retention of adequate numbers of participants who are representative of the target population remains a significant challenge for researchers. For example, despite patient participation being the highest in clinical trials in oncology, they attract no more than 3–5% of eligible patients as research participants. For other indications, participation is much lower (Rojavin, 2009). When recruiting a sample, it is important to ascertain the characteristics of those who accept or decline to participate in a study and the reasons for declining. If there are substantial and systematic patterns of non-participation it may be difficult to determine to whom the results apply. Characterisation of the responders and non-responders allows the breadth and limitations of the obtained sample to be evaluated. Ease of recruitment indicates the feasibility of the study design and the appeal of the intervention for potential participants, and from a public policy perspective, low participation could be indicative of an incongruity between the intervention and the target population or community (Prinz et al., 2001).

Retention is also important as low rates may compromise the scientific quality of your research. Therefore the maintenance of adequate retention rates requires careful planning and sufficient resources. Retention issues are most relevant for research involving multiple data collection points, such as those employing follow-up data collection or longitudinal designs. Significant attrition can erode the impact and value of a trial by creating non-representative groups or by reducing the statistical power. Differential attrition by treatment group can be a serious threat to the internal validity of the study design because some of the characteristics of the intervention (or comparison condition) might be influencing retention versus attrition. Although statistical techniques can mitigate some of the problems with missing data and differential attrition problems, it remains vital to utilise recruitment and retention methods that optimise, and not impair, participation.

Aims for successful recruitment and retention

- Your sample is characteristic of the target population, including adequate representation of sex, ethnicity, and so on.
- Shows good external validity.
- Maintains statistical power.
- Avoidance of type II errors.
- Recruitment is within the timescale.
- Identification of characteristics of those who decline to participate as well as those who do.
- Avoidance of differential attrition.
- Enrolment is at a constant rate to maintain study power and avoid excessive workload.

Recruitment and retention and research design

Choosing your site

It is important to select the right investigator sites at the earliest stages of trial design in order to ensure that trials are completed within the specified timelines, on budget, and to the highest standards. You may need to have more than one site involved depending on your power calculation, and the actual numbers of patients with the disease or condition and the number of those that would meet the eligibility criteria at each site (this will indicate how many sites you need). You also need to ascertain the ability of the site to deliver the care as specified by the protocol. Time spent planning and setting realistic expectations based on the evidence will be rewarded when the trial recruits on time and with fewer drop-outs.

Sites are usually recruited via key clinicians who can provide the largest number of eligible patients in the required time period. However, it is also important to identify and recruit investigators who are motivated and competent to conduct the trial in accordance with the protocol and good clinical practice guidelines. Health professionals who are more likely to be involved in trials and to recruit participants are those who are more research oriented, which is generally correlated with research experience and research involvement. Doctors who believe trial participation affects patient–doctor relationship or that it restricts their ability to individualise care, are less likely to recruit patients into trials (Tooher et al., 2008). Identifying suitable clinicians is often done through your and your colleagues' network of contacts or through national research networks, for example, UK Clinical Research

Network. A search of the published literature may also identify potential investigators with relevant research interests and can be an indicator of their previous experience of successfully delivering clinical trials (please see Chapter 2: 'Finding the Evidence to Support your Research Question'). Other sources of information on leading clinicians in a specific disease area are the authors and contributors to national and international guidelines; the clinicians on the editorial boards of journals; and the speakers at conferences and congresses. Another way of identifying clinicians is through databases which many companies and large commercial research organisations have developed in which investigators are listed by area of therapeutic interest, geographical location, research experience and the facilities they have at their site. These databases are designed to quickly and effectively match trials with potential investigator sites. Some of these databases are available both on a complimentary (TrialWatch) and fee for service basis.

Following the identification of potential investigators, it is important to consider the selection criteria on which your decision to include a site will be based. There is little point in recruiting sites that are not going to remain in the study or, worse, do not recruit. The following factors should be taken into consideration:

- Investigator qualifications and experience;
- Enrolment potential, access to the required population with the disease condition being studied;
- Current competing trials at that site;
- Willingness to recruit (investigators must have equipoise without strong beliefs in one treatment, otherwise they may either not recruit or not follow the protocol);
- Other time commitments of the investigator;
- Availability of co-investigators and other research staff at the site;
- Basic infrastructure at the site.

Having identified potential sites, the next stage is to assess each potential site against your defined selection criteria. This can be achieved by performing a visit or phone call to assess if the site meets all of your requirements. This final stage of site recruitment should begin as close to the initial recruitment of participants as possible; if too much time elapses sites may drop out or develop other interests.

Research design

Randomised controlled trials (RCT) are the gold standard for the evaluation of the effectiveness and safety of health care interventions, principally because they protect against selection bias (Kunz et al., 2007) (please see Chapter 11: 'Clinical Trials'). However, recruiting participants to randomised trials can be extremely difficult and it has been estimated that less than 50% of trials meet their recruitment target, or meet their target without extending the length of the trial (Treweek et al., 2010). The recruitment and retention of an adequate number of participants who are representative of the population is essential for the successful completion of an RCT.

Another design for which an appropriate recruitment and retention strategy is imperative is in the prospective longitudinal study. Here a sample is studied in successive waves over time, and provides us with an opportunity to assess change as people move through developmental and transitional experiences (please see Chapter 10: 'Epidemiology'). The confidence with which we can rely upon and generalise this type of study's findings depends on how representative the initial and final samples are of the target population. Poor recruitment rates at baseline are a potential source of bias, since non-responders are likely to differ from respondents in important characteristics. Attrition in longitudinal studies may introduce further bias, particularly if loss to follow-up is differential with regard to important participant characteristics. There is no assurance that a sample that is initially representative will remain so over time. It can be difficult to discriminate between changes in sample parameters due to a longitudinal process, for example, ageing, disease stage, etc., and changes due to attrition. The issue is particularly challenging if one of the purposes of your study is to compare differences between two or more groups over time, because there may be differential attrition across groups. It is therefore important to distinguish between the two types of changes in longitudinal studies, i.e. selective survival and selective drop-out (Gregson et al., 1997). Baltes (1968) described selective survival as something that changes the population's composition over time, due to survival correlating with variables. For example, cognitive ability is positively associated with age in the older population, i.e. the better the cognitive ability, the longer the life (Perls et al., 1993; Siegler et al., 1982). Therefore if your longitudinal research was with a geriatric population, you may want to do a cognitive function test to ascertain whether survival was due to your intervention, or their cognitive ability. Selective drop out on the other hand, applies only to the research sample and may bias your results, such as in weight loss programmes there might be drop out of participants who do not reach their goals (Kaplan and Atkins, 1987).

Challenges in recruitment and retention

An inadequate number of participants recruited and/or retained is widely recognised as a threat to the success of a research project. One of the major causes of ineffective recruitment is due to a phenomenon called Lasagna's law or the 'funnel effect' of recruitment (Gul and Ali, 2010). This phenomenon relates to the tendency of the researcher who, on the basis of the prevalence of a disease, overestimates the pool of available participants who both meet the inclusion criteria and who would be willing to take part in a trial. It has been suggested that only 1–10% of the eligible target population participate in studies due to this over-estimation (Hunninghake et al., 1987). As the consent rate for intervention studies can be as low as 1% (Cooley et al., 2003), researchers much recognise the many factors that can influence the decision to participate in a study. Such factors could include personal, contextual or research/researcher-related factors. These factors can be identified during the design process with appropriate patient involvement so that an appropriate recruitment and retention strategy can be drafted (please see Chapter 16: 'Patient and Public Involvement').

Participant-related factors

Demographics

It is well recognised that factors such as age, sex, income and education are strong predictors of recruitment and retention in studies (Gul and Ali, 2010; Hunninghake et al., 1987; Sangi-Haghpeykar et al., 2009). High rates of refusal and attrition are more pronounced among multi-ethnic, low-income populations (Barnett et al., 2012) and in those with low education and poor health awareness (Gul and Ali, 2010). The barriers to successful study involvement for marginalised groups include language factors, economic constraints, transient living situations, unreliable contact information, transportation difficulties, cultural differences, distrust of the medical community, and negative patient experiences (Barnett et al., 2012). Such reports have given rise to the belief among the medical community that the recruitment and retention of such groups in intervention studies may be demanding (Sangi-Haghpeykar et al., 2009; Tooher et al., 2008). These perceptions in turn may lead to a lower enrolment of these populations, which leaves study populations atypical.

Gender can also influence recruitment, especially low-income women who may have specific constraints on their time due to work and child care commitments or feel risk-averse if pregnant (Tooher et al., 2008). Research has suggested that willingness to participate may relate to the perceived importance of the study topic for women. For example, high retention rates have been shown in studies on childhood asthma (Nicholson et al., 2011), a chronic disease that can have severe symptoms. More benign topics however are less well recruited, perhaps because the study is not perceived to be important to mothers (Nicholson et al., 2011).

The lack of representation of ethnic minorities in research studies is an issue of particular concern, particularly in countries with a large ethnic population. For example, whilst racial and ethnic minorities represent over a third of the US population, they represent less than a 10% of clinical trial participants in the US (Sangi-Haghpeykar et al., 2009). Adequate representation of minority populations in clinical trials is crucial in eliminating the disparities that are present in health outcomes and health care between whites and non-whites (Sangi-Haghpeykar et al., 2009). Racial and ethnic minorities are particularly susceptible to some health issues but are often underrepresented in studies which target that particular issue. For instance, racial and ethnic minorities in the US suffer disproportionately from obesity and its associated co-morbidities, yet intervention study literature lacks sufficient attention to these populations, with 86% of weight management studies conducted between 1966 and 2003 failing to even report the race/ethnicity balance of recruited participants (Brown et al., 2012). Sufficient minority involvement is required in all types of studies. This can be achieved by specifically drawing samples from geographic areas in which substantial numbers of one or more minority groups reside, or oversampling to produce proportions of ethnicities beyond their levels of representation in a population (Yancey et al., 2006). For further information, the National Institutes of Health (NIH) in the United States and other scientific groups publish guidelines regarding the inclusion of minorities and women in research (Barnett et al., 2012).

Psychosocial and motivational

Identification of the factors that motivate participants whether to join a study or not, should be considered in order to identify ways to enhance recruitment. Psychosocial factors such as values and beliefs, influence of family members, and negative perceptions about the study have also been shown to influence recruitment and retention of participants (Gul and Ali, 2010). Other high impact factors have to do with a predominantly negative perception of the funders of studies, such as pharmaceutical industries, and the diminished level of trust in clinical research professionals (Rojavin, 2009). In research studies that deal with sensitive issues, it may be particularly important to consider participants' fear of emotional distress (Dimattio, 2001).

Contextual and environmental factors

Contextual factors that may inhibit study recruitment and retention include culture, and community practices, and political issues. For example, in some Asian cultures, women may not be able to travel alone, creating clear barriers to study participation. In some communities, people's decisions are not only influenced by members of their family, but also by trusted members of the community (Gul and Ali, 2010). Political and media-related factors may also influence study participation, due to the increasing accessibility of health care information, consumer empowerment and a mistrust of research (Gross and Fogg, 2001). Environmental factors include qualities of the research site such as the hospital or clinic structure, such as their clinic hours; the interdisciplinary care team; lack of continuity of care; and competing priorities of clinical care providers such as teaching and research. There can also be institutional factors which act as significant barriers to trial involvement among health professionals. These may include lack of time, lack of managerial support, lack of expert support staff to coordinate recruitment and data management, lack of financial reward, either for individuals or departments involved in trials, together with the expense and financial implications involved in trial participation. A positive organisational culture, involvement of a dedicated clinical trial manager and material support for trial activity increases health professional participation (Tooher et al., 2008).

Research-related factors

Problems, demands and discomforts associated with the research design could also have an effect on participants' decision to consent to, or remain in a study. The act

of randomisation in an RCT may cause resistance and an unwillingness to participate if participants have a strong treatment preference (Gul and Ali, 2010). Also the
time taken to participate may interfere with their work or private lives and require
participants to change their daily routine, thus disrupting their everyday lives. Such
factors may reduce recruitment and lead to early withdrawal; over 40% of study
participants withdraw consent after study enrolment (Sangi-Haghpeykar et al.,
2009). Care should be taken to provide appropriate guidance about the nature of the
requirements of the study prior to consent (Sangi-Haghpeykar et al., 2009) and cus-
tomised patient-specific follow-up approaches should be devised, including limiting
the number of visits or having flexible scheduling to accommodate participants
with full-time jobs, small children or those with transportation problems.

There is evidence to suggest that many potential trial participants may have difficulty understanding the nature of randomisation and equipoise in RCTs and often
show signs of misunderstanding the basis of their treatment allocation, and of wrongly
assuming that one treatment is already known to be better than the other or others.
Failure to understand random allocation and equipoise could occur if trial information
is too complex for the participant to comprehend, or if the participant is not given sufficient time to think about it (Robinson et al., 2004). Therefore accessible information
about the scientific benefits of randomisation should be given to potential participants
at recruitment. Research-related barriers to clinician participation in trials include the
use of aggressive treatments or placebo, complex protocols, strict eligibility criteria and
relevance (particularly to the local population) of the trial (Tooher et al., 2008).

Strategies for effective recruitment and retention

It now well recognised that active recruitment strategies are more effective for both
recruitment and retention than passive methods like mass media and direct mailing. A Cochrane review of strategies to improve recruitment to randomised controlled trials has identified several interventions that look promising and appear to
be effective in increasing recruitment (Treweek et al., 2010). The most promising of
these are telephone reminders to non-responders (Harris et al., 2008; Nystuen and
Hagen, 2004), as is sending text messages containing anonymised quotes from other
participants (Free et al., 2010), particularly in populations where mobile phones are
widely used. Text messages informing potential participants of attempts to contact
them appears to make them more receptive to answering their phone when next
contacted about the study. Opt-out is another promising method, where potential
participants are required to contact the research team if they do not want to be
contacted about a study, rather than the standard opt-in procedures, whereby
potential participants contact the research team if they are interested in taking part
in the project (Trevena et al., 2006).

Another method which may help with your recruitment is by using an open
design for your trial, where participants and research staff know the treatment allocation rather than the more traditional blinded studies, as this design has been
shown to improve recruitment (Avenell et al., 2004; Hemminki et al., 2004). This

kind of design however diminishes the scientific rigour of the randomised study and careful consideration should be given to the risk associated with a greater potential for bias and high attrition rates in individuals who have a strong preference for one intervention over another, especially if assigned to a placebo or usual care intervention, versus the benefit of better recruitment. The effects on recruitment of other design and delivery strategies, including participant preference design where participants can choose which arm to go into if so wished (Cooper et al., 1997), the use of active controls rather than placebo controls (Leader and Neuwirth, 1978), such as an alternative therapy, and increasing the regular contact between the coordinating centre and research sites, are encouraging, although less clear.

Minimising participant-related barriers

To minimise barriers that could prevent participation, you need to consider the practical difficulties associated with the study and visit schedule to ensure that they are not burdensome or costly for the participants. Needing to miss work, needing to change their usual routine, not having child care, treatment side effects and being treated like a guinea pig have all been cited as reasons not to participate in a study (Kennedy and Burnett, 2007). To overcome this, some studies have visits at suitable times for the participant, such as after work or on the weekends and in locations such as the participant's home or child care centre (Corrigan and Salzer, 2003; Gross and Fogg, 2001; Gross et al., 2001). Monetary incentives may overcome the barrier of the perception that it will be costly to participate and has been shown to improve recruitment (Bentley and Thacker, 2004; Free et al., 2010; Halpern et al., 2004) compared to no monetary incentive (Martinson et al., 2000). There is no recognised formula to assist in calculating how much compensation to give, however it 'should be sufficiently high so as to encourage participation but not so high as to be coercive' (Gross and Fogg, 2001: 532). Although monetary incentives achieve higher recruitment rates, their impact on retention has not been established. Gross et al. (2001) identified that participants who consented because of the monetary compensation showed poor follow-up attendance. Therefore incentives could also be used to increase study retention such as giving gift vouchers (Voyer et al., 2008).

Cultural and contextual barriers

Consideration to the participants' cultural background should be taken when presenting a trial. Western European and North American cultures may be more inclined to find individual benefits appealing, while Asian American cultures may see benefits for the community or society as more inviting (Lee and Zane, 1998). Increased racial, ethnic and language diversity among research staff is also important. A trial of African American men (Ford et al., 2003) showed an increase in recruitment when they used a research team with similar backgrounds to the participants. In a similar trial of Hispanic women (Larkey et al., 2002), lay advocates who were women already enrolled in the trial were more successful in enrolling participants than Anglo women.

There have been a number of studies that have evaluated strategies for improving recruitment and retention in hard-to-reach groups such as ethnic minorities and people of low income. Successful minority engagement depends on conveying respect, trustworthiness and importance of diversity throughout a trial, not just at the point of recruitment (Brown et al., 2012). Brown and team found that simple modifications to recruitment letters can have a meaningful impact on minority reach and initial engagement. For example, direct mail has been shown to be more effective than mass media for recruiting minorities (Robinson et al., 2007), with some studies showing an additional benefit of a significant number of participants being referred to the study by friends/family who were sent a letter, i.e. snowball sampling (Sangi-Haghpeykar et al., 2009). Recruitment materials with pro-diversity statements (where ethnicity is valued) increased trust among African Americans more than 'colour-neutral' materials (where ethnicity is immaterial) (Purdie-Vaughns et al., 2008). An ethnically targeted statement in direct mail letters noting health disparities among multiple ethnic groups has also been shown to increase response rates (Brown et al., 2012). Whether personalisation, i.e. addressing the recipients by name, is effective in recruitment letters is open to debate. Personalisation is costly and time consuming with some studies showing a benefit whilst others have not (Brown et al., 2012). Brown and team suggest that, given the proliferation of computerised direct mail marketing, recipients may be increasingly indifferent to seemingly disingenuous personalisation. Bilingual study coordinators and medical translators as well as study videos or printed material in the patient's own language are also essential when targeting racial and ethnic minorities (Sangi-Haghpeykar et al., 2009).

Case study

Barnett et al. (2012) conducted a study with low-income multi-ethnic women in the Bronx, New York, which had a 98.1% retention rate at the 29-month follow-up. Their recruitment and retention 10-point plan maximised study staff access and availability to the participant, and facilitated strong support staff rapport with participants, and in doing so addressed the barriers to participation in this population with resultant optimal follow-up rates. Qualitative assessment of participants' experience of the study suggested that the high retention rates were due to the strong rapport between participants and researchers, the data collection via short interviews required little time commitment and the participants' perception of the study was informative. All staff were bilingual and study materials produced in Spanish (New York's unofficial second language) and English.

The 10-point recruitment–retention plan used to recruit and retain participants was:

1. During recruitment, participants were required to provide contact information for themselves as well as two other contact persons. Participants were asked for their address, mobile, home and work phone numbers, and email addresses.

2. For each of the three telephone interviews spread over the 29 months, participants would receive an additional $20 gift card via the mail to encourage retention.

3. Participants were provided with study labelled materials, such as logo branded magnets and brochures, which provided the participant with the study's contact information.

4. Study staff obtained bi-weekly updates of changes in participant contact information from electronic medical records.

5. Research staff mailed logo branded postcards to participants to remind them of upcoming interviews, approximately 10 days before, as well as study contact information.

6. Research assistants (RAs) conducted weekday evening and weekend calls for participants that were consistently unreachable during normal working hours, i.e. 9am to 5pm.

7. Participants were provided with a business card containing the RAs' mobile phone numbers.

8. RAs sent out personalised letters and emails to alert participants that they were unable to reach them to conduct the interview. Study contact information was provided in this correspondence.

9. A list was compiled weekly that recorded details of participants who were deemed difficult to reach. RAs utilised the electronic medical record system to obtain new contact information for them.

10. RAs searched participants' medical records for upcoming clinic visits for the hard-to-reach participant. RAs would meet them at their visits to either issue an in-person reminder of the upcoming interview, or to conduct the interview then and there. Updated contact information was also obtained at this time.

Minimising research-related barriers

It is essential that there is an understanding of what drives enrolment success. Factors which are known to impact on recruitment and retention rates are:

- The number of patients at a site that would meet the inclusion exclusion criteria. Projected recruitment numbers should therefore be based on retrospective data from recruiting sites over a specified time period.

- Number of recruiting sites, although more is not always better and can prolong the project.

- Percentage of poor recruiting sites, although this should be limited based on your rigorous selection process, particular consideration should be given to ensuring that resources are available for the trial, including sufficient time and staff to commit to the identification and recruitment of suitable candidates.

- Site initiation rates, these need to be planned ahead of time to ensure the availability of both site and coordinating centre staff for the initiation visit.
- Predicted drop-out rates, carefully considering the length and frequency of study visits, types of assessments needed, and test and intervention regimes which need to be comparable to usual care wherever possible to limit the burden of participation.

It is therefore advised that significant thought and time is given to developing a comprehensive recruitment strategy, including evidence-based recruitment prediction graphs, comprehensive data management planning and ensuring adequate levels of data management staff for the close monitoring and rapid identification of recruitment, retention and adherence problems, to guarantee the timely implementation of corrective actions and protocol changes where necessary.

In studies with long-term follow-up or longitudinal studies, there is the additional complexity of maintaining engagement with participants over extended periods of time. Particular consideration should be given to the geographical location, and the demographics of participants, whether they are transient, and making sure you collect sufficient contact information, which may include personal information, for example, national identity numbers (Lyons et al., 2004) to assist in locating them in cases where their address or phone number changes. Asking participants for a backup contact, perhaps a relative or friend, may also be a good idea, however this will require written permission from the named person in order to keep their contact information on file.

Case study

Your trial team are planning a small complex group intervention study of 324 patients due to start in August 2014 and need to predict the time it will take to recruit this number into the study. Recruitment to the trial will be managed in a series of time-limited recruitment phases: initial identification, consent and randomisation (maximum of 2 weeks), assessments (2 weeks), intervention (12 weeks group treatment or usual care). The team know that the minimum treatment group size is 6 participants and the maximum 10. Sites will therefore need to identify a minimum of 12 participants during the initial identification phase to ensure there are adequate numbers consenting to meet the minimum group size. There are 3 sites selected for the study. Each site has 4 eligible participants per month and can run one group per quarter; based on this information, sites will identify, consent and randomise every 2.5 months. The trial team have produced a recruitment graph that predicts the trial will take 2 years to recruit (Figure 18.1).

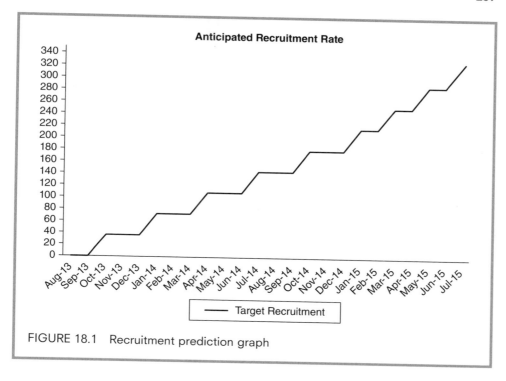

FIGURE 18.1   Recruitment prediction graph

Education of site personnel

The education of site staff on both the general principles of research, and study-specific training on the protocol, is the foundation of successful recruitment and retention and should be undertaken in person, on an individual basis in the form of a site initiation visit, or en masse in the form of an investigator meeting. The individual site initiation visit is preferable, remembering that collaboration may last for several years and establishing good relationships with investigators and site staff from the beginning is of vital importance to the success of the study. However, the investigator meeting provides the opportunity for the site staff to share ideas, reinforce timelines, and identify potential problems with the design, recruitment or retention of participants and can be a good motivational and team-building exercise.

During the initial education of the site, it is of paramount importance that all study-specific aspects that are non-negotiable and procedures that must be complied with are made absolutely clear and emphasised throughout the training. Investigators and staff must understand clearly the importance of adhering to these procedures for maintaining scientific validity. The agenda for any site education whether individually or in large groups should include the following:

- Description and/or demonstration of the study intervention, including background and development, administration and risks.
- Review of the study protocol making sure the sites are familiar with the objectives of the study, eligibility criteria, treatment allocations, randomisation procedure, schedule of events, outcome measures, adverse event reporting, enrolment phase, treatment phase and follow-up phase.
- Strategies for recruitment, including recruitment target and timelines, pathways for identifying potential participants, how they will be approached and by whom and whether the site will recruit in cohorts or individually.
- Roles and responsibilities, defining, agreeing and documenting who is responsible for which procedures based on qualifications and role within the study e.g. pharmacist, research nurse, etc.
- Good clinical practice and regulatory requirements including the informed consent process and documentation regarding the protection of the rights, safety and well-being of trial participants.
- Data collection requirements, including identifying what needs to be collected and when, the method of collection which can be paper-based or electronic and how to make corrections and resolve queries.

Role of the pilot study

It is now recognised that preparatory feasibility or pilot work is needed to identify and address both practical difficulties and recruitment and retention issues (Van Teijlingen et al., 2001). Therefore, it is advisable to undertake a feasibility or pilot study before the main study to provide evidence-based estimates of the many unknowns associated with recruitment and retention rates. The objective of these studies is to identify parameters that could affect successful study conduct and reduce uncertainties such as: the number of patients meeting the eligibility criteria; ease of identifying patients; willingness of patients and clinicians to randomise; adherence with treatment; completeness of data; retention rates, and to identify the degree of burden for participants, while obtaining suggestions to make the trial design or intervention more acceptable (Conn et al., 2001) and to answer the generic question can this study be done?

Summary

- Enhancing the conditions to ensure optimal participation is a key aim in research studies and the recruitment and retention of adequate numbers of participants who are representative of the target population remains a challenge.
- Should recruitment procedures and/retention measures fail, study findings may be skewed, underpowered or the study's external validity may be threatened.
- Failure to adequately plan a recruitment and retention strategy may have negative time and financial implications on the study, its participants and its investigators.
- Good recruitment and retention strategies consider factors relating to the choice of research site; participant-related factors; and research-related factors.

- Strategies to improve recruitment and retention include flexibility of design, monetary compensation, ensuring cultural sensitivity, community consultation and staff education.

Questions for Discussion

1. If you were planning a randomised controlled trial of two treatments for a rare skin disease that is predominately associated with an elderly population, what challenges would you need to consider when planning the strategies for effective recruitment?

2. Your study has a three-year follow-up, with annual postal questionnaires and a visit in the third year. What strategies would you employ to maintain an adequate retention rate?

Further Reading

Campbell, M.K., Snowdon, C., Francis, D., Elbourne, D., McDonald, A.M., Knight, R., Entwistle, V., Garcia, J., Roberts, I. and Grant, A. (the STEPS group) (2007) 'Recruitment to randomised trials: strategies for trial enrolment and participation study. The STEPS study', *Health Technology Assessment*, 11: 48.

Hewison, J. and Haines, A. (2006) 'Overcoming barriers to recruitment in health research', *British Medical Journal*, 333: 300–2.

Macleod, M., Craigie, A.M., Barton, K.L., Treweek, S., Anderson, A.S. and on behalf of the WeighWell team (2012) 'Recruiting and retaining postpartum women from areas of social disadvantage in a weight-loss trial: an assessment of strategies employed in the WeighWell feasibility study', *Maternal and Child Nutrition*. doi: 10.1111/j.1740–8709.2011.00393.x.

National Institute of Mental Health (2005) *Points to Consider about Recruitment and Retention while Preparing a Clinical Research Study*: www.nimh.nih.gov/research-funding/grants/recruitment-points-to-consider-6-1-05.pdf (accessed Dec. 2012).

Nwaru, B.I., Parkkali, S., Abacassamo, F., Salomé, G., Chilundo, B., Augusto, O., Cliff, J., Dgedge, M., Regushevskaya, E., Nikula, M. and Hemminki, E. (2012) 'A pragmatic randomised controlled trial on routine iron prophylaxis during pregnancy in Maputo, Mozambique (PROFEG): rationale, design, and success', *Maternal and Child Nutrition*. doi: 10.1111/mcn.12006.

Penckofer, S., Byrn, M., Mumby, P. and Ferrans, C.E. (2011) 'Improving subject recruitment, retention, and participation in research through Peplau's theory of interpersonal relations', *Nursing Science Quarterly*, 24: 146–51.

References

Avenell, A., Grant, A.M., McGee, M., McPherson, G., Campbell, M.K. and McGee, M.A. (2004) 'The effects of an open design on trial participant recruitment, compliance and retention: a randomized controlled trial comparison with a blinded, placebo-controlled design', *Clinical Trials*, 1: 490–8.

Baltes, P.B. (1968) 'Longitudinal and cross-section sequences in the study of age and gereation effects', *Human Development*, 11: 145–70.

Barnett, J., Aguilar, S., Brittner, M. and Bonuck, K. (2012) 'Recruiting and retaining low-income, multi-ethnic women into randomized controlled trials: successful strategies and staffing', *Contemporary Clinical Trials*, 33 (5): 925–32.

Bentley, J.P. and Thacker, P.G. (2004) 'The influence of risk and monetary payment on the research participation decision making process', *Journal of Medical Ethics*, 30: 293–8.

Brown, S.D., Lee, K., Schoffman, D.E., King, A.C., Crawley, L.M. and Kiernan, M. (2012) 'Minority recruitment into clinical trials: experimental findings and practical implications', *Contemporary Clinical Trials*, 33 (4): 620–3.

Conn, V.S., Rantz, M.J., Wipke-Tevis, D.D. and Maas, M.L. (2001) 'Designing effective nursing interventions', *Research in Nursing and Health*, 24: 433–42.

Cooley, M.E., Sarna, L., Brown, J.K., Williams, R.D., Chernecky, C., Padilla, G. and Danao, L.L. (2003) 'Challenges of recruitment and retention in multisite clinical research', *Cancer Nursing*, 26: 376–84; quiz 385–6.

Cooper, K.G., Grant, A.M. and Garratt, A.M. (1997) 'The impact of using a partially randomised patient preference design when evaluating alternative managements for heavy menstrual bleeding', *British Journal of Obstetric Gynaecology*, 104: 1367–73.

Corrigan, P.W. and Salzer, M.S. (2003) 'The conflict between random assignment and treatment preference: implications for internal validity', *Evaluation and Program Planning*, 26: 109–21.

Dimattio, M.J. (2001) 'Recruitment and retention of community-dwelling, aging women in nursing studies', *Nursing Research*, 50: 369–73.

Ford, M.E., Havstad, S.L. and Tilley, B.C. (2003) 'Recruiting older African American men to a cancer screening trial (the AAMEN Project)', *Gerontologist*, 43: 27–35.

Free, C., Hoile, E., Robertson, S. and Knight, R. (2010) 'Three controlled trials of interventions to increase recruitment to a randomized controlled trial of mobile phone based smoking cessation support', *Clinical Trials*, 7: 265–73.

Green, B.L., Partridge, E.E., Fouad, M.N., Kohler, C., Crayton, E.F. and Alexander, L. (2000) 'African-American attitudes regarding cancer clinical trials and research studies: results from focus group methodology', *Ethn Dis*, 10: 76–86.

Gregson, B.A., Smith, M., Lecouturier, J., Rousseau, N., Rodgers, H. and Bond, J. (1997) 'Issues of recruitment and maintaining high response rates in a longitudinal study of older hospital patients in England: pathways through care study', *Journal of Epidemiology and Community Health*, 51 (5): 541–8.

Gross, D. and Fogg, L. (2001) 'Clinical trials in the 21st century: the case for participant-centered research', *Research in Nursing and Health*, 24: 530–9.

Gross, D., Julion, W. and Fogg, L. (2001) 'What Motivates Participation and Dropout among Low-Income Urban Families of Color in a Prevention Intervention?', *Family Relations*, 50: 246–54.

Gul, R.B. and Ali, P.A. (2010) 'Clinical trials: the challenge of recruitment and retention of participants', *Journal of Clinical Nursing*, 19 (1–2): 227–33.

Halpern, S.D., Karlawish, J.H.T., Casarett, D., Berlin, J.A. and Asch, D.A. (2004) 'Empirical assessment of whether moderate payments are undue or unjust inducements for participation in clinical trials', *Archives of Internal Medicine*, 164: 801–3.

Harris, T.J., Carey, I.M., Victor, C.R., Adams, R. and Cook, D.G. (2008) 'Optimising recruitment into a study of physical activity in older people: a randomised controlled trial of different approaches', *Age and Ageing*, 37: 659–65.

Hemminki, E., Hovi, S.L., Veerus, P., Sevon, T., Tuimala, R., Rahu, M. and Hakama, M. (2004) 'Blinding decreased recruitment in a prevention trial of postmenopausal hormone therapy', *Journal of Clinical Epidemiology*, 57: 1237–43.

Hunninghake, D.B., Darby, C.A. and Probstfield, J.L. (1987) 'Recruitment experience in clinical-trials: literature summary and annotated-bibliography', *Controlled Clinical Trials*, 8 (4): S6–S30.

Kaplan, R.M. and Atkins, C.J. (1987) 'Selective attrition causes overestimates of treatment effects in studies of weight loss', *Addictive Behaviour*, 12 (3): 297–302.

Kennedy, B.M. and Burnett, M.F. (2007) 'Clinical research trials: factors that influence and hinder participation', *Journal of Cultural Diversity*, 14: 141–7.

Kunz, R., Wegscheider, K., Guyatt, G., Zielinski, W., Rakowsky, N., Donner-Banzhoff, N., et al. (2007) 'Impact of short evidence summaries in discharge letters on adherence of practitioners to discharge medication: a cluster-randomised controlled trial', *Quality and Safety in Health Care*, 16 (6): 456–61.

Larkey, L.K., Staten, L.K., Ritenbaugh, C., Hall, R.A., Buller, D.B., Bassford, T. and Altimari, B.R. (2002) 'Recruitment of Hispanic women to the Women's Health Initiative. The case of Embajadoras in Arizona', *Controlled Clinical Trials*, 23: 289–98.

Leader, M.A. and Neuwirth, E. (1978) 'Clinical research and the noninstitutional elderly: a model for subject recruitment', *Journal of American Geriatrics Society*, 26: 27–31.

Lee, L.C. and Zane, N.W.S. (1998) *Handbook of Asian American Psychology*. Thousand Oaks, CA: SAGE.

Lovato, L.C., Hill, K., Hertert, S., Hunninghake, D.B., Probstfield, J.L. (1997) 'Recruitment for controlled clinical trials: literature summary and annotated bibliography', *Controlled Clinical Trials*, 18 (4): 328–52.

Lyons, K.S., Carter, J.H., Carter, E.H., Rush, K.N., Stewart, B.J. and Archbold, P.G. (2004) 'Locating and retaining research participants for follow-up studies', *Research in Nursing and Health*, 27: 63–8.

Martinson, B.C., Lazovich, D., Lando, H.A., Perry, C.L., Mcgovern, P.G. and Boyle, R.G. (2000) 'Effectiveness of monetary incentives for recruiting adolescents to an intervention trial to reduce smoking', *Preventive Medicine*, 31: 706–13.

Nicholson, L.M, Schwirian, P.M., Klein, E.G., Skybo, T., Murray-Johnson, L., Eneli, I., et al. (2011) 'Recruitment and retention strategies in longitudinal clinical studies with low-income populations', *Contemporary Clinical Trials*, 32 (3): 353–62.

Nystuen, P. and Hagen, K.B. (2004) 'Telephone reminders are effective in recruiting nonresponding patients to randomized controlled trials', *Journal of Clinical Epidemiology*, 57: 773–6.

Perls, T.T., Morris, J.N., Ooi, W.L. and Lipsitz, L.A. (1993) 'The relationship between age, gender and cognitive performance in the very old: the effect of selective survival', *Journal of American Geriatrics Society*, 41 (11): 1193–201.

Prinz, R.J., Smith, E.P., Dumas, J.E., Laughlin, J.E., White, D.W. and Barron, R. (2001) 'Recruitment and retention of participants in prevention trials involving family-based interventions', *American Journal of Preventive Medicine*, 20 (1): 31–7.

Purdie-Vaughns, V., Steele, C.A., Davies, P.G., Ditlmann, R. and Crosby, J.R. (2008) 'Social identity contingencies: how diversity cues signal threat or safety for African Americans in mainstream institutions', *Journal of Personality and Social Psychology*, 94 (4): 615–30.

Robinson, E.J., Kerr, C., Stevens, A., Lilford, R., Braunholtz, D. and Edwards, S. (2004) 'Lay conceptions of the ethical and scientific justifications for random allocation in clinical trials', *Social Science and Medicine*, 58 (4): 811–24.

Robinson, E.J., Kerr, C.E.P., Stevens, A.J., Lilford, R.J., Braunholtz, D.A., Edwards, S.J., et al. (2005) 'Lay public's understanding of equipoise and randomisation in randomised controlled trials', *Health Technology Assessment* 9 (8): III–+.

Robinson, J.L., Fuerch, J.H., Winiewicz, D.D., Saivy, S.J., Roemmich, J.N. and Epstein, L.H. (2007) 'Cost effectiveness of recruitment methods in an obesity prevention trial for young children', *Preventive Medicine*, 44 (6): 499–503.

Rojavin, M. (2009) 'Patient recruitment and retention: from art to science', *Contemporary Clinical Trials,* 30 (5): 387.

Sangi-Haghpeykar, H., Meddaugh, H.M., Liu, H. and Grino, P. (2009) 'Attrition and retention in clinical trials by ethnic origin', *Contemporary Clinical Trials,* 30 (6): 499–503.

Siegler, I.C., McCarty, S.M. and Logue, P.E. (1982) 'Wechsler Memory Scale Scores, Selective Attrition, and Distance from Death', *Journal of Gerontology,* 37 (2): 176–81.

Tooher, R.L., Middleton, P.F. and Crowther, C.A. (2008) 'A thematic analysis of factors influencing recruitment to maternal and perinatal trials', *BMC Pregnancy and Childbirth,* 8: 36.

Trevena, L., Irwig, L. and Barratt, A. (2006) 'Impact of privacy legislation on the number and characteristics of people who are recruited for research: a randomised controlled trial', *Journal of Medical Ethics,* 32: 473–7.

Treweek, S., Pitkethly, M., Cook, J., Kjeldstrom, M., Taskila, T., Johansen, M., Sullivan, F., Wilson, S., Jackson, C., Jones, R. and Mitchell, E. (2010) 'Strategies to improve recruitment to randomised controlled trials', *Cochrane Database of Systematic Reviews.*

Van Teijlingen, E.R., Rennie, A.M., Hundley, V. and Graham, W. (2001) 'The importance of conducting and reporting pilot studies: the example of the Scottish Births Survey', *Journal of Advanced Nursing,* 34: 289–95.

Voyer, P., Lauzon, S., Collin, J. and Cousins, S.O. (2008) 'Research method issue: recruiting and retaining subjects in a research study', *Nurse Research,* 15: 12–25.

Yancey, A.K., Ortega, A.N. and Kumanyika, S.K. (2006) 'Effective recruitment and retention of minority research participants', *Annual Review of Public Health 2006,* 1–28.

Part V

ANALYSIS AND DISSEMINATION

19

QUANTITATIVE ANALYSIS

Nick Taub and Dawn-Marie Walker

- To appreciate the role of quantitative analysis
- To understand what the different types of data are: numerical and categorical
- To be aware of the importance of getting data ready for analysis, including coding and handling missing data
- To know what standard deviations, confidence intervals and p-values are
- Understand the purpose of some common methods of analysis of numerical data

Introduction

Quantitative analysis, also known as statistical analysis, is the process used by researchers to obtain results from data – that is, to get 'facts from figures' (Moroney, 1975). This process is needed in almost all quantitative studies because their aim is usually to answer questions related to a very large group of people, i.e. the target population, using data collected on just a small sample (please see Chapter 17: 'Sampling'). The overall purpose of an analysis is to answer the questions, including testing hypotheses, that the study sets out to answer, and it should be done in a way that is systematic, understandable and accepted as valid by readers.

Case study

Some researchers were conducting a small quantitative project. The first step in the project was collecting survey data:

1. What is your age in years?
2. What sex are you? Female........☐ Male.......☐
3. What is your weight in kilograms?
4. What colour are your eyes?
    Blue ☐   Green ☐   Brown ☐   Grey ☐   Black ☐   Hazel ☐
    Other ☐ (Please specify) _____
5. Do you carry out more than 2 hours of exercise per week, on average?
    No.......☐   Yes........☐
6. What kind of organisation do you work for?
    Primary Care ☐   Hospital ☐   University ☐   Local authority ☐
    Other ☐ (Please specify)...............................
7. Which blood group do you belong to?
    A ☐   B ☐   O ☐   AB ☐   Don't know ☐

Types of data

The choice of the information requested in the questionnaire in the case study illustrates the different forms of data. The type of data affects both the best ways of summarising and describing it, and also the best ways of analysing it. The most important distinction is between numerical data and categorical data (please see Figure 19.1).

Numerical data

Numerical data consist of values that can be measured and thus the data are numbers. In the case study, for example, age and weight would be numerical data. Numerical data come in two main forms:

- Counted data are data obtained from counting, such as the number of visits made to a family doctor last year, or the number of acute episodes of an illness that occurred during a trial.

- Continuous 'interval' data are derived from measurements on a continuous scale, such as in the case study, age in years, or weight in kilograms. The word 'interval' indicates that there is equal spacing between each unit of measurement. For example a difference of 1kg in bodyweight has the same meaning, whether it is from 50kg to 51kg or from 65kg to 66kg.

Categorical data

Data are regarded as categorical when there is a set of categories defined, and each individual is assigned to just one of the categories. For instance, in the case study, sex, eye colour, exercising, work organisation and blood group should all be regarded as categorical. Categories need to be chosen carefully since inappropriate choices can bias the results. Every value should belong to one, and only one, category, and there should be no doubt as to which one. A common mistake is to have categories overlapping, such as defining age groups 20–30, 30–40 years, etc. If you were 30 which one would you choose? You should also provide an 'other' category if you have any doubt that your list of choices is exhaustive.

Categorical data comes in three main forms:

- Binary data are data where there are only two possible values given, such as 0=no and 1=yes, or 0=survive and 1=die, or as in the case study, Sex (1=female and 2=male). We usually come across binary data when our real interest is the proportion of a sample having a certain characteristic or event.

- Nominal data are where the categories are differentiated by a naming system, with no particular meaningful order. The purpose of nominal data is to indicate some characteristic that all those individuals in the same category have in common, such as having in common that their eye colour is brown.

- Ordinal data are where there is an obvious progressive order to the categories, such as the severity of a disease, where there is a clear gradient from 'none', to 'mild' and then on through 'moderate' to 'severe'. The values given to the categories are arbitrary and thus we cannot assume that the progression between categories 1 to 2 is the same 'amount' as from 2 to 3. Therefore, although the codes '1', '2', '3' and '4' may appear to be numerical data, they are not treated as numerical data if we cannot make the assumption of 'equal spacing' between the categories. Another common example of this is the Likert scale commonly used in behavioural research where, as a response to a statement such as 'Physical exercise is an important part of my daily routine', the five categories of response might be labelled: 1=Strongly Disagree, 2=Disagree, 3=Neutral, 4=Agree and 5=Strongly Agree.

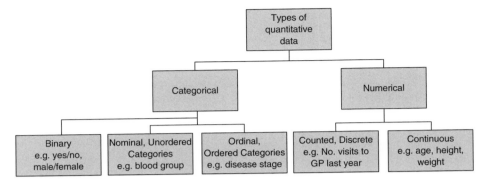

FIGURE 19.1   The different types of quantitative data

Preparation of quantitative data

Once you have collected your data, you need to think about coding any categorical data into a numerical form to enable analysis, then entering the data into a database and cleaning it prior to analysis. There are many statistical software packages, such as SPSS, SAS and Stata, which provide you with a data table or spreadsheet in which you can enter your data, check it and correct any errors, and then produce tables and charts, before carrying out analyses to test hypotheses and estimate certain proportions and other quantities of interest. The software will do the calculations at your command, but you still need to understand the rationale for your choice of methods of analysis, and be able to explain and justify them in any reports that result from the study. Good statistical software is not usually free, and so it is worth checking which reputable packages your institution has a licence for. Using the software can also initially require some training or tuition. Examples of good guides to software packages, including SPSS and SAS, are Field 2013; Field and Miles, 2010.

Case study

A coding form was designed for the categorical questions on the questionnaire indicating the numerical code for each possible answer category.

Question	Variable name	Code	Value
2. What sex are you?	sex	1	Female
		2	Male
4. What colour are your eyes?	eyes	1	Blue
		2	Green

Question	Variable name	Code	Value
		3	Brown
		4	Grey
		5	Black
		6	Hazel
		7	Other
5. Do you carry out more than 2 hours of exercise per week, on average?	exercise	0	No
		1	Yes
6. What kind of organisation do you work for?	work	1	Primary Care
		2	Hospital
		3	University
		4	Local Authority
		5	Other
7. Which blood group do you belong to?	Bloodgp	1	A
		2	B
		3	O
		4	AB
		5	Don't know

Once you have coded all of your categorical answers, you are ready to enter all of your data into your database. Usually, the columns of the database represent the variables or outcomes, and each row represents one participant.

Case study

Of the 80 questionnaires distributed, 62 were returned. Therefore a response rate of 78% was achieved. Each respondent was given a unique ID (first Column, in Table 19.1), as the data should not be identifiable in accordance with ethical guidance. The link between the IDs and participant details should be held securely elsewhere (please see Chapter 15). After coding the categorical responses using the coding form, the data were entered into a database (please see Table 19.1).

(Continued)

(Continued)

TABLE 19.1 Data from the questionnaire

ID	age	gender	weight	eyes	exercise	work	bloodgp
1	27	1	51	1	1	3	5
2	36	2	52	3	0	1	5
3	39	2	46	3	0	2	5
4	38	2	55	1	1	3	3
5	29	1	73	5	0	2	1
6	40	2	50	4	1	2	5
7	58	2	102	3	0	2	1
8	40	2	999	3	1	2	1
9	43	2	62	6	1	2	1
10	47	2	56	1	1	2	1
11	35	2	58	4	1	2	3
12	38	2	64	2	1	3	1
13	45	2	70	1	0	1	3
14	29	2	75	3	1	3	1
15	42	1	999	3	1	1	5
16	25	2	68	2	1	999	5
17	42	2	55	3	0	2	3
18	33	2	67	6	1	1	5
19	36	2	59	6	1	3	2
20	36	2	67	1	1	2	1
21	45	2	68	6	0	1	3
22	38	2	63	3	1	2	5
23	45	2	63.5	1	1	2	3
24	35	2	56	6	1	3	1
25	27	2	55	1	0	4	5
26	51	2	60	6	1	5	2
27	45	2	65	6	0	3	3
28	30	2	55	3	1	2	4
29	29	2	64	1	1	2	5
30	38	2	999	3	0	4	2
31	39	1	84	3	1	2	4
32	43	2	63	1	1	2	1
33	54	1	85	1	0	3	2
34	44	2	80	5	0	2	3
35	24	2	120	1	0	1	3
36	45	2	68	3	1	3	3
37	26	2	61	1	1	1	5
38	25	2	65	1	1	3	5
39	53	2	76.2	6	0	3	1
40	27	2	65	3	0	3	5

ID	age	gender	weight	eyes	exercise	work	bloodgp
41	44	2	999	1	1	1	1
42	48	2	999	2	0	1	3
43	44	2	77	1	1	5	5
44	30	2	58	1	1	3	2
45	30	1	70	1	0	2	1
46	25	2	44.45	3	1	2	5
47	39	1	70	3	1	4	4
48	26	2	55	1	0	3	1
49	46	2	65	2	1	2	5
50	31	2	60	1	1	1	3
51	47	2	74	1	0	2	2
52	27	2	999	6	0	3	3
53	47	2	51	1	1	5	1
54	48	2	70	2	1	3	1
55	33	2	45	1	0	2	5
56	37	1	65	4	1	3	5
57	29	2	60	3	0	2	5
58	54	2	60.7	3	1	2	3
59	31	1	52	5	0	3	3
60	28	2	56	1	1	3	3
61	41	2	63	1	1	2	3
62	41	2	58	4	1	2	1

Missing data

You may have noticed that there were some 999s in Table 19.1. This code was chosen to represent missing data so that, when conducting analysis, it is straightforward to make sure that the software understands that this code represents missing data. No field, i.e. space allocated for a particular piece of information, should be left blank in a database. By using 999 it will be easier to see at a glance if you have accidentally missed typing some data in. You can then calculate the number/proportion of missing values for each variable to assess the size of the problem. For example, in the case study 'weight' was unrecorded for six (10%) of the participants. It is also important to look systematically for patterns in the missing data, such as older people having less/more missing data than younger people, as this might warn you that the lack of data could be introducing bias into your study results.

When you are designing a study, all reasonable measures should be taken to maximise the completeness of the data collected, especially regarding the primary outcome measures and those variables suspected of influencing the outcomes. However, some missing data are unavoidable. You can handle missing data either by including in the analysis only those participants where all of the important variables were recorded, known as the complete case approach, or you could use some form of data imputation where a reasonable estimate is substituted for each missing value. For example, you might choose to take the value from another participant who is similar in age and sex (please see Allison, 2002). It is often preferable, however, to use the complete case approach, making clear which data are missing, and discussing the likely reasons for it and the implications this may have in interpreting the main study results.

Standard deviation

The standard deviation (SD) is a measure of how spread out the data are from the mean value, and shows the relation that a set of scores has to the mean of the sample. A common-sense measure of variability could be defined as the mean distance between each individual score and their sample's mean score. However, this quantity is difficult to handle in statistical theory, so instead we calculate the mean of the squared, i.e. that number multiplied by itself, difference between each score and the mean value, and call this the variance. The SD is the square root of the variance, i.e. the number which if squared would be equal to the variance. The SD is the most generally useful measure of the variability within the sample. Figure 19.2 shows the shape of the normal distribution, with vertical lines indicating one SD away from the mean in either direction (in dotted lines), and two SDs away from the mean in each direction. It can be seen that 68% (34% + 34%) of the values lie within 1 SD either way of the mean, and 95% ($13^{1}/_{2}$% + 34% + 34% + $13^{1}/_{2}$%) of the values will be within 2 SDs, either way.

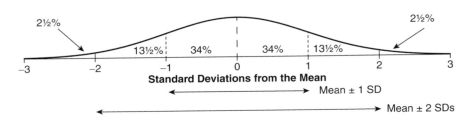

FIGURE 19.2   The distribution of some normally distributed data, showing the proportion of individuals to be expected in each section

Standard error

The SD tells us how variable the individual values are around their mean value, with a small standard deviation telling us that most of the data are closely clustered around the mean, and a large standard deviation telling us our data are scattered away from the mean. However, remember that the mean has been calculated from a sample of data taken from the target population, and that the aim of most analyses

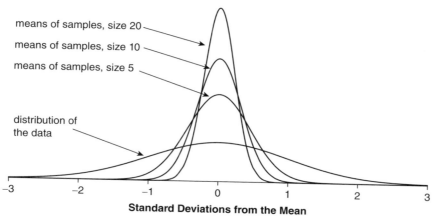

means of samples, size 20

means of samples, size 10

means of samples, size 5

distribution of
the data

-3   -2   -1   0   1   2   3

Standard Deviations from the Mean

FIGURE 19.3   The normal distribution, together with the distribution of mean values
from samples of size 5, 10 and 20

is to generalise from our sample to the population (see Chapter 17: 'Sampling'). If
we repeatedly took various samples of individuals from the same population, then
the mean values would all be slightly different, due to the samples coming from
different people, i.e. sampling variation. If we were then to calculate the SD of the
means for all of the different samples, this would then give us an indication of the
variability between the sample means, i.e. *the standard error of the mean*. In practice,
we will only have one sample of data available to us, and then the simple way of
estimating the standard error of the mean is by dividing the SD by the square root
of the sample size. From this formula, we see that the standard error (SE), increases
as the SD increases. Also, as can be seen in Table 17.5 (p. 280) (and also in Figure
19.3 above), as the sample size gets larger, error decreases as a larger sample gives
less opportunity for random variation. Where the sample sizes are not very small
(say at least 30, though some people would set a higher limit) the distribution of the
sample means will be a reasonable approximation to the normal shape, even if the
shape of the data's own distribution is not close to normal.

Confidence intervals

Suppose that we wanted to know the mean body weight of people in the target
population from which the sample in our case study were recruited. It is easy to
calculate the mean body weight in those 56 participants in our sample who had
their weight recorded (all of the weights added up together and divided by 56),
which gives us a mean weight of 64.3kg, but how precise is our estimate? To put it
another way, what is the margin for random error that we should allow?

We have already seen that the standard error of the mean, SE, may be useful for
this purpose – and we calculate the 95% margin for random error as multiplier ×
SE, where the multiplier will be a number close to 2.0, and always ≥ 1.96 (equal to
or greater than 1.96). The exact value of the multiplier is taken from the relevant 't'

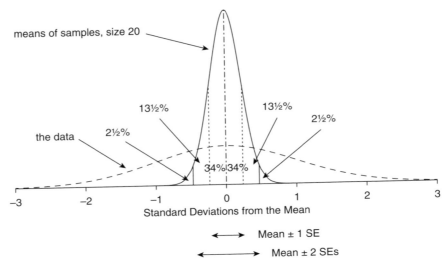

FIGURE 19.4 The normal distribution, together with the distribution of mean values from samples of size 20*

distribution, which has a very similar shape to the normal distribution (details on this can be found in Field, 2013), but in practice you are likely to use a statistical package for these calculations.

Using the 95% margin for random error we can work out our 95% confidence intervals which will range from (i) the lower limit, i.e. sample mean –95% margin for random error, to (ii) the upper limit, i.e. sample mean + 95% margin for random error. Referring to our case study again, Figure 19.4 shows the distribution we would expect to see if mean body weight was taken many times from samples of 20 individuals, in comparison with the wider and much more variable distribution of the target population's data (dashed line). It shows also where we would expect the middle 95% of these sample mean values to lie, calculated as the mean plus or minus twice the standard error. The 95% confidence interval for a mean value can therefore be usefully thought of as the range of values within which we are '95% confident' that the true population mean will lie. The width of a confidence interval for a mean from a sample of 20 individuals reflects the distance between the tail-regions where the 'unusual' 5% of the sample's values lie (see the arrowed horizontal line at the bottom of Figure 19.4, labelled 'Mean ± 2 SEs').

The above example is regarding a numerical variable. We might on the other hand want to analyse binary data. For example in our case study, 39 of the total 62 participants exercised on average more than two hours a week. The summary of this, which is equivalent to calculating the mean value of a numerical quantity is $39 \div 62 = 0.629$. Therefore 62.9% were high exercisers. Similar to when we calculated the standard error of the mean using numerical data, here we calculate the standard error of the proportion = square root of (proportion × (1 – proportion) ÷ sample size). In our case study example, the proportion of high exercisers = 0.629, so that the SE of the proportion is $\sqrt{(0.629 \times (1 - 0.629) \div 62)} = \sqrt{0.00376} = 0.061$.

*The percentages indicate the proportion of values for the sample mean to be expected in each section.

We can now calculate the approximate 95% confidence interval for the proportion to tell us how precise our estimate of 63% high exercisers is of the target population, in a similar way to how you would calculate the 95% confidence intervals for numerical data, i.e. (i) lower limit which is the proportion minus (1.96 times SE of the proportion), and (ii) upper limit which is the proportion plus (1.96 times SE of the proportion). Therefore in our case study example, the corresponding margin for random error in each direction is $1.96 \times 0.061 = 0.120$, and therefore the approximate 95% confidence interval for our estimate is from (i) lower limit: $0.629 - 0.120 = 0.509$ thus our lower limit is 50.9%, up to (ii) upper limit: $0.629 + 0.120 = 0.749$ thus our upper limit is 74.9%. As before, we interpret this loosely as saying that we have '95% confidence' that the proportion in the population lies between 50.9% and 74.9%. This is a good example of statistics telling us that the margin for random error, from a sample of more than 60 people, is wider than we might have guessed.

Hypothesis tests and p-values

The usual aim of a hypothesis test, also often called a significance test, is to compare the mean value of a specific variable, say body weight, between two separate groups of individuals. The way a hypothesis test works is we first state our 'null hypothesis', such as that the mean body weight for the high exercisers is equal to that of the low exercisers, using our case study question. The answer to this test will be given in the form of a probability value (p-value). The p-value is the probability that we would observe the same difference as observed, or larger (relative to the SE), if there really was no difference between the groups. If the p-value is small, then the results are unlikely to have arisen by chance, and thus we can reject the null hypothesis, as we now have reason to believe that there is a true difference. What p-values represent is not only useful for your own research, as you will need to report them in any publications, but are also useful when critically appraising quantitative papers to inform your own clinical practice (please see Chapter 3: 'Critical Appraisal'). However the p-value is not directly connected with the clinical importance of the results, but rather reports the possibility of a result having occurred due to chance.

By convention, we usually regard an observed difference as statistically significant if the p-value is <0.05 (less than 0.05) meaning that there is a less than 1 in 20 possibility that a difference as big as the one seen in the study (relative to the SE) could have arisen by chance if there was no real true difference, and describe this as a result 'significant at the 5% level'. A p-value of <0.01 (less than 0.01) is conventionally called 'highly significant' because it indicates that there is less than 1 in 100 possibility that a difference as big as the one seen in the study could have arisen by chance, if there really was no true difference. However, if the p-value is relatively large, ≥ 0.05 (greater than or equal to 0.05), we don't reject the null hypothesis as the statistic is telling us that the results could plausibly be due to chance. It is important to be aware that a non-significant result, say, in a comparison test, tells us that we have no evidence from the data that the groups are different, but it does not tell us that the groups are the same. It may be just that the sample was too small to detect a clinically important difference (see Chapter 17: 'Sampling').

Comparing two groups

Often a project will be comparing two or more groups, such as in a clinical trial comparing two different interventions. The most important variables for comparison will already have been defined in the study protocol and reflected in the statistical analysis plan as the primary outcome measures, followed by the secondary outcome measures if appropriate, bearing in mind that the study might not be powered for these (please see Chapter 11: 'Clinical Trials').

T-test

The t-test is a very useful and widely used method for comparing numerical data between two groups of individuals. It compares the mean values of a numerical data variable by taking into account the observed difference in mean values between the two groups, relative to the SD of the data within each group. The diagrams in Figure 19.5 represent visually how distributions of normal data may be

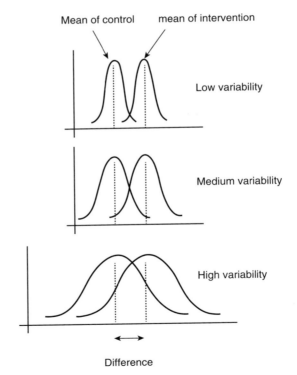

FIGURE 19.5   Diagram showing three contrasting situations when comparing two groups of normally distributed outcome variables

separated from each other to a greater or lesser degree. The first one shows there is a small standard deviation, thus there is hardly any overlap with the distribution. This would indicate that the two groups look different on this variable. In the last diagram, there is a large standard deviation, but although the means are different between the groups, due to the large overlap, the two groups look like they may not be so different in outcome.

It is important to know in advance which of two versions of the t-test you need to use. The paired t-test should be used when it is possible to pair observations from two related samples. This might be the case where you are collecting data from the same participants at two different time points, such as in a before-and-after study, or if you were comparing two different methods of measurement using the same participant. When you have paired samples like this, you would choose a paired t-test. If, on the other hand, you wanted to compare two different samples, such as in a randomised controlled trial when you have two different groups of participants, then you would chose an independent t-test (also known as the 'unpaired t-test').

Another choice you need to make is whether to choose a 'two-tailed' (or 'two-sided') t-test or a 'one-tailed' (or 'one-sided') t-test. A one-tailed t-test is chosen only if, before carrying out a study, your only interest is in (say) seeing whether the mean of your intervention group is at least as large as the mean of your control group – with no interest at all in the opposite happening. However, the usual and safest form of the test is the two-tailed, in which we consider the difference between the groups in either direction. For example, in the case study, the high exercisers having either a higher or lower mean body weight when compared to the low exercisers is equally important to detect. One-tailed tests would *ignore* a difference in the direction not expected, such as if the high exercisers had the higher mean body weight.

It is a general rule that, when comparing two groups of data with a two-tailed test, the results should be significant at the 5% level, i.e. the p-value will be less than 0.05, if and only if: the corresponding 95% confidence interval for the mean difference is either entirely above 0 or entirely below 0. If 0 is inside the 95% confidence interval, then we cannot reasonably reject the possibility that our results were obtained by chance, and so the result is non-significant at the (corresponding) 5% level. This is different when it is the odds ratio or risk ratio between the two groups that is being compared, as what matters for a ratio is whether the 95% confidence interval is entirely above or entirely below 1.0 (please see Chapter 10: 'Epidemiology').

Case study

The research team have already gathered data regarding weight and exercise habits and now would like to compare the weight of the high exercisers (more than two hours per week, on average), against the low exercisers (the rest). They choose an independent t-test as the comparison is between two separate groups of people. In

(Continued)

(Continued)

the statistical software package that they were using (SPSS) they chose 'exercise' as the grouping variable. The researchers then chose 'weight' as the test variable, since this represents the participant's body weight. Of the 56 participants with their body weight recorded – the mean weight of the 36 high-exercisers was 62.0kg (SD 7.8kg), and that of the low-exercisers was 68.4kg (SD 18.6kg). The researchers carried out a special version of the independent t-test (see Field, 2013) that allows for the standard deviation to differ substantially between the two groups (7.8kg as against 18.6kg). The result showed a two-tailed p-value of 0.155, which is non-significant at the 5% level (since 0.155 is greater than 0.05). The statistical package also calculated the corresponding 95% confidence interval for the estimated difference in body weight between the groups which showed that the mean weight of the low exercisers was 6.4kg higher than that of the high exercisers, 95% confidence interval -2.6kg to 15.4kg.

   The researchers now need to use their medical knowledge to interpret the confidence interval – for example, what would be the public health implications of a group difference as little as -2.6kg, or as large as 15.4kg? The conclusion is likely to be that this range is too wide to answer the researchers' original question – thus a larger sample is required for this study in order to attain a more precise estimate, with a narrower 95% confidence interval that has a less ambiguous interpretation. The researchers should also make clear that, from a cross-sectional survey of this kind, they could not in any case tell whether exercise might be affecting body weight, or that a person's body weight might affect their likelihood of choosing to exercise.

Descriptive statistics

Once the data have been 'cleaned' (please see Chapter 12: 'Surveys' for a description), the first aim of analysis is usually to describe the most relevant demographic and other baseline characteristics of the sample of participants. Descriptive statistics can either be univariate analysis or bivariate.

Univariate analysis

The study data are usually first described taking one variable at a time, the 'univariate' approach. Univariate analysis describes just one variable (whether numerical or categorical) and can ascertain the frequency distribution, i.e. a summary of how often the different scores occur in the sample. This allows you to note any outliers (which are atypical scores and which might indicate error) and to assess whether the shape of the distribution is symmetrical or skewed. The centre of the frequency distribution can be described by the mean or the median. The median is the middle score in the list after all the scores have been sorted into ascending order – the median value of body weight in the case study example is 63kg, close to the mean value.

   For presenting numerical data, a histogram is a graph with the scores along the horizontal line of the x axis, and the frequency on the vertical line of the y axis (an easy way to remember this is 'y points to the sky'). Histograms allow you to observe

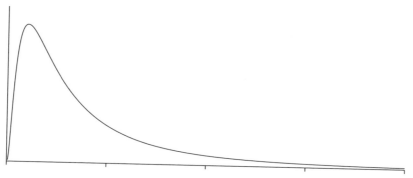

FIGURE 19.6   A diagram of a frequency distribution for a positively skewed variable

any potential outliers. You need to think carefully whether a possible outlier might really be a realistic value, however, and if possible check the raw data to see if it is due to a typing error. It is important that, if you do exclude any outliers, then these exclusions are recorded, and that all changes to the study data are traceable. An example of a histogram can be seen in the next case study which graphically illustrates the frequency distribution for weight (Figure 19.7).

In a highly 'positively skewed' distribution such as that shown in Figure 19.6, there is a 'tail' of data towards the right-hand end of the graph, indicating a small number of high values. If you have a highly positively skewed distribution, then the mean may not be a good estimate of the centre of the frequency distribution, as it can be dominated by the few very large values (or by very small values in a negatively skewed distribution), which may not be typical of the majority. In cases such as this the 'median' is a better summary of the centre of the distribution. Judging whether the distribution is normal can also be important in influencing the approach to the analysis that you will use, i.e. parametric tests are based on normal distributions, whereas non-parametric tests are not.

The variability of highly skewed data is best shown by calculating the first quartile and the third quartile (collectively known as the inter-quartile range, IQR). Having sorted the values into ascending order, as when calculating the median, the first quartile is the value that is one-quarter the way up the list (starting from the lowest value), and the third quartile is the value that is three-quarters way up the list. For the body weight in the case study data, the first and third quartiles are 56kg and 69kg respectively.

Case study

A histogram was produced for the weight of the respondents. You can observe that the body weight of the great majority of participants lies between 40kg and 85kg, with most being near the middle of this range. As you can see in the text to the right of the

(Continued)

(Continued)

graph (Figure 19.7), the mean weight was 64.3 kg. However the standard deviation is large at 12.9kg, meaning that there is a large amount of variability. This is partly due to the two participants who have substantially higher body weights than the rest, as is shown by the two isolated bars on the right-hand side of the graph, i.e. two potential outliers. By removing these, the SD falls to 9.23 – and the distribution would be less skewed.

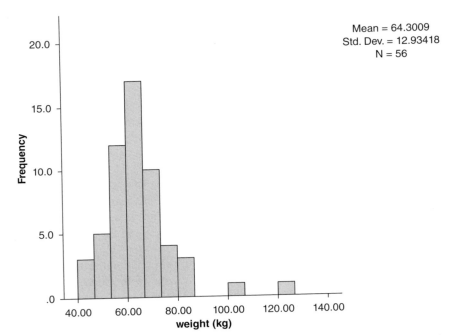

FIGURE 19.7   Histogram showing the frequency distribution of body weight, using data from the questionnaire

However the researchers decide not to remove the two outliers as they know from previous literature that body weight naturally has a positively skewed distribution, and that a few high values are to be expected.

Bivariate analysis

This analysis can be used to describe relationships between pairs of variables (rather just looking at one variable at a time, as in univariate descriptive analysis). You could look at associations via scatterplots, or by the computation of a correlation coefficient (please see Chapter 10: 'Epidemiology'). To decide on the type of analysis you want to use you need to determine the type of data the variables contain. If you are comparing two variables that hold interval data, Pearson's correlation coefficient could be used. Correlation measures the strength of the linear association between two normally distributed variables, and indicates the degree to which two variables increase or decrease together (positive correlation in the range 0 to +1), or go in opposite directions (negative correlation in the range 0 to -1), or appear to be unrelated to each other (zero or close to zero correlation). A perfect correlation is 1, either positive or negative. In the case study, the researchers not only collected weight via the survey, but they also measured the participant's height. As these are both interval data, they used a Pearson's correlation coefficient resulting, in a correlation coefficient of 0.21 with p-value 0.128 (for the 55 participants who had both weight and height recorded), therefore the association is not statistically significant. However, suppose that the researchers wanted to look whether there was an association between exercise and place of work: these are both nominal variables and thus a different analysis is needed. Here the chi-squared test may be used (see Field, 2013, for details).

Regression

A regression analysis enables us to calculate the average amount of change caused to the outcome variable (also referred to as the 'dependent' variable) by a change in the explanatory variable (also referred to as the 'independent' variable). The explanatory variable is the input, whilst the outcome variable is the effect or output. For example, if you were conducting a trial to ascertain the effectiveness of different medication regimes for antidepressants, your explanatory variable is your regimes, whilst your outcome variable would be an outcome measure such as a depression scale. An easy way to remember the difference between these variables is that the explanatory variable (e.g. regime) might plausibly cause a change in outcome variable (e.g. depression) score measured after treatment but it is not possible, the outcome variable (e.g. depression scale) could cause a change in the explanatory variable (e.g. regime).

A regression equation enables us to predict the value of the outcome variable from knowing the value of the explanatory variable. It is important to note that the relationship is dependent on there being a genuine linear relationship (or something close), and also is valid only for an individual whose value of the explanatory variable (such as height) is well within the range for which we have data.

Case study

Using the weight data from the survey and the height data from the objective measurements, the researchers calculate the change in weight (outcome variable) in association with height (explanatory variable) via a regression. As you can see from Figure 19.8, a 'best fit' line has been drawn over the scatterplot, and from this

(Continued)

(Continued)

model you could predict the amount of change in weight associated with a change in height.

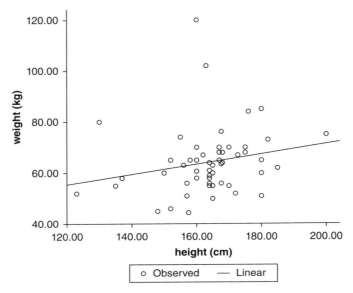

FIGURE 19.8   Scatterplot of body weight against height, including the linear regression line of best fit

The researchers also calculate the R^2, the statistic which indicates the goodness of fit of the line to the data. It is the square of the Pearson correlation and therefore is a number between 0 and 1.0. An R^2 near 1.0 indicates that a regression line fits the data well, while an R^2 closer to 0 indicates the regression line does not fit the data very well. The R^2 in Figure 19.8 is 0.043 which tells us that height accounts for 4.3% of the change in weight. Therefore, over 95% of the variability is due to inherent unpredictability and/or one or more other variables, i.e. possible confounders (please see Chapters 6 and 10 for description). Therefore you would not rely on height to predict weight.

Multiple regression

As you can see from the above case study, little of the variability in body weight is explained by the variability in height, and in general, it is rare that the explanatory variable accounts for all of the variability in the outcome variable. Life is more complicated than that! Thus, we may want to add another explanatory variable to the model which we think could be a good predictor, i.e. a multiple regression. A multiple regression allows us to study the relationship simultaneously between the outcome (outcome variable) and two or more predictors (explanatory variables). Suppose that the researchers in our case study had previously noticed that there seemed to be a positive association between the more fried food eaten and the heavier the person.

They then asked the participants to keep a record of how much fried food they eat in one week, with the assumption that this could influence their weight. Thus, they could run a multiple regression with the explanatory variables of height and consumption of fried foods. From this data suppose they obtained an R^2 of 0.97, this would indicate that variability in height and fried food consumption accounts for 97% of the variability in weight! Thus we could predict weight from height and eating fried foods. In practice it is unusual to see an R^2 value so close to 1.0 – generally 0.7 is regarded as high and therefore of good value in health-related research, but there is no general rule of interpretation.

Summarising the results

The first data we usually present are descriptive data which, together with a report of how the data were collected, help the reader decide your result's generalisability and whether they apply to their own clinical practice. This summary of the sample data is usually presented as the first table in a medical journal paper, and will contain one row for each measurement, such as body mass index or blood pressure, or an assessed characteristic, such as the severity of disease. When summarising categorical data (as calculated with univariate analysis), it can be presented in the form of a frequency table where the number, or percentages, of participants in each category are presented. However, to make an impact during a conference presentation, it may be more suitable to show these frequencies in a pie chart. Otherwise, if you need to summarise numerical data such as age, it is best summarised graphically in the form of a histogram (see Figure 19.7 which shows a histogram of weight). If, on the other hand, you are interested in presenting the association between two variables (as calculated with bivariate analysis), then a scatterplot or a multiple bar chart is more suitable.

Case study

Our researchers are now ready to present their findings via a conference presentation and a report for their employers. To summarise the categorical data they decide to use a pie chart. Figure 19.9 shows the pie chart they produced with the frequencies of the workplaces of the respondents.

The researchers would also like to present some of their bivariate analyses, in particular the association between participant's work organisation and whether they

(Continued)

(Continued)

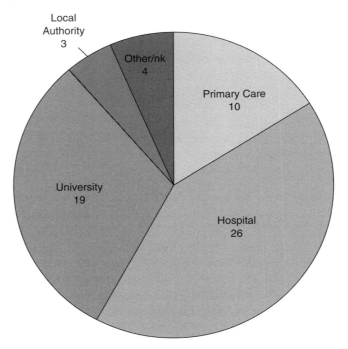

FIGURE 19.9   Pie chart showing the breakdown of participants by their work organisation

were a 'high exerciser', defined as doing more than two hours of exercise per week. As they would like to present this association as a bar chart, they first obtain a cross-tabulation table which displays the joint distribution of two or more variables. Their cross-tabulation table shows the percentage of participants according to their work organisation who are high exercisers (Table 19.2), from which their bar chart is drafted (Figure 19.10).

TABLE 19.2   Number and percentage of high exercisers, by participant's work organisation

Place of work	Total	High exercisers (%)
Primary Care	10	5 (50)
Hospital	26	17 (65)
University	19	12 (63)
Local Authority	3	1 (33)
Other/not known	4	4 (100)
Total	62	39 (63)

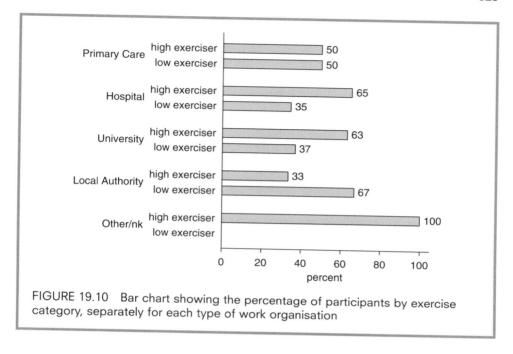

FIGURE 19.10   Bar chart showing the percentage of participants by exercise category, separately for each type of work organisation

When presenting the results of the hypothesis tests that you have carried out, it is important to mention every test, and to make clear which tests were specified in advance in the study protocol and which, if any, were 'post-hoc' tests that were suggested by observation of the data and other results as they were found. (Please see Chapter 1: 'Asking the Right Questions' for a discussion of the danger of making many 'multiple comparisons', which may lead to apparently significant results being found by chance.) It is also vital that all non-significant results, as well as the significant results, are reported in journal papers, so that a future systematic review gets a true and unbiased view of all relevant research (please see Chapter 14: 'Systematic Reviews').

Summary

- The main value of quantitative analysis in health research is to describe patterns of data, and to provide estimates of defined quantities together with a measure of their precision.

- Data take two forms: numerical (counted and interval data); and categorical (binary, nominal and ordinal). Each form requires different analytical techniques.

- There are steps to take to get data ready for analysis, including coding and handling missing data.

- A good first step in analyses is to explore your data, such as with the use of univariate analysis with histograms that can help identify outliers and skewness.

- Bivariate analysis and regression can identify associations between two variables – or more, if using multiple regression.

- T-tests are a versatile method for comparing two samples of numerical interval data, either the paired t-test (for paired samples) or the independent t-test (for separate samples).

Questions for Discussion

1. For each variable collected in the case study (from the survey, and also the height measurements and the fried food diary) decide which type of data it contains, according to Figure 19.1.

2. A research team has developed a new medication that they hypothesise will increase a user's intelligence by 50 IQ points when compared to a placebo group. They will measure the effectiveness with an IQ test and a quality of life scale measured at baseline and again at the end of the study.

    i.   Which is the outcome (dependent) variable?

    ii. Which are the exploratory (independent) variables?

    iii. If they analysed with a t-test, would they use a paired t-test or an independent t-test and why?

Further Reading

Altman, D.G. (1991) *Practical Statistics for Medical Research*. London: Chapman & Hall.
Petrie, A. and Sabin, C. (2009) *Medical Statistics at a Glance* (3rd edn). Chichester: Wiley-Blackwell.
Van Belle, G. (2008) *Statistical Rules of Thumb* (2nd edn). Chichester: Wiley.

References

Allison, P.D. (2002) *Missing Data*. London: SAGE.
Field, A. (2013) *Discovering Statistics Using IBM SPSS* (4th edn). London: SAGE.
Field, A. and Miles, J. (2010) *Discovering Statistics Using SAS*. London: SAGE.
Moroney, M.J. (1975) *Facts from Figures*. Harmondsworth: Penguin.

20

QUALITATIVE ANALYSIS

Caitlin Notley, Gill Green and Louise Marsland

Learning Objectives

- To appreciate the continuum between qualitative data collection and analysis
- To understand the key approaches to qualitative data analysis, recognising the commonalities and differences between them
- To enable you to make an informed choice of analysis between grounded theory and framework analysis, the most commonly applied analytical approaches within health services research, and be able to justify your choice

Introduction

Decisions about which qualitative data analysis approach to choose should always be guided by the research question which, if it is clear and well defined, will guide you towards a particular analytical approach (please see Chapter 1: 'Asking the Right Question'). It is also critical that approaches to qualitative data analysis be considered as part of a methodological continuum, where data collection and data analysis 'fit' the research question. For these reasons it is important when deciding on a qualitative analytical approach that this chapter be read in conjunction with Chapter 7: 'Qualitative Methodology'.

When selecting a qualitative approach, and specifically an approach to analysis, the researcher should be prepared to justify that choice. Although qualitative approaches are being increasingly valued as an important part of comprehensive health services research, there are still frequent misunderstandings regarding the qualitative approach. A common criticism is that findings are not 'generalisable', as analysis may be based on a small, non-representative, or even a 'biased' sample. However, it should be emphasised that it is not the aim of qualitative analysis to be generalisable, but rather that findings may be transferable to similar situations or populations (Lincoln and Guba, 1985). This argument recognises the unique and socially situated nature of qualitative research. It celebrates the detailed and nuanced understanding that can be gained from close and detailed analysis of a small number of cases, and suggests that lessons that can be drawn from a small number of cases could be transferable to other similar cases. However, an important caveat to this is that the uniqueness of human experience does not lend itself to the formation of generalised messages, applicable to all people, across all times, and all cultures.

A second criticism often levelled at qualitative analysis is that it is subjective, or inherently biased, as results are based on individual (or team) interpretations of data. This means that analysis is not necessarily replicable or 'reliable', as others may have interpreted the data differently. However, qualitative data analysis does not aim to be replicable. The uniqueness of the situated experience is emphasised, and the subjectivity of the researcher is reflected upon and fully acknowledged in an open manner in any written reports or publications. It is possible to ensure that data analysis is trustworthy however. This is achieved through careful and transparent analysis, and requires reflexivity on the part of the researcher. It also includes a process of checking and verifying the results, which may involve patients (please see Chapter 16: 'Patient and Public Involvement'), participants or other independent researchers.

Qualitative approaches to data analysis

Until recently there were only a limited number of approaches to qualitative analysis which were primarily based upon the ethnographic methods of observation and participation (please see Chapter 7: 'Qualitative Methodology'). However, there has been a proliferation of new approaches emerging as qualitative data have become increasingly accepted and valued by health research and other disciplines, such as psychology. The framework approach (which will be discussed later in this chapter), discourse analysis, narrative analysis, case studies and interpretive phenomenological analysis are just some of the qualitative analytic approaches that have recently emerged and which are now widely used. Although these different approaches have varied theoretical underpinnings, there are many features that most qualitative methods have in common:

Context-rich

All approaches are demonstrably context-rich, which is perhaps the defining feature of all qualitative analysis as it struggles to make sense of 'the complex, rich and messy nature of qualitative findings' (Finlay, 2006: 6).

Inductive

Most qualitative approaches are inductive rather than deductive, i.e. they aim to generate rather than test theory. For example, a qualitative study about accessing health care may collect narratives focusing on people's pathways to treatment, and then seek to develop a theory about the key factors that either encourage or discourage access. This could then be used to structure an intervention which can be tested using quantitative methods to see if this changes the number of people seeking treatment.

Small purposively selected samples

Sample sizes are generally smaller than those required in quantitative research. Usually some form of purposive sampling is used, where you deliberately select participants who have characteristics of interest to the research. For example, if you were looking at the relationship people with type 2 diabetes have with food, you may wish to include some participants who do their own cooking, and some who are looked after, e.g. younger participants. You may also wish to include some cultural variation, as this disease is more prevalent in the south Asian population (please see Chapter 17: 'Sampling'). In practice, however, what researchers aim to do and what actually happens, may not be the same as it is not always possible to recruit the sample you want for practical reasons or because some samples are 'hard to reach'. For instance, if your study was about children's relationships with their parents, you may identify absent fathers to be particularly important to include, but you may have trouble accessing this population from which to collect data.

There are, however, some differences in sample selection between approaches. The framework approach, for example, can involve quite large, heterogeneous samples in an attempt to get a broad representation of the population of interest, whereas grounded theory uses a form of purposive sampling known as theoretical sampling, where the sample is selected on the basis of the emerging data and analysis.

Inclusive

Although sample sizes are generally small in qualitative research, analysis incorporates data obtained from all participants, whereas in quantitative analysis, those who are not within the normal distribution are classified as 'outliers' and can be excluded from statistical analysis (please see Chapter 19: 'Quantitative Analysis'). Qualitative analysis embraces those participants who 'buck the trend' as they are generally valuable in developing the analysis and subsequent theory: in the example above about accessing treatment, a participant who has never sought health care of any type would provide a unique perspective.

Interpretative and reflexive

In qualitative research, text is the main unit of analysis and the analysis process usually involves the researcher first developing themes derived from the data, and then progressing to interpretive analysis to show how these themes link to each other and to existing theory. To do this the researcher assigns codes and themes subjectively, interpreting the text within their own belief structure. Thus, bias is inherent in any qualitative analysis and reflexivity is important in order to acknowledge what bias or influence the researcher believes was pertinent during the data collection and analysis stages.

Data processing

Qualitative data may take a number of forms. Although it is predominantly text from transcriptions of one-to-one interviews or focus groups, it may also include researchers' field notes, or visual data such as photographs or film. It is usual for qualitative data collected from interviews/focus groups to be digitally recorded, uploaded into an audio file (or .wav), and then transcribed verbatim to provide a text version of the data for analysis. Recording the data has a number of advantages over note-taking as it provides a complete record of the information provided. Note-taking, on the other hand, may introduce bias as attempting to take handwritten notes inevitably involves a level of selection. A digital recording also retains intonation and expression which are invaluable for interpretation during analysis. For example, it is only through intonation or laughter that what is said may be interpreted as sarcasm, whereas in written form, the same words could have a very different meaning. Even with exceptional shorthand skills, taking notes may impede the flow of the interview. A recording device allows the interviewer to pay full attention to the interviewee and the interview process, so helping ensure the fullest possible account is obtained. Digital recording does have a number of drawbacks however. Some participants may be reluctant to take part if they are going to be recorded, or feel inhibited by the presence of a microphone. Permission to record must be included as part of the consent process, and detailed information about what will happen to the recordings after data collection should help allay any anxieties of those considering taking part. Within the interview, a 'matter of fact' approach to the recorder usually ensures interviewees quickly forget about its presence. It is therefore essential to be familiar with the recorder's operating instructions in order to minimise fuss and to ensure you obtain a good-quality recording. Always take a spare set of batteries, and try to minimise any background noise. For example, if the interview room overlooks a busy road, keep the windows closed.

One of the greatest challenges produced by the recording of interviews is the volume of data obtained; a one-hour interview will generate approximately 10,000 words. The time taken to transcribe interviews is considerable, and it is generally advised to allow up to six times the actual length of the interview for this process. Transcription is therefore an important consideration when estimating project timescales. Despite the time involved in transcribing interviews/focus groups, there are advantages to doing this yourself; it is likely to increase accuracy, and also allows you to relive the interview/focus group and begin the process of immersion. Through the mechanical act of converting the verbal recordings to written word, you will inevitably start identifying themes and sub-themes, and begin making links between the data. In this way, then, transcribing can form an important part of the analysis process.

For many researchers, however, the time required to transcribe the interviews themselves is simply too great. A pragmatic compromise is to have a third party undertake the transcribing (if your budget will allow) and then to listen to the interview recording while reading the transcripts, checking for accuracy and reliving the interview in this way. Using transcription services clearly has time-saving advantages, but it is essential that they are provided with clear instructions, such as whether verbatim transcripts or summaries are required, and whether exclamations such as sighs, laughs or pauses should be noted. The involvement of a third party who has access to the interview data needs to be included in any ethics applications, and to ensure safe keeping of the data, you may wish to use a reputable transcription company and get them to sign a confidentiality agreement which outlines what to do with the audio files and copies of the transcriptions upon completion of the work. The personal nature of qualitative data means that, even in an anonymised form, individuals may be identifiable from their interviews. Secure storage of data, both hard and electronic copies, is therefore especially important. You also have a duty of care to the transcriber if the interviews contain issues for which they may need emotional support.

Computer-Aided Qualitative Data Analysis Software (CAQDAS)

There are a number of computer programmes known as CAQDAS (Computer-Aided Qualitative Data Analysis Software) currently available to assist with qualitative data analysis. Those most commonly used at the time of writing are NVivo, Ethnograph, Nudist, ATLAS.ti or MaxQDA. Each has somewhat different functions and levels of complexity but essentially all are a means of storing and retrieving textual data and some also have capacity to include visual, audio or quantitative data.

The widespread use of CAQDAS has led to much debate about the role of technology and computer software in qualitative data analysis. Some researchers feel that

CAQDAS is an indispensable aid as it simplifies the process of storing and retrieving data, therefore assisting in the process of locating key words, phrases or quotations as well as storing the data in the given categories. These programmes do not do the analysis, but they help with the organisation of the data. The traditional way of organising the data was to manually cut and paste data segments from printed copies of the transcripts into categories. With CAQDAS you can chop up large amounts of lengthy text into more manageable bite-size chunks. Many of the programmes also facilitate more sophisticated analysis, such as producing diagrams and illustrations to help you make comparisons between cases, and links between key themes. However, some researchers feel that CAQDAS is contrary to the spirit of qualitative data analysis. Dissecting the text into chunks in a mechanistic way may distance the data and the researcher from the contextual richness of the setting in which the data were collected. In addition, some of the programmes (but not all) take some time to master and thus may not save time, particularly if your data set is small. Some qualitative researchers thus prefer to avoid CAQDAS altogether, although agencies funding applied health research may expect CAQDAS to be used in a funded study. If you want to find out more about how to use CAQDAS, Lewins and Silver (2007) have produced a guide. Whether or not you choose to use CAQDAS, the essence of the analytic process remains the same. Computers cannot identify categories, interpret data, theorise or reflect, all of which are key to the analysis of qualitative data and must come from you as the researcher.

Thematic analysis

Thematic analysis is a term used to denote the identification of categories emerging from the data and is the vehicle by which a large amount of textual data is condensed to identify the most salient points and, generally as the analysis progresses, patterns and links between them. It is a key part of the analysis, with the process often starting while data are being collected. Thematic analysis involves first coding (i.e. assigning labels to) small chunks of data. Codes with similar meaning are then grouped together to form themes, which may include data such as quotes from many participants. This stage of descriptive analysis may start with predetermined codes or themes, but more often is an inductive process whereby themes emerge through your engagement with the data.

Robson (2011) identifies several phases of thematic analysis:

- Familiarisation with the data whereby the researcher reads, and rereads, interview transcripts and field notes.
- Generation of initial codes often using a coding tree, or hierarchical coding. This is a process where some codes are grouped with others to form a 'branch'. Codes which remain alone, are the sub-codes, similar to twigs, they branch off from their 'parent' branch which they relate to in some way. This tree then is used to code all the data set and may be refined during this process.

- Identification of themes by collating codes. It is often at this stage that the analysis moves from description to interpretation (please see Table 20.1 for an example of a tree).

- Constructing thematic networks, which identify patterns and linkages between the themes for commonalities and differences across the sample as a whole.

- Integration and interpretation, which is the reflexive stage of the thematic analysis. While interpreting the data you will reflect on the potential bias you may be introducing, and will record it so you can be as transparent as possible when you report the findings.

Thematic analysis can be 'stand-alone' as a straightforward and pragmatic approach to analysing qualitative data descriptively (which can be useful in a mixed-methods study to offer explanations for quantitative findings), or can be an integral part of a more specialised analytic approach. The level of description/interpretation is variable, dependent upon why the analysis is being conducted. Some research is more interested in description to inform policy, whereas others are more focused on searching for meaning of an experience and strive for a more interpretive level of understanding. The analysis chosen may reflect *a priori* thinking, as in the framework approach, or it can be predominantly inductive and used to generate theory, as in grounded theory, or most commonly, a combination of both. An example of research with *a priori* thinking could be a study exploring reasons some women fail to attend an appointment for breast screening. In this case, the researcher has some preformed ideas and uses these to generate an interview schedule including questions about, for example, logistical obstacles, for example, timing of the appointment, location of the screening clinic, and emotional barriers, for example, fear. The subsequent coding tree will then

TABLE 20.1   Part of the coding tree based on a study relating to the mental health of young ex-soldiers (Green et al., 2010)

Theme	Code	Subcode
Stress from combat	Cause	Fear
		Bereavement
		Horror
	Symptoms	Depression
		Aggression
		Alcoholism
'Lack of fit' with civilian life	Soldier identity	Camaraderie
		Discipline
		Hierarchy
	Social exclusion	Homelessness
		Unemployment
		Lack of life skills

reflect the interview schedule and the researcher's *a priori* thinking. This is appropriate, although if the themes that emerge are purely a mirror image of the interview schedule then it suggests that the data have produced little information not previously known by the researcher and no new insights have emerged. This is rarely an issue for more inductive methods which tend to set out with few preconceptions and build up the coding tree and themes directly from the data. An example of this may be research that seeks to explore the experience of living with a chronic illness. Rather than making assumptions about how this may affect people, the researcher may simply ask the participants one question such as 'What impact does this illness have on your life?' or 'Tell me about your experience of living with this condition'. The rest of the interview follows on from what the participant says, i.e. an unstructured interview, and the coding tree will be created from these emerging data.

Thematic analysis is used in most qualitative analysis methods to categorise data, and is thus the basis of a range of different qualitative methods. Some methods are less structured in approach such as grounded theory, whereas others are more structured and collect data about specific topics systematically, such as the framework approach.

Grounded theory

Grounded theory is an approach to analysis that follows a number of well-defined stages which take the analysis from simple descriptions, and summaries of themes as in thematic analysis, to a more interpretive analysis which is useful for developing substantive theory or hypotheses. This entails moving away from the context of the actual qualitative data in order to generate new insights. Therefore this approach is an excellent choice for data analysis in areas of research where little is currently known, and thus, where it is not yet possible to form focused research questions.

Grounded theory methodology has a long historical tradition, being first formulated by Glaser and Strauss (1967) in their seminal work *The Discovery of Grounded Theory*. As the approach developed, a divide became apparent between a more objective perspective, drawing on quantitatively orientated concerns such as limiting researcher bias, and a more realist approach recognising the subjective and reflexive role of the researcher (Strauss and Corbin, 1990, 1998). This realist approach also recognised the important role of researcher's *a priori* knowledge, whether this is drawn from personal experience, or academic understanding such as through published literature. Most recently, Charmaz (2003, 2006) has developed a 'constructivist' approach to grounded theory which takes a pragmatic approach to recognising and taking into account the role of the researcher and his/ her prior knowledge and understanding of the clinical area, therefore allowing interpretative analysis to develop whilst simultaneously acknowledging this prior knowledge.

The idea of an 'iterative' approach to data collection and analysis, as processes that occur simultaneously and cyclically, is integral to the grounded theory approach. Once an initial sample has been defined, data are collected, usually following an

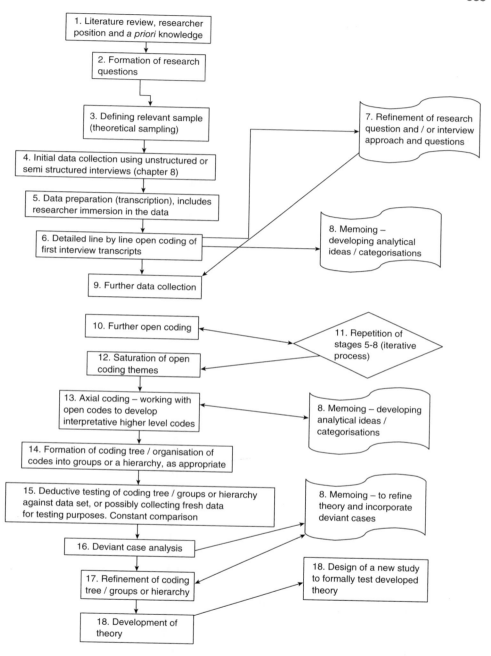

FIGURE 20.1   Grounded Theory process

unstructured interview guide, in order that the participant can discuss experiences, views, thoughts and feelings about the topic under discussion in a manner that is personally meaningful to them. This allows for inductive analysis of the data via open coding, which involves reading the interview transcript line by line, word by word, whilst coding the meaning of what the interviewee has said. These open codes are therefore derived directly (or 'grounded') in the data from which they have emerged (please see Figure 20.1).

Initial open coding (step 6 in Figure 20.1) may direct you towards focusing on particular themes as key areas of further study, as participants may discuss certain experiences and views not previously envisaged. Following this, the interview schedule may be refined to specifically focus on these important areas for future interviews (step 7 in Figure 20.1). This process continues in a cyclical manner until a stage of 'theoretical saturation' is reached, which is when no new themes, issues, views or experiences arising from the interviews emerge (step 12 in Figure 20.1). Reaching theoretical saturation is somewhat of a judgement call on the part of the researcher, and may be an imperfect concept, especially in the complex field of health services research, as you may have to indicate how many people you will interview prior to collecting data in order to secure appropriate funding and ethical approval.

The point where grounded theory moves towards a more interpretative approach is in the undertaking of the further stages of 'axial' coding (step 13 in Figure 20.1). This involves working with the mass of open codes generated from the data to develop 'higher level' codes that encapsulate, group together or interpret the 'lower level' open codes, which are themselves closer to the original data. Working with these axial codes, the researcher, who by this stage is completely immersed in the data, may see patterns and groupings of codes that work together to begin explaining the phenomenon being studied. Thus axial codes may be organised into groups or a coding tree or hierarchy (step 14 in Figure 20.1). Ideally, this hierarchy is then tested back against the data set, or tested against fresh data collected on the same topic, to ensure 'fit' with all of the data (step 15 in Figure 20.1). The idea of 'deviant case analysis' becomes important at this point, as specific outlying (deviant) cases that do not easily fit with the emergent theory must be incorporated into the explanatory theory (step 16 in Figure 20.1). This may result in alteration or further refinement of the theory (step 17 in Figure 20.1). In reality, many studies do not reach this advanced stage of analysis, but halt at the stage of axial coding. This is often very informative however, and offers a depth of explanation and understanding usually sufficient to meet the research aims. According to the formal grounded theory method, however, ideally the emergent coding tree or theory is then formally tested in a new study (step 18 in Figure 20.1).

At all stages of the research process, the concept of memoing is central to the grounded theory approach (step 8 in Figure 20.1). This involves the researcher recording field notes, thoughts, feelings and hunches about the data, rather like keeping a research diary (you can do this within most CAQDAS). It may be that certain ideas are defined within memos and then tested out against subsequent data analysis. This process of memoing shapes the direction that the researcher takes in their data collection and analysis, and forms the basis of the emergent theory. For example, you may notice certain groupings that seem to be emerging during the open coding stage, which may then be subsequently tested during the axial coding stage to see if these groups 'fit' with your original idea. This process of constant comparison and verification of emergent theoretical ideas is central to the grounded theory method. Verification can be further ascertained by a process of triangulation. This might involve a team of researchers undertaking independent coding of the data, and then cross-checking their analysis with the analyses from the other team members to ensure that there is a consistent approach to coding, which is not overly subjective. You may also involve others outside of your immediate research team in this process, such as patients or members of the public (please see Chapter 16: 'Patient and Public Involvement'), which will ensure that the analysis makes sense and is applicable to the target population, such as a specific patient group.

Case study

A grounded theory project was designed as a qualitative sub-study of a randomised controlled trial examining the effectiveness of an opiate maintenance treatment delivery method for patients being treated for heroin addiction. The maintenance treatment delivery method was supervised consumption, which is a standard UK practice whereby community pharmacists 'watch' patients consume their medication. However, the research team were concerned that this may impinge on an individual's privacy as little was known about patient experiences of supervised consumption. Therefore the grounded theory sub-study sought to answer the question: 'What is the patient experience of supervised consumption?'

A theoretical sampling approach was pursued whereby as much variation in patient characteristics within the sample as possible was sought. The in-depth, face-to-face interviews were semi-structured, covering the key themes around treatment experiences whilst allowing participants to 'tell their stories' of their drug treatment. Open coding was completed alongside the data collection, and the interview schedules were subsequently refined to specifically ask patients about the issues of stigma, and how they developed relationships with their community pharmacists, two key areas that emerged from the early analysis stage. Saturation of analytical themes was reached in the 29th interview, upon which data collection was concluded. Eventually, axial coding was able to organise the open codes into individual, social and medication related themes that appeared to impact upon the patient's experience of supervised consumption, offering an explanatory framework of the experience. This explanatory framework was tested against the data set and further refined. The qualitative study was able to conclude that patients accepted supervision in the short term despite privacy and stigma being difficult issues, due to a positive relationship with the pharmacist. However, it was important for participants to move on to unsupervised treatment as early as possible.

The framework approach

Framework is a matrix-based approach to analysing qualitative data which was devised by Ritchie and Spencer (1994) for analysing data generated in studies which they term 'applied policy research', and which lies at the more structured end of the qualitative research continuum.

Unlike grounded theory, where the interview is largely participant-led and tends to be exploratory in nature, framework analysis seeks to answer specific (usually policy-related) research questions. This means that it is appropriate to use a structured interview schedule to keep the data collection focused (please see Chapter 7: 'Qualitative Methodology'). Consequently, the analysis process incorporates this *a priori* thinking, while allowing newly emerging themes to be included. Another difference is that in grounded theory data collection and analysis occur concurrently, but for framework analysis it is usual for all interviews to have been completed before the formal process of analysis is started. Although, as with most qualitative analysis methods, framework incorporates elements of thematic analysis, the value of framework is the opportunity it provides to move the data beyond description. Ritchie and Spencer (1994: 176) identify six directions framework analysis may take depending upon the specific research question(s):

- Defining concepts
- Mapping the range, nature and dynamics of the phenomena
- Creating typologies
- Finding associations
- Seeking explanations
- Developing new ideas, theories and strategies

The framework approach to analysis has six stages and, although they are presented linearly in Figure 20.2, involves moving backwards and forwards between the stages. Equally, although it is presented as a step-by-step approach, in no way is it a mechanical, guaranteed formula. As with all approaches to qualitative analysis, it relies upon the intuitive thinking and interpretative skills of the researcher.

Familiarisation (step 1 in Figure 20.2) is the initial stage where the researcher reads a selection of transcripts to begin identifying key themes (and some sub-themes) that will form the basis of the framework. The transcripts selected for this would ideally reflect some variation within the sample. For example, it may have become apparent during the interviews that certain participants were expressing different views from others. Therefore you would include transcripts to reflect these differences. If the interviews and analysis are undertaken by the same researcher, this process of familiarisation will actually have begun during the interview process.

As the process of familiarisation progresses, the researcher then begins to structure the themes and sub-themes into a thematic framework (step 2 in Figure 20.2). As this framework is developed, the themes and sub-themes are numbered to create an index. To some extent the index will resemble the interview schedule or topic guide – it would be strange if it did not – but it will also include some newly emerging themes. Furthermore, the index may not necessarily be structured in the same way as the interview schedule as it may already be apparent that aspects of the data

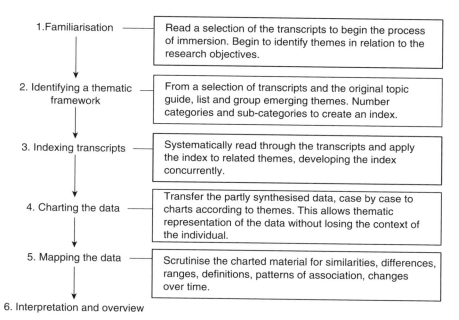

1.Familiarisation —— Read a selection of the transcripts to begin the process of immersion. Begin to identify themes in relation to the research objectives.

2. Identifying a thematic framework —— From a selection of transcripts and the original topic guide, list and group emerging themes. Number categories and sub-categories to create an index.

3. Indexing transcripts —— Systematically read through the transcripts and apply the index to related themes, developing the index concurrently.

4. Charting the data —— Transfer the partly synthesised data, case by case to charts according to themes. This allows thematic representation of the data without losing the context of the individual.

5. Mapping the data —— Scrutinise the charted material for similarities, differences, ranges, definitions, patterns of association, changes over time.

6. Interpretation and overview

FIGURE 20.2 Framework approach to analysing qualitative data in applied policy research (developed from Ritchie and Spencer, 1994)

relate to one another in unanticipated ways. At this stage the themes will be quite broad. Once the skeleton of the index has been created, it is possible to begin indexing (or coding) the transcripts (step 3 in Figure 20.2). This involves reading each transcript in detail and, for each theme identified in the text, applying the appropriate numerical code from the index by writing it in the margin. At the same time as indexing the transcripts, the researcher continually develops the index to incorporate new themes as they arise.

The next stage of the framework approach is the creation of charts to facilitate detailed scrutiny of the data (step 4 in Figure 20.2). The charts are actually grids or tables, most commonly with themes and sub-themes across the top, and interviewees down the side (although this can be reversed). Through the earlier process of indexing, the researcher may have become aware of various relationships within the data and wish to explore these further. The organisation of the themes and sub-themes in the charts therefore reflects the researcher's developing thinking as s/he becomes increasingly immersed in the data. For ease, each of the headings on the chart includes the index number(s) of the themes and sub-themes it incorporates. Once the charts are created, partially synthesised data and quotes from the transcripts are recorded in each cell. The page number of the transcript from which it originated is also noted to allow the full data or quote to be revisited, both for accuracy and to enable it to be considered in context. Whilst the physical process of synthesising and transferring the data can be labour intensive, it allows you to become fully immersed in the data, and far from a mechanical process, it is the stage where much of the analytical thinking occurs.

Case study

A qualitative interview study undertaken in Sydney, Australia, explored how education and health literacy affects individuals' involvement in their health decision-making (Smith et al., 2009). The sample of 73 men and women was selected to reflect diversity in educational attainment (with or without a university degree), and participants were subsequently scored for health literacy. The in-depth interviews were semi-structured, and based upon a topic guide which discussed participants' involvement in their health decision-making, including their views on the advantages and disadvantages of being involved, their health information-seeking habits and strategies for understanding health information.

The authors describe how three team members (SS, KM, and AD) were involved in the five stages of framework analysis (mapping and interpretation were combined). Familiarisation was undertaken by all three members, who each read a sample of transcripts and used these as a basis for discussion to identify the key themes. A provisional thematic framework was then developed by SS, after which SS and AD independently indexed the transcripts, meeting regularly to refine the thematic framework or coding index. A chart was then created using the final coding index, into which data which were synthesised by SS and AD were noted. The three team members then met to interpret the chart.

The framework approach facilitated a comparison between three groups of participants, those with:

- higher education and higher health literacy
- lower education and higher health literacy
- lower education and lower health literacy

From the chart, three overarching themes were identified:

- understanding the experiences of involvement in health care decision-making
- influence of the patient–practitioner relationship
- the perceived function of health information

The findings indicated that people with different levels of education and health literacy conceptualise their involvement in health care decisions in different ways, although greater differences emerged in relation to education than to health literacy. In particular, participants with a higher education appeared to perceive their involvement in health care decision-making as a shared responsibility with the doctor (including verifying the credibility of information and exploring alternative options). Whereas those with a lower education appeared to perceive their involvement in health care decision-making in terms of consenting to (or rejecting) an option recommended by the doctor. In addition, the higher educated participants described wanting respect for their professional status, whereas those with a lower education valued doctors who conveyed empathy and had a genuine interest in their personal circumstances.

Once all the data are charted, the charts can then be scrutinised, to obtain a 'picture' of the data which will show links between themes. Ritchie and Spencer (1994) advocate transferring the information from the themed charts to central maps to facilitate further interpretation (step 5 in Figure 20.2). However, an alternative approach is to begin by considering the data within each of the chart columns – this equates to thematic analysis and facilitates some basic description. It may also provide sufficient evidence for answering policy-related questions. To move beyond this, and to exploit the data at an analytic level, it is then possible to look for groups of interviewees who are similar to each other (and different from others) according to some theme of interest, and then to explore the other columns or themes to see if there are other ways in which these individuals differ from the others, thus exposing associations and possible explanations for the phenomena of interest.

Summary

- The choice of qualitative analysis needs to be carefully justified to ensure 'fit' with the research question, aims of the research and the method of data collection.

- All qualitative analysis approaches tend to be context-rich, inductive, inclusive, and use smaller sample sizes than quantitative methods. Qualitative analysis covers the spectrum from description to interpretation, and emphasises the reflexive role of the researcher.

- Thematic analysis is a broad, descriptive approach to qualitative analysis, and forms the basis of a range of qualitative methods.

- Grounded theory is a detailed, iterative approach to qualitative data collection and analysis and is especially informative in the development of new theory. It is ideal for exploring areas of health care where there is little existing evidence.

- A structured method for qualitative data analysis is the framework approach. This was developed for, and used in, the field of applied policy research. It is particularly useful for research questions that are less exploratory and where applied findings are required.

Questions for Discussion

1. How might you counter criticism that qualitative analysis is not statistically generalisable to the wider population?

2. What approach to analysis might best suit a research question which seeks to explore the experiences of adolescents at high risk for developing long-term mental health conditions?

3. How might a researcher respond to the criticism that their analysis is biased by their own interpretation?

Further Reading

Richards, L (2010) *Handling Qualitative Data: A Practical Guide* (2nd edn). Chippenham: SAGE.

Ritchie, J., Spencer, L. and O'Connor, W. (2003) 'Carrying out qualitative analysis', in J. Ritchie and J. Lewis (eds), *Qualitative Research Practice: A Guide for Social Science Students and Researchers*. London: SAGE, pp. 219–62.

Saldana, J. (2009) *The Coding Manual for Qualitative Research*. Chippenham: SAGE.

Schreier, M. (2012) *Qualitative Content Analysis in Practice*. Croydon: SAGE.

References

Charmaz, K. (2003) 'Grounded theory – objectivist and constructivist methods', in N.K. Denzin and Y.S. Lincoln (eds), *Strategies of Qualitative Inquiry* (2nd edn). Thousand Oaks, CA: SAGE.

Charmaz, K. (2006) *Constructing Grounded Theory: A Practical Guide through Qualitative Analysis*. London: SAGE.

Finlay, L. (2006) 'Going exploring: the nature of qualitative research', in L. Finlay and C. Ballinger (eds), *Qualitative Research for Allied Health Professionals*. Chichester: John Wiley & Sons.

Glaser, B.G. and Strauss, A.L. (1967) *The Discovery of Grounded Theory: Strategies for Qualitative Research*. London: Weidenfeld & Nicolson.

Green, G., Emslie, C., O'Neill, D., Hunt, K. and Walker, S. (2010) 'Exploring the ambiguities of "masculinity" in accounts of emotional distress in the military among young ex-servicemen', *Social Science and Medicine*.

Lewins, A. and Silver, C. (2007) *Using Software in Qualitative Research: A Step-by-Step Guide*. London: SAGE.

Lincoln, Y.S. and Guba, E.G. (1985) *Naturalistic Inquiry*. Beverley Hills. CA: SAGE.

Ritchie, J. and Spencer, L. (1994) 'Qualitative data analysis for applied qualitative research', in A. Bryman and B. Burgess (eds), *Analysing Qualitative Data*. London: Routledge, pp. 173–94.

Robson, C. (2011) *Real World Research* (3rd edn). Chichester: John Wiley & Sons.

Smith, S., Dixon, A., Trevena, L., Nutbeam, D. and McCaffery, K.J. (2009) 'Exploring patient involvement in healthcare decision making across different education and functional health literacy groups', *Social Science and Medicine,* 69 (12): 1805–12.

Strauss, A. and Corbin, J. (1990) *Basics of Qualitative Research – Grounded Theory Procedures and Techniques*. Newbury Park, CA: SAGE.

Strauss, A. and Corbin, J. (1998) *Basics of Qualitative Research: Techniques and Procedures for Developing Grounded Theory* (2nd edn). Newbury Park, CA: SAGE.

21

DISSEMINATION

Carol Rivas and Raksha Pandya-Wood

Learning Objectives

- Appreciate the priorities when developing a dissemination strategy
- Understand the rationale behind, and need for, a cohesive, well-thought-out dissemination strategy
- Consider the advantages of staged dissemination
- Develop an analytical approach to determining your audiences, considering their needs and the most appropriate ways of disseminating to them
- Critically consider the use of different dissemination platforms and styles
- Be aware of ways of measuring the impact of your dissemination and the importance of doing so

Introduction

Dissemination is 'a process of sharing information and knowledge. The challenge of dissemination is to improve the accessibility of research findings to those we are trying to reach' (Saywell et al., 2007: 1). Therefore a well-planned dissemination strategy is important for any piece of research. Historically, the emphasis of dissemination was on developing an evidence base in health research and it was often sufficient in research plans to say that you would publish in one or two high-impact, peer-reviewed journals. Latour and Woolgar (1979) argued that the primary focus of a science laboratory was the production of papers for publication; discoveries were almost a means to this end. Nowadays, with the focus on translational research with measurable clinical impact, patient-centred care and value for money, this is no longer the case. Time is needed to think through a much more inclusive, but at the same time carefully targeted, dissemination strategy that will be effective in getting your research known by the people who matter, which in turn will inform clinical practice.

It is increasingly acknowledged that academics and funders may not be the most important research stakeholders and that it is good practice to share research plans and findings routinely with the local community, research participants, patients and also government, health services and policy-makers. This ensures the results are relevant and become embedded into clinical practice, and enables examination of their generalisability in other settings. It can also be argued that all researchers have a moral, ethical and professional obligation to disseminate their research, as dissemination enables other researchers to build on your work, rather than working to answer the same questions. This avoids unethical experimentation where participants are included in a study which is redundant as the answer is already known, i.e. consequentialism (please see Chapter 15: 'Designing and Conducting an Ethical Research Study'). Dissemination can also help other researchers decide on an appropriate methodology if they are conducting a similar study to yours, especially if you have shared issues and problems that have arisen when undertaking your research. For these reasons, some research organisations, such as the Economic and Social Data Service in the UK, and the Australian National Health and Medical Research Council, make it a requirement of funding that researchers deposit their data and any publications arising from their project in an appropriate subject and/or institutional archive or repository which are usually free access to all (please see Chapter 2: 'Finding the Evidence'). Dissemination is also vital to building up, establishing and sustaining a research career, whether you are a health professional or an academic. It is a demonstration of your research abilities to examiners, employers or the scientific community at large. Funders may be reluctant to support someone whose research experience is not evident in publications, and employers may not recruit or promote you if you do not have an active research profile assessed by your dissemination activity.

To ensure that your dissemination strategy is appropriate and thorough, it should be planned prior to your research commencing, and many funding bodies ask for your intended dissemination strategy prior to financial award. Dissemination should be considered as an iterative, long-term venture, adapted and refined through feedback regarding its effectiveness. The four main questions you need to answer when devising your dissemination strategy are:

- Who is my audience?
- Why do I need to inform them (and what should they be told, or need to know)?
- When should they be told?
- What medium, or platform, and style should I use?

You will find yourself jumping back and forth between these, but at all times your guiding factors should be who your audiences are, and what outcomes you desire from your dissemination.

Case study

This case study is based upon a piece of research by Pandya (2006). Pandya had found that there was anecdotal evidence to suggest that HIV positive mothers who were asylum seekers or refugees would only access specialist HIV services at key points in their lives, such as during pregnancy or immediately after disclosing to a family member, but would not continue using the services once these key points had passed. Therefore, Pandya conducted some qualitative research to explore this issue using interviews.

The study aims were to identify:

- services the women were currently accessing and what services they wanted;
- barriers they had experienced in accessing services;
- any further issues to inform future HIV service provision.

The main stakeholders to disseminate to were:

- refugee or asylum-seeking women with HIV;
- families of these women, including their children;
- specialist HIV service providers;
- youth services;
- medical service providers to the refugee or asylum-seeking communities;
- academic community at large to expand on the research further;
- policy-makers and budget holders.

Who is my audience?

There are many potential audiences for you to disseminate to (see case study); each with their own values, concerns and needs. Understanding what each audience

TABLE 21.1   Details for one potential stakeholder for our case study

Stakeholder and conduit	Setting for dissemination	Stakeholder			Opportunities and benefits	Problems and issues
		Values	Concerns	Needs		
Women with HIV who are refugees or asylum seekers. Need creative conduits that they will take notice of.	Via local groups and networks in the community.	Want to protect their families from stigmatisation.	Worried about costs for services and health care.	Reassurance that it is safe, free with removal of perceived barriers to services.	Need to ensure they are engaged with the study recommendations and likely to take advantage of any change in service.	The women may not want to attend a dissemination event due to fear of stigmatisation.

is like and what benefits you are most likely to derive from them, and they from you, will help you communicate your results effectively and so you need to spend time reflecting on these.

When you design your dissemination strategy we recommend that you brainstorm an exhaustive list of stakeholders, as eventually you will have to disseminate something to each one. Write this list of stakeholders in the first column of a table, and use the other columns to write down what you understand their values, concerns, and needs to be, and what opportunities and other benefits are likely to result from disseminating to them. Your last column will contain any anticipated problems or issues you may have with disseminating to this stakeholder (an example can be seen in Table 21.1). Try not to be too general when listing the stakeholders or your message will be unfocused Specify the settings across which dissemination will occur, the type of person you wish to reach, the conduit of the information and, if you know it, an individual or group's name as your main contact. This is more obvious with academic and clinical audiences but needs to be carefully thought out for patients and the public too (for further information an patient and public involvement in research please see Chapter 16).

Why do I need to inform them, and what should they be told, or need to know?

Now you have your list, you need to consider not what you want your audiences to know, but rather what you want them to do with your results. In other words, you need to work backwards from your desired outcomes. Just as in advertising, the aim is not simply to get people to take notice of what you are saying at the time that you say it, but to remember what is said, by whom and to use the product/results (Figure 21.1). Therefore as in advertising, you need your strapline, and up to three key messages. These should convey and build on your research's 'unique selling points'. Begin with a generic strapline and key messages which you should refer to whenever you disseminate to ensure that your messages remain consistent (see case study).

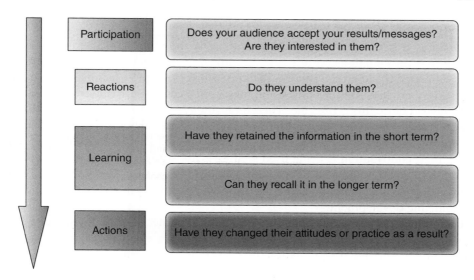

FIGURE 21.1   A hierarchy of effects model

When you are happy with these, and have checked them with your team and organisation, develop supporting messages to provide the facts, and explanations that reinforce these key messages. Supporting messages can vary in detail and scientific sophistication depending on your target audience, so you need to develop different sets for each audience. These supporting messages are what you actually disseminate. It is best to write these at the start of your dissemination to ensure a cohesive and well-structured campaign. Spell out the advantages, or disadvantages, your research results show, and what problems, if any, you are targeting or have solved for the reader/observer. *Make it clear why they should take notice of them.* It is likely that you will need to refer to the usefulness of your research, and probably also the viability, acceptability to end users and cost effectiveness which could be conferred upon the adoption of your recommendations.

Case study

Based upon the obtained interview data, the dissemination strategy's key messages for policy-makers, health care and service providers in relation to service provision were:

1. HIV services should ensure a link with existing mainstream youth services so that children affected by maternal HIV are supported.
2. Specialist HIV and mainstream services should work closely together to provide a more coordinated package of care.
3. Existing HIV services should consider avenues such as self-help/training courses/workshops that tackle ways that HIV positive women may disclose their HIV status to family members.

Information about a range of issues regarding HIV needs to be promoted widely across all routes of HIV testing so that people infected, or affected, by HIV know where to get help.

When should they be told?

Sometimes it is better to produce scientific outputs, such as academic papers, or conference presentations/posters first, or publish your literature review if you have not completed the analysis. You can then refer to these in any ensuing dissemination such as lay articles. At other times, you may need to make sure the local community is involved before this is possible. Therefore, you need to develop an action plan that lists messages, activities and optimal timings for dissemination for each audience (Baeyaert, 2005). Regular newsletters for stakeholders should be routine so they know their contribution is being used well (see case study). Keeping them informed will also encourage them to adopt your findings, by keeping them primed for the main message, which can be delivered after analysis via events such as training, or by guideline development.

Dissemination is an ongoing task and does not necessarily finish when the research project is complete, as a single dissemination event is quickly forgotten. After all the official dissemination processes are complete, researchers should always aim to keep the messages of their work alive, both formally and informally. Keeping abreast of new knowledge as it emerges that affects your research will add to your body of knowledge forming on the topic, and enables you to respond with letters to the editor citing your own work and therefore further promoting it. Do not disseminate materials before they are ready however. If they have taken longer than you have timetabled, invest more time and resources in getting them finalised rather than releasing something half-finished and unprofessional. If your evidence is weak, limit your dissemination; be wary of overstating its importance or generalisability, and instead recommend further research.

Case study

The proposed dissemination strategy should lead to better care for the women with greater access to services and a clear care pathway. However, as mentioned before, the opportunities and benefits arising from the results are tempered by the women's engagement with the changes. Therefore, this needs to be tackled with the women, together with suggested solutions, as well as the key messages, when disseminating to them. To ensure that they adopt the results, some dissemination was undertaken before data analysis to keep the women engaged with the study. For example, the participants were kept informed about the progress of the research via regular newsletters, were asked for feedback throughout the study and were involved in planning some of the later dissemination.

What medium or platform should I use?

Often the first wave of dissemination is by presentation, be it academic conferences, seminars or workshops, as these often occur prior to fully completing the project/analysis, and ensuing feedback can help with later dissemination, such as further defining your key messages. Your audience will then also be primed for your main message. Do try to follow up, or back up, any presentations with peer-reviewed texts or other articles that can be cited if you have any, or your message may only last as long as your presentation. Presentations at public open days using creative outputs such as plays and songs can be very effective in delivering your messages to the community in a way that is comprehensible and has meaning to those with little knowledge of science. Drama groups have been set up specifically to disseminate research messages to patients and the public.

The second wave of dissemination, most often after the project is complete and the data fully analysed, is the more traditional route, i.e. dissemination through the written word, in particular through academic journals and technical reports. To maximise the impact of articles in peer-reviewed publications, you should consider the status and reputation of the journal or publisher, the speed of their peer-review process (will their decision timeframe enable your dissemination to be timely?), and their audience. Do not neglect practitioner broadsheets, or if you are developing or evaluating instrumentation or equipment, trade magazines, as these will reach the people most likely to adopt your findings into everyday practice. To disseminate to patients or the public, different media and platforms need to be used. Consider producing leaflets and giving them out at local events (such as health fairs), or get your research adopted by the Department of Health, or relevant charities for national coverage in their newsletters, websites or press releases. It is often helpful to get the press interested in your research as this can increase citations (Phillips et al., 1991). Contact your local radio or TV stations to see if they are interested in covering your research, and approach national radio or TV if you think your story is big enough. If trying to disseminate via mainstream media, you need to show your research is novel, interesting, current, relevant to the audience (including geographically), and affects either a significant number of people or significant people (celebrities). If the story release coincides with a current hot topic such as obesity, or there is some associated event happening such as an international congress, so much the better. Your institution may have a public relations office which can help you with mainstream media coverage if required.

The internet can also be a powerful medium for dissemination using interfaces such as blogs, podcasts, project websites and other social media sites. Internet-based options reach more people than any other form of dissemination, but make sure your platform is appropriate for your target audience. You can increase visitors by 'liking' or linking your web-based dissemination from other websites that may be relevant to your work, such as relevant charities' webpages. Other media outputs may also cite your work. An example is a *British Medical Journal* blog written by Walker (2011a), which was later to be found reproduced in the *Wall Street Journal* (Walker, 2011b)! However this form of dissemination is out of your control and carries the risk of becoming inaccurate. To minimise the chance of this occurring, there is little you can do beyond subscribing to RSS feeds about mentions of your work, and ensuring that you have a home page or other official web-based research page that spells out your key messages simply and unambiguously. Make sure that your email signature and your business card have the URL to these pages and that your site and all your media output (and articles on others' sites) point back to you and your official project pages.

Dissemination style and content

Consider what information is potentially most useful to your different audiences. Do they need to know all of it in general terms, or sections of it at a time in detail? For example, emphasise the 'big picture' when addressing lay audiences, or policy-makers. For conference presentations or academic publications, consider splitting your results to answer individual aims in detail, which also increases the number of publications you get from your project.

Conventions already exist regarding style and content. Scientific reports and papers, for example, tend to use a structure based around the sequence of: abstract, introduction, method, results, discussion and conclusion, with rhetoric in scientific language (see Kirkman, 2005). Figures and tables are often included in publications as they allow others to inspect your analysis. Always provide the data that enable your reader to convert percentages back into raw data if they so wish. Consider the arrangement of rows and columns in tables, or axes, bars or pie slices in graphs. Choose the one that gets your message across accurately and in the most useful and obvious way. Historically, qualitative papers have been difficult to write due to the word limit imposed by publications, which impedes the richness of the data published. However, many publications have associated websites where it is sometimes possible to upload your data for any interested readers. For a good idea of what style to use and content to write, read a couple of papers and the authors' guidance in the journal you hope to submit to (please see Rivas, 2012, for more discussion of this).

To present your findings to a non-academic or clinical audience, it is useful to use other styles such as images or cartoons. One very creative example is the multiple sclerosis Big Knit in which the public were encouraged to knit multiple sclerosis genes and other objects relevant to the illness (www.immunology.org/msthebigknit). Also using metaphors and analogies reflecting the experiences that your audience may be familiar with, such as playing sports, can be very helpful in getting your message understood. However, their use may encourage imprecision and loss of meaning, so state the accurate version first, and then give the metaphor or analogy as a way of explanation. The UK National Health Service digest of current health research (www.nhs.uk/news/Pages/NewsIndex.aspx) provides excellent examples of the way technical research can be presented in a manner which is comprehensible to the lay person. You may also get some ideas for style and content by reviewing leaflets designed for patients and the public. Good examples will be easy to read, informative and may use figures or pictures to break up the text. Use a similar style to produce your newsletter or articles for local groups and also for practitioner publications or other broadsheets and magazines aimed at professionals.

Authorship and involvement in dissemination

If you are submitting to a peer-reviewed publication, there may be more than one author involved in producing the paper. These co-authors should be people who have been part of the research project, *and* who have helped write the article. This can be useful as each team member can write a section of the paper pertaining to their area of expertise, such as statistics. Journals now require signed declarations about each author's involvement in the research and in the preparation of the paper. If someone has been part of the research project but not the writing, they should be named in acknowledgements instead. It may also be that the article is written by ghost-writers, who are professional writers not part of the research team. They are not acknowledged on the paper, but are just paid to write the article (this practice is more prevalent in papers published by pharmaceutical companies). This practice is frowned upon, as it results in a lack of accountability for the paper itself and its data and results within. It was assumed that the signed declarations required by most journals would reduce these practices, however, in a recent cross-sectional survey sent to the corresponding authors of all papers published in a selection of high-impact journals in 2008, the prevalence of ghost authorship was 21.0%. Although showing a decrease from 1996, when it was 29.3%, this is still a significant percentage (Wislar et al., 2011).

Dissemination which actively involves lay groups is often required by funders and ethical approval committees, and is good practice as it can help with the transition of your research results into practice (Schneider et al., 2004; for further information an patient and public involvement in research please see Chapter 16). Depending upon the method of involvement, support and training may be required as there is a danger of messages from the research being lost though poor delivery, poor preparation and poor presentation skills (McLaughlin, 2006).

Measuring impact

Since the primary aim of dissemination is to ensure that your research has impact, it is helpful to assess this, whether negative or positive, and it may be a requirement of your stakeholders, for example, funders, employers (Petrie et al., 2006). Assessment can be based upon measures such as citation scores, the number of people who have contacted you about your research, number of people who have visited your project website, references in the trade press, policy documents or the mass media, with the ultimate impact being a change to practice or behaviour. When assessing impact you may want to consider Figure 21.2.

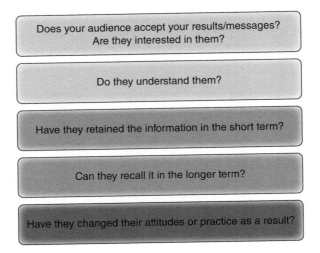

FIGURE 21.2   Assessing impact of your dissemination strategy

You might also contact stakeholders for feedback, for example with short questionnaires or focus group sessions (please see Chapter 7: 'Qualitative Methodology') as these might reveal obstacles to the uptake of your findings as well as successes. An example of this is a project conducted by Professor Keith Hawton and his team (2012) who held a series of focus groups and interviews with various stakeholders to gain feedback on a self-help booklet developed for those bereaved by suicide (Hawton et al., 2008). They then forwarded this feedback to the Department of Health who produce the booklet, to enhance its usefulness and appropriateness for its audience. Evaluating the success of your dissemination efforts is an iterative process therefore, with monitoring over time. Davies et al. (2005: 2) raise some useful questions for researchers when evaluating impact:

> Research may directly influence changes in policy, practices and behaviours. Or it may, in more subtle ways, change people's knowledge, understanding and attitudes towards social issues. Tracking these subtle changes can be difficult, but it is perhaps more important in the long run. Additional problems include knowing where to look for research impacts (who are the research users?); knowing when to look for these impacts (how long is sufficient for research to take effect?); and knowing how to assess the specific contributions made by research (was the research really the key factor in any changes observed?).

By addressing these points you will also be demonstrating the activities and achievements of your research to show value for money of benefits over cost to funders.

Summary

- Researchers have a moral, ethical and professional obligation to disseminate their research.

- Time is needed to think through an inclusive, targeted dissemination strategy that will be effective in getting your research known, accessed and used by the people who matter.

- Consider who your audiences are and understand their needs and values to fully engage them. Assess the benefits and problems of disseminating to them.

- Plan to disseminate information out to different audiences at different times to suit particular purposes. This gives your message longevity. Consider dissemination as a long-term activity that does not end with your project.

- Be creative in your use of platforms and media. Do not forget the internet, and mainstream media.

- Assess that your dissemination is having an impact on practice or attitudes. If not, revise your strategy.

Questions for Discussion

Vignette

You have undertaken some research regarding HIV with a focus on female sex workers and men who pay for their services. You believe your findings could reduce the spread of the disease if you could reach your target audiences effectively.

1. Complete the following table (21.2) detailing your dissemination strategy for the above vignette.

2. What might be the most effective ways of reaching the key audiences?

3. What would be inappropriate ways to disseminate?

TABLE 21.2   Table to complete for the vignette

Stakeholder and conduit	Setting for dissemination	Stakeholder			Opportunities and benefits	Problems and issues
		Values	Concerns	Needs		

Further reading

Albert, T. (2000). *Winning the Publications Game* (3rd edn). Oxon: Radcliffe Publishing.

Becker, L. and Denicolo, P. (2012) *Publishing Journal Articles*. London: SAGE.

Broitman, R. (2009) *100+ Resources to Boost Your Social Media Savvy in 2009: Top Tips and Advice from the Experts*. Reston, VA: Interactive Insights Group: www.interactiveinsightsgroup.com/blog1/100-resources-to-boost-your-social-media-savvy-top-tips-advice-from-the-experts (accessed April 2012).

Carpenter, D., Nieva, V., Albaghal, T. and Sorra, J. (2005) 'Dissemination Planning Tool', in *Development of a Planning Tool to Guide Dissemination of Research Results. Advances in Patient Safety: From Research to Implementation,* vol. 4, *Programs, Tools and Practices*. Rockville, MD: Agency for Healthcare Research and Quality: www.ahrq.gov/qual/advances/planningtool.htm (accessed April 2012).

Day, R.A. (2012) *How to Write and Publish a Scientific Paper* (7th edn). Cambridge: Cambridge University Press.

Dunn, E., Norton, P.G., Stewart, M., Tudiver, F. and Bass, M. (eds) (1994) *Disseminating Research/Changing Practice*. London: SAGE.

Kirkman, J. (2005) *Good Style: Writing for Science and Technology* (2nd edn). Abingdon: Routledge.

Nelson, D.E., Brownson, R.C., Remington, P.L. and Parvanta, C. (2002) *Communicating Public Health Information Effectively: A Guide for Practitioners*. Washington, DC: American Public Health Association.

Rivas, C. (2012) 'Writing a research report', in C. Seale (ed.), *Researching Society and Culture* (3rd edn). London: SAGE.

Robinson, E.T., Baron, D., Heise, L.L., Moffett, J. and Harlan, S.V. (2010) *Communications Handbook for Clinical Trials: Strategies, Tips, and Tools to Manage Controversy, Convey Your Message, and Disseminate Result*: www.fhi360.org/en/RH/Pubs/booksReports/comm_handbook.htm (accessed April 2012).

Sullivan, T.M., Strachan, M. and Timmons, B.K. (2007) *Guide to Monitoring and Evaluating Health Information Products and Services*. Washington, DC: Center for Communication Programs, Johns Hopkins Bloomberg School of Public Health: www.infoforhealth.org/hipnet/MEGuide/MEGUIDE2007.pdf (accessed April 2012).

Welch-Ross, M.K. and Fasig, L.G. (2007) *Handbook on Communicating and Disseminating Behavioral Science*. Thousand Oaks, CA: SAGE.

References

Baeyaert, P. (2005) 'Developing an external communications strategy', presentation at Communicating European Research, 14 Nov.: http://ec.europa.eu/research/conferences/2005/cer2005/presentations/14/h1_communications_strategy_cer2005.pdf (accessed April 2012).

Davies, H., Nutley, S. and Walter, I. (2005) 'Assessing the impact of social science research: conceptual, methodological and practical issues', ESRC Symposium on Assessing Non-Academic Impact of Research, 12–13 May.

Hawton, K., Simkin, S. and Rees, S. (2008) 'Help is at hand for people bereaved by suicide and other traumatic death', *Psychiatric Bulletin*, 32: 309–11.

Hawton, K., Sutton, L., Simkin, S., Walker, D.-M., Stacey, G., Waters, K., and Rees, S. (2012) 'Evaluation of a resource for people bereaved by suicide', *Crisis*, 33 (5): 254–64.

Kirkman, J. (2005) *Good Style: Writing for Science and Technology* (2nd edn). Abingdon: Routledge.

Latour, B. and Woolgar, S. (1979) *Laboratory Life: The Construction of Scientific Facts.* Princeton, NJ: Princeton University Press.

McLaughlin, H. (2006) 'Involving Young Service Users as Co-Researchers: possibilities, benefits and costs', *British Journal of Social Work,* 36 (8): 1395–410.

Pandya, R. (2006) *Exploring the Support Needs of HIV Positive Mothers with Uninfected Children: An Account of Speaking with Ten Local Women about Life, Motherhood and HIV*: www.faithinpeople.org.uk/Documents/4651%20Main%20Report%20red.pdf (accessed April 2012).

Petrie, S., Fiorelli, L. and O'Donnell, K. (2006) 'If we help you what will change? Participatory research and young people', *Journal of Social Welfare and Family Law,* 28 (1): 31–45.

Phillips, D.P., Kanter, E.J., Bednarczyk, B. and Tastad, P.L. (1991) 'Importance of the lay press in the transmission of medical knowledge to the scientific community', *New England Journal of Medicine,* 325: 1180–3.

Rivas, C. (2012) 'Writing a research report', in C. Seale (ed.), *Researching Society and Culture* (3rd edn). London: SAGE.

Saywell, D., Cotton, A. and Woodfield, J. (2007) *Spreading the Word: Disseminating Research Findings Synthesis Note*: www2.eastwestcenter.org/research/popcomm/pdf/2_Selected_Readings/spreading_the_word.pdf (accessed April 2012).

Schneider, E.F., Lang, A., Shin, M. and Bradley, S.D. (2004) 'Death with a story: how story impacts emotional, motivational, and physiological responses to first-person shooter video games', *Human Communication Research,* 30: 361–75.

Walker, D.-M. (2011a) 'The emergence of online research methods', *British Medical Journal Group Blogs*: *http://blogs.bmj.com/bmj/2011/10/28/dawn-marie-walker-the-emergence-of-online-research-methods/* (accessed April 2012).

Walker, D.-M. (2011b) 'The emergence of online research methods', *Wall Street Journal*: http://onespot.wsj.com/health/2011/10/28/7633e/dawn-marie-walker-the-emergence-of-onlin (accessed April 2012).

Wislar, J.S., Flanagin, A., Fontanarosa, P.B. and DeAngelis, C.D. (2011) 'Honorary and ghost authorship in high impact biomedical journals: a cross sectional survey', *British Medical Journal,* 343: d6128.

INDEX